Cancer Screening and Genetics

Editor

CHRISTOPHER L. WOLFGANG

SURGICAL CLINICS
OF NORTH AMERICA

www.surgical.theclinics.com

Consulting Editor
RONALD F. MARTIN

October 2015 • Volume 95 • Number 5

ELSEVIER

1600 John F. Kennedy Boulevard • Suite 1800 • Philadelphia, Pennsylvania, 19103-2899

http://www.surgical.theclinics.com

SURGICAL CLINICS OF NORTH AMERICA Volume 95, Number 5
October 2015 ISSN 0039–6109, ISBN-13: 978-0-323-40106-7

Editor: John Vassallo, j.vassallo@elsevier.com
Developmental Editor: Colleen Viola

Surgical Clinics of North America (ISSN 0039–6109) is published bimonthly by Elsevier Inc., 360 Park Avenue South, New York, NY 10010-1710. Months of publication are February, April, June, August, October, and December. Business and Editorial Offices: 1600 John F. Kennedy Blvd., Suite 1800, Philadelphia, PA 19103-2899. Periodicals postage paid at New York, NY and additional mailing offices. Subscription prices are $370.00 per year for US individuals, $627.00 per year for US institutions, $180.00 per year for US students and residents, $455.00 per year for Canadian individuals, $793.00 per year for Canadian institutions, $510.00 for international individuals, $793.00 per year for international institutions and $250.00 per year for Canadian and foreign students/residents. To receive student/resident rate, orders must be accompanied by name of affiliated institution, date of term, and the *signature* of program/residency coordinator on institution letterhead. Orders will be billed at individual rate until proof of status is received. Foreign air speed delivery is included in all *Clinics* subscription prices. All prices are subject to change without notice. POSTMASTER: Send address changes to *Surgical Clinics*, Elsevier Health Sciences Division, Subscription Customer Service, 3251 Riverport Lane, Maryland Heights, MO 63043. **Customer Service (orders, claims, online, change of address): Telephone: 1-800-654-2452 (U.S. and Canada); 314-447-8871 (outside U.S. and Canada). Fax: 314-447-8029. E-mail: journalscustomerservice-usa@elsevier.com (for print support); journalsonline support-usa@elsevier.com (for online support).**

Reprints. For copies of 100 or more, of articles in this publication, please contact the Commercial Reprints Department, Elsevier Inc., 360 Park Avenue South, New York, New York 10010-1710. Tel. 212-633-3874, Fax: 212-633-3820, E-mail: reprints@elsevier.com.

The *Surgical Clinics of North America* is also published in Spanish by McGraw-Hill Interamericana Editores S.A., P.O. Box 5-237 06500 Mexico D.F. Mexico; and in Portuguese by Interlivros Edicoes Ltda., Rua Comandante Coelho 1085, CEP 21250, Rio de Janeiro, Brazil; and in Greek by Paschalidis Medical Publications, Athens Greece.

The *Surgical Clinics of North America* is covered in *MEDLINE/PubMed (Index Medicus)*, *EMBASE/Excerpta Medica*, *Current Contents/Clinical Medicine*, *Current Contents/Life Sciences*, *Science Citation Index*, and *ISI/BIOMED*.

Contributors

CONSULTING EDITOR

RONALD F. MARTIN, MD
Staff Surgeon, Department of Surgery, Marshfield Clinic, Marshfield, Wisconsin; Clinical Associate Professor, University of Wisconsin School of Medicine and Public Health, Madison, Wisconsin; Colonel (ret.), Medical Corps, United States Army Reserve

EDITOR

CHRISTOPHER L. WOLFGANG, MD, PhD
Chief, Hepatobiliary and Pancreatic Surgery, Paul K. Neumann Professor of Pancreatic Cancer Research, Professor of Surgery, Pathology and Oncology, Johns Hopkins University, Baltimore, Maryland

AUTHORS

ROBERT ABOUASSALY, MD, MSc
Assistant Professor, Urology Institute, University Hospitals Case Medical Center, Cleveland, Ohio

NITA AHUJA, MD
Professor of Surgery, Oncology and Urology, Department of Surgery, Johns Hopkins University School of Medicine, Baltimore, Maryland

ANDREW V. BIANKIN, MD, PhD
Wolfson Wohl Cancer Research Centre, Institute of Cancer Sciences, University of Glasgow, Glasgow, United Kingdom; The Kinghorn Cancer Centre, Darlinghurst, New South Wales, Australia; Cancer Research Program, Garvan Institute of Medical Research, Darlinghurst, Sydney, New South Wales, Australia; Department of Surgery, Bankstown Hospital, Bankstown, Sydney, New South Wales, Australia; Faculty of Medicine, South Western Sydney Clinical School, University of NSW, Liverpool, New South Wales, Australia

LODEWIJK A.A. BROSENS, MD, PhD
Department of Pathology, University Medical Center Utrecht (H04-312), Utrecht, The Netherlands; Department of Pathology, Johns Hopkins University School of Medicine, Baltimore, Maryland

ANDREW M. CAMERON, MD, PhD
Director of Liver Transplantation; Associate Professor, Johns Hopkins Hospital, Baltimore, Maryland

DAVID K. CHANG, MD, PhD
Wolfson Wohl Cancer Research Centre, Institute of Cancer Sciences, University of Glasgow, Glasgow, United Kingdom; The Kinghorn Cancer Centre, Darlinghurst,

New South Wales, Australia; Cancer Research Program, Garvan Institute of Medical Research, Darlinghurst, Sydney, New South Wales, Australia; Department of Surgery, Bankstown Hospital, Bankstown, Sydney, New South Wales, Australia; Faculty of Medicine, South Western Sydney Clinical School, University of NSW, Liverpool, New South Wales, Australia

MARK E. DEFFEBACH, MD
Division of Hospital and Specialty Medicine, Pulmonary and Critical Care Medicine, Portland VA Health Care System; Department of Medicine, Oregon Health and Science University, Portland, Oregon

PHILIP A. DI CARLO, MD
Instructor, Department of Radiology, Johns Hopkins Hospital, Johns Hopkins University, Baltimore, Maryland

DAVID EUHUS, MD
Professor of Surgery, Department of Surgery, Johns Hopkins Hospital, Johns Hopkins University, Baltimore, Maryland

KJETIL GARBORG, MD
Department of Transplantation medicine, Oslo University Hospital, Oslo; Department of Medicine, Sørlandet Hospital HF, Kristiansand, Norway

FRANCIS M. GIARDIELLO, MD
Department of Medicine, Oncology Center; Department of Pathology, Johns Hopkins University School of Medicine, Baltimore, Maryland

JIN HE, MD, PhD
Assistant Professor, Department of Surgery, Johns Hopkins University School of Medicine, Baltimore, Maryland

LINDA HUMPHREY, MD, MPH
Division of Hospital and Specialty Medicine, Portland VA Health Care System; Department of Medicine, Oregon Health and Science University, Portland, Oregon

NIGEL B. JAMIESON, MD, PhD
Wolfson Wohl Cancer Research Centre, Institute of Cancer Sciences, University of Glasgow; Academic Unit of Surgery, School of Medicine, College of Medical, Veterinary and Life Sciences, Glasgow Royal Infirmary, University of Glasgow; West of Scotland Pancreatic Unit, Glasgow Royal Infirmary, Glasgow, United Kingdom

NAGI F. KHOURI, MD
Associate Professor, Department of Radiology, Johns Hopkins Hospital, Johns Hopkins University, Baltimore, Maryland

GWEN A. LOMBERK, PhD
Assistant Professor, Laboratory of Epigenetics and Chromatin Dynamics, Gastroenterology Research Unit, Departments of Biochemistry and Molecular Biology and Biophysics; Division of Gastroenterology and Hepatology, Department of Medicine, Mayo Clinic, Rochester, Minnesota

G. JOHAN A. OFFERHAUS, MD, PhD, MPH
Department of Pathology, University Medical Center Utrecht (H04-312), Utrecht, The Netherlands

PAUL F. PINSKY, PhD
Division of Cancer Prevention, National Cancer Institute, Bethesda, Maryland

YUN-SUHK SUH, MD, MS
Department of Surgery, Cancer Research Institute, Seoul National University College of Medicine, Seoul, Korea

WILLIAM TABAYOYONG, MD, PhD
Urology Institute, University Hospitals Case Medical Center, Cleveland, Ohio

KYOICHI TAKAORI, MD, PhD, FACS, FMAS(H)
Division of Hepato-Biliary-Pancreatic Surgery and Transplantation, Department of Surgery, Kyoto University Graduate School of Medicine, Sakyo-ku, Kyoto, Japan

L. WILLIAM TRAVERSO, MD, FACS
St. Luke's Center for Pancreatic and Liver Disease, Boise, Idaho

RAUL URRUTIA, MD
Professor, Laboratory of Epigenetics and Chromatin Dynamics, Gastroenterology Research Unit, Departments of Biochemistry and Molecular Biology, Biophysics, and Medicine, Mayo Clinic, Rochester, Minnesota

KEITA WADA, MD, PhD
Department of Surgery, Teikyo University School of Medicine, Tokyo, Japan

HAN-KWANG YANG, MD, PhD, FACS
Department of Surgery, Cancer Research Institute, Seoul National University College of Medicine, Seoul, Korea

Contents

> There is now compelling evidence that the molecular heterogeneity of cancer is associated with disparate phenotypes with variable outcomes and therapeutic responsiveness to therapy in histologically indistinguishable cancers. This diversity may explain why conventional clinical trial designs have mostly failed to show efficacy when patients are enrolled in an unselected fashion. Knowledge of the molecular phenotype has the potential to improve therapeutic selection and hence the early delivery of the optimal therapeutic regimen. Resolution of the challenges associated with a more stratified approach to health care will ensure more precise diagnostics and enhance therapeutic selection, which will improve overall outcomes.

> Pancreatic adenocarcinoma is painful, generally incurable, and frequently lethal. The current progression model indicates that this cancer evolves by mutations and deletions in key oncogenes and tumor suppressor genes. This article describes an updated, more comprehensive model that includes concepts from the fields of epigenetics and nuclear architecture. Widespread use of next-generation sequencing for identifying genetic and epigenetic changes genome-wide will help identify and validate more and better markers for this disease. Epigenetic alterations are amenable to pharmacologic manipulations, thus this new integrated paradigm will contribute to advance this field from a mechanistic and translational point of view.

> Cancer screening has long been an important component of the struggle to reduce the burden of morbidity and mortality from cancer. Notwithstanding this history, many aspects of cancer screening remain poorly understood. This article presents a summary of basic principles of cancer screening that are relevant for researchers, clinicians, and public health officials alike.

Screening for lung cancer in high-risk individuals with annual low-dose computed tomography has been shown to reduce lung cancer mortality by 20% and is recommended by multiple health care organizations. Lung cancer screening is not a specific test; it is a process that involves appropriate selection of high-risk individuals, careful interpretation and follow-up of imaging, and annual testing. Screening should be performed in the context of a multidisciplinary program experienced in the diagnosis and management of lung nodules and early-stage lung cancer.

Colorectal cancer (CRC) is a leading cause of cancer morbidity and mortality in the Western world. Advances in surgical and medical management have led to improved outcomes; however, the prognosis of CRC is often poor when detected at a symptomatic stage. Most cases of CRC develop over years from removable well-defined precursor lesions, and asymptomatic, curable disease may be detected by convenient noninvasive tests. These features make CRC a suitable candidate for screening, and several options are available. This article outlines the evidence for established CRC screening tests along with a discussion on newer tests and ongoing research.

Breast cancer screening has become a controversial topic. Understanding the points of contention requires an appreciation of the conceptual framework underpinning cancer screening in general, knowledge of the strengths and limitations of available screening modalities, and familiarity with published clinical trial data. This review is data intense with the intention of presenting enough information to permit the reader to enter into the discussion with an ample knowledge base. The focus throughout is on striking a balance between the benefits and harms of breast cancer screening.

Accurate tests for at-risk populations are available for hepatitis B virus, hepatitis C virus (HCV), and hepatocellular carcinoma (HCC). Effective treatments for all three diseases exist if diagnosed early. New antivirals are making a significant impact on HCV. Liver transplant is curative for early HCC and is prioritized by the United Network for Organ Sharing in the United States. Screening and surveillance for deadly disease only makes sense if there are identifiable populations at risk for the condition, there are sensitive and specific low-cost tests available for the condition, and there are effective treatments for the condition.

William Tabayoyong and Robert Abouassaly

Prostate cancer is the most common malignancy diagnosed in men and the second leading cause of cancer death for men in the United States. Widespread use of prostate-specific antigen (PSA) screening led to a decrease in mortality; however, PSA screening may have led to overdiagnosis and overtreatment of clinically insignificant cancers. The US Preventive Services Task Force (USPSTF) released a statement recommending against the use of PSA, which was met with concern from professional organizations. This article reviews the epidemiology of prostate cancer, data from the largest screening trials, USPSTF recommendation statement, and current strategies used to improve overdiagnosis and overtreatment.

Keita Wada, Kyoichi Takaori, and L. William Traverso

Neither extended surgery nor extended indication for surgery has improved survival in patients with pancreatic cancer. According to autopsy studies, presumably 90% are metastatic. The only cure is complete removal of the tumor at an early stage before it becomes a systemic disease or becomes invasive. Early detection and screening of individuals at risk is currently under way. This article reviews the evidence and methods for screening, either familial or sporadic. Indication for early-stage surgery and precursors are discussed. Surgeons should be familiar with screening because it may provide patients with a chance for cure by surgical resection.

Yun-Suhk Suh and Han-Kwang Yang

Low ratio of mortality over incidence of gastric cancer in Asian countries including Korea and Japan could be explained by early detection after screening, different treatment strategy, or genetic disparity between the East and West. Early detection after screening program for gastric cancer and subsequent surgical treatment including appropriate lymph node dissection has been developed successfully in high-risk areas such as East Asian countries. Even in countries with a low prevalence of gastric cancer, a specific screening program is recommended for any high-risk population.

Lodewijk A.A. Brosens, G. Johan A. Offerhaus, and Francis M. Giardiello

Colorectal cancer (CRC) is the third most common cancer and the third leading cause of cancer death in men and women in the United States. About 30% of patients with CRC report a family history of CRC. However, only 5% of CRCs arise in the setting of a well-established mendelian inherited disorder. In addition, serrated polyposis is a clinically defined

SURGICAL CLINICS
OF NORTH AMERICA

THE CLINICS ARE AVAILABLE ONLINE!
Access your subscription at:
www.theclinics.com

Foreword

Cancer Screening and Genomics

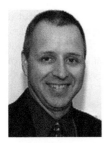

Ronald F. Martin, MD
Consulting Editor

Shortly before the turn of the century, somebody told me that 500 years from now the only two names people would remember from the millennium were Christopher Columbus and Neil Armstrong. I have no idea if that will turn out to be true, but the proposition has been nagging at me for fifteen years. Not because I really care all that much about who actually remembers whom, but rather because I wonder what causes people or things to be important enough to be specifically remembered at all. Certainly, in the cases of Columbus and Armstrong—both of whom were or are probably remarkable people—they will be remembered for what they famously did and not for who they were.

I, as I suspect you do, encounter many items on a daily basis that are important and that I *must* remember (digital devices set off alarms to tell me so). The e-mails with exclamation points, the urgent pages to page someone who doesn't want to wait by a phone for me to answer their page, the ever-present warnings to comply with this or that very important dictate or mandate—probably none of them are important enough to remember for even a few days let alone a few centuries. So, does any task I do or that anybody else does really matter? Well, of course it does. It may not matter to collective humanity, but it matters to somebody, however briefly.

There is, however, something that we all do that does matter, even over the millennia—we store, process, and pass on information. The information we pass on may be in many forms, some of which are more durable than others. The facts have their place, as do the data and the analyses, but what really matters is passing along the ability to keep asking the questions and to reframe inquiry. We program ourselves, and we program one another.

This issue of the *Surgical Clinics of North America* is devoted to cancer, specifically, screening for cancer and genomics. It may not immediately seem like the usual fare for general surgeons, but it should be. Dr Blake Cady once opined in a presidential address that when it comes to cancer, "Biology is king." He was right then, and he always will be. Our version of what biology means will change. Our knowledge of how to intervene or redirect the biological behavior of cancer will change. But Blake's sentiments about biology will always be right despite our refinement of knowledge. That is an enduring principle. That needs to be passed along.

Surg Clin N Am 95 (2015) xiii–xiv
http://dx.doi.org/10.1016/j.suc.2015.07.002
0039-6109/15/$ – see front matter © 2015 Published by Elsevier Inc.

surgical.theclinics.com

When people have limited tools, they do the best they can with what they have. For centuries, we have thought of cancer as a disease to be cut out. Perhaps somewhat surprisingly, that actually works pretty well sometimes. About 60 years ago, we were given a clearer understanding of DNA, and since then, our knowledge of the genetic nature of cancer has evolved in ways that would have been hard to imagine. Yet, we still treat cancer in many circumstances with knives and string, and we cut it out—and it still works, to some degree. To be fair, we accompany with operative management all that we have learned about manipulating the biological behavior of tumor cell, as well. We have designed studies and tested this form or that form of ways of destroying cancer cells to keep people alive or improve their lives. We measure outcomes, and we have made some progress but not nearly enough.

People with unlimited resources can worry about outcomes. People with limited resources need to worry about indications. You have to put your limited material and efforts into those things that will give you bang for your buck. It is the fundamental value equation. Operations cost money, time, and resources and have unintended consequences even when they go well. Nonoperative management has exactly the same set of concerns. If we want to do better things for people and fewer bad things to people, we need to have a better understanding of who is likely to benefit from what we do and how we pick the right therapy for those who need it. Targeted therapy and screening are more likely to yield value than nondirected approaches. Basing medical therapy on genetic profiles is likely to increase the percentage of persons who benefit from potentially toxic therapy. The days of one size fits all are over.

Dr Wolfgang and his colleagues have compiled an excellent collection of articles on the genetics and screening of cancer as well as information on genomics and targeted therapy. I encourage you to read it, think about it, and pass along what you have learned to others.

An evolutionary biologist once told me a woman is an egg's way of making another egg. Parenthetically, she also told me that men were basically biologically disposable. Not to demean either gender, but the idea is that, individually, we aren't that important in the grand scheme of things, but the information that we pass along, in the form of DNA, is important—at least in the aggregate. Cells and multicellular organisms (that's you and me) are really around to pass along the genetic information. That being said, somebody has to pass along the intellectual information as well because it doesn't seem to want to pass itself along.

One day, people will probably look back on our most sophisticated efforts in surgery and medicine today and regard them much the way we feel about cupping and leeches. And if that day comes about, it will be okay, because the only reason they will be that much smarter than we are will be because we built them a better foundation than the one we had. If they can remember that, they may not think we were all that stupid after all. Also, perhaps it's a reminder to look back with a bit of kindness on the cuppers and leech handlers, even if they were way off track. They thought they were enlightened once upon a time as well.

Ronald F. Martin, MD
Department of Surgery
Marshfield Clinic
1000 North Oak Avenue
Marshfield, WI 54449, USA

E-mail address:
martin.ronald@marshfieldclinic.org

Preface

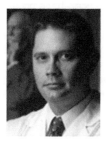

Christopher L. Wolfgang, MD, PhD
Editor

The instruction book for an individual is written in their DNA. Physical stature, cognitive skills, personality traits, and likely even longevity are determined by our genetic code. It would follow that many diseases also have a genetic basis, and this is certainly the case for cancer. Despite all of the complexities of cancer biology, it is inherently a genetic disease. The genetic origin of cancer can either be passed from generation to generation through germline alterations that predispose individuals to risk or through somatic alterations acquired during the lifetime of a person. These alterations can arise by chance or be initiated by environmental factors, such as tobacco, radiation, or UV light. Although it is conceptually easy to think of cancer development as a simple manifestation of genetic alterations, in actuality, the molecular events and interplay among host tissues are complex. Acquired alterations occur at a relatively high rate in dividing cells, but most are corrected by an elaborate editing system or programmed cell death and are never realized by the organism. Those alterations that persist through this first layer of protection, but create a phenotype that provides no growth advantage, are also eliminated or remain silent. Those rare events that lead to a phenotypic advantage may ultimately develop into a cancer. The manner in which this occurs is complex since the genetic code is simply the instruction book, and numerous events in the implementation of the instructions also come into play. Alterations in normal epigenetic and micro-RNA control of gene expression, RNA processing, posttranslational modification of proteins, among numerous other events, are all necessary for tumorigenesis.

Recent developments have made a basic understanding of the genetic and molecular basis of cancer more than academic. The first report of the human genome in 2003 and the continued refinement of these data have set the stage for new approaches to treat cancer. The ability to sequence germline and tumor DNA has grown at an unprecedented pace mainly through the development of next-generation sequencing techniques. It is now theoretically possible to sequence an individual's entire genome in about a week and at a cost that rivals that of routine imaging or diagnostic testing. Industry has rapidly embraced this technology and numerous companies now offer both targeted and global genetic testing. This growth has been paralleled by growth in proteomics and metabolomics. How clinicians use and

Surg Clin N Am 95 (2015) xv–xvi
http://dx.doi.org/10.1016/j.suc.2015.07.001
0039-6109/15/$ – see front matter © 2015 Published by Elsevier Inc.

surgical.theclinics.com

understand this information has implications to clinical care. Certain cancers, such as lung and colorectal, can harbor relatively prevalent specific mutations that can alter the choice of systemic therapy. Others, such as pancreatic cancer, have no predominant targetable alteration but have markers of biological behavior that may direct management. In some cancer types, molecular profiling has become standard to guide treatment practice, while this information may be of little use in others. In addition, it is not uncommon for a patient to walk into a clinic with self-initiated genetic germline or somatic genetic analysis. For these reasons, it is important for surgeons caring for patients with cancer to have a basic understanding of cancer genetics and screening.

Screening for early cancers is thought to have made a positive impact on survival for certain cancer types, such as breast, colorectal, and prostate. However, many aspects of screening remain controversial and in some instances have been thought to be counterproductive. The addition of genetic status to the screening of high-risk individuals has added additional complexity to the process. Thus, a basic understanding of cancer screening is also important for surgeons caring for patients with cancer.

The purpose of this issue is to provide surgeons with a basic understanding of the genetic and molecular basis of cancer and how this impacts management. In addition, several articles in this issue also focus on the benefits and limitations of cancer screening.

Christopher L. Wolfgang, MD, PhD
Department of Surgery
Johns Hopkins Hospital
685 Blalock Building
600 North Wolfe Street
Baltimore, MD 21287, USA

E-mail address:
cwolfga2@jhmi.edu

Cancer Genetics and Implications for Clinical Management

Nigel B. Jamieson, MD, PhD[a,b,c], David K. Chang, MD, PhD[a,d,e,f,g], Andrew V. Biankin, MD, PhD[a,d,e,f,g],*

KEYWORDS

- Genomics • Next-generation sequencing • Pancreatic cancer
- Stratified medicine • Translational medicine

KEY POINTS

- Molecular heterogeneity of cancer leads to disparate molecular phenotypes with variable disease outcomes and responses to therapy in histologically indistinguishable cancers.
- There are opportunities for potential rapid improvements in cancer outcomes by adopting a more selective or stratified approach to therapy.
- Analysis of genomic data is identifying candidate actionable molecular phenotypes with existing therapeutics (repurposing) approved for use in other cancers.
- Successful translation of genomic discoveries necessitates a shift in cancer trial design and clinical service delivery to incorporate low-prevalence actionable phenotypes across multiple cancer types.
- Whole-genome sequencing has revealed that genomic aberrations in addition to point mutations in coding sequences have the potential to provide clinically useful biomarkers.
- Analysis of exceptional responders may inform how current therapeutics decision-making can be improved, and provide a mechanism for development of novel therapies.

Disclosure: The authors have nothing to disclose.
[a] Wolfson Wohl Cancer Research Centre, Institute of Cancer Sciences, University of Glasgow, Garscube Estate, Switchback Road, Bearsden, Glasgow G61 1BD, UK; [b] Academic Unit of Surgery, School of Medicine, College of Medical, Veterinary and Life Sciences, Glasgow Royal Infirmary, University of Glasgow, Alexandra Parade, Glasgow G31 2ER, UK; [c] West of Scotland Pancreatic Unit, Glasgow Royal Infirmary, Alexandra Parade, Glasgow G31 2ER, UK; [d] The Kinghorn Cancer Centre, Garvan Institute of Medical Research, 370 Victoria Street, Darlinghurst, New South Wales 2010, Australia; [e] Cancer Research Program, Garvan Institute of Medical Research, 384 Victoria Street, Darlinghurst, Sydney, New South Wales 2010, Australia; [f] Department of Surgery, Bankstown Hospital, Eldridge Road, Bankstown, Sydney, New South Wales 2200, Australia; [g] Faculty of Medicine, South Western Sydney Clinical School, University of NSW, Goulburn St, Liverpool, New South Wales 2170, Australia
* Corresponding author. Wolfson Wohl Cancer Research Centre, Institute of Cancer Sciences, University of Glasgow, Garscube Estate, Switchback Road, Bearsden, Glasgow G61 1BD, UK.
E-mail address: andrew.biankin@glasgow.ac.uk

Surg Clin N Am 95 (2015) 919–934
http://dx.doi.org/10.1016/j.suc.2015.05.003
0039-6109/15/$ – see front matter © 2015 Elsevier Inc. All rights reserved.
surgical.theclinics.com

INTRODUCTION

The concept that chromosomal abnormalities may result in cancer was initially proposed a century ago,[1] but only 40 years have passed since Sakurai and Sandberg[2] more definitely published an original report suggesting that certain tumor genomic changes could influence the clinical management of cancer. Their karyotype aberration classification represented the first example of how the genetic information of cancer cells could inform clinical decision making.

It is now well accepted that most cancers are driven by genomic alterations that dysregulate key molecular pathways influencing cell growth, survival, and other hallmarks of cancer. Cancer genomics refers to the study of tumor genomes at multiple levels, including changes in DNA sequence, structure, the epigenome (methylation, histone modification), and the transcriptome (messenger RNA and noncoding RNA). The spectrum of genetic dysregulation promoting tumorigenesis includes gene activation or inactivation, and changes in gene expression.[3] These advances have begun to challenge traditional clinical approaches in oncology, in which patients' treatment is focused exclusively on the tumor tissue of origin. The ability to harness the full clinical potential of tumor genetic information has only recently become manifest and although the primary site of origin matters, so too do its genomic characteristics.

Aberrations playing crucial roles in tumorigenesis and progression, described as driver events, may confer critical tumor dependencies, with addiction of a cancer cell to one or several specific molecular pathways. Identification of biologically important genes and pathways commonly disrupted across different cancer types can generate clinically relevant diagnostic, predictive, prognostic, and therapeutic information.[4]

Technology has redefined the field, with the advent of large-scale genomic surveys systemically capturing cancer genomic information orchestrated by collectives including the International Cancer Genome Consortium (ICGC)[5] and The Cancer Genome Atlas (TCCA),[6] replacing serial investigation of genetic defects. Systematic and scalable methods of genetic analysis, captured by the term genomic sequencing, have facilitated the characterization of thousands of cancer genomes. Translating this systematic knowledge from individuals and their tumors may improve clinical outcomes for patients with cancer; however, rigorous evaluation of this genomics-driven cancer medicine hypothesis will require logistical transformation and innovation guided by conceptual advances in pretherapy and posttherapy tissue acquisition, specimen processing, tumor genomic profiling, data interpretation, clinical trial design, and the ethical return of genetic results to clinicians and their patients.

This article outlines aspects of recent progress in cancer genomics and provides a perspective for potential clinical applications of genomic research to advance personalized medicine and oncologic strategies.

UNDERSTANDING THE CANCER GENOME LANDSCAPE AND TRANSLATING ADVANCES FOR THERAPEUTIC GAIN

As clinicians better understand the molecular pathology of cancer, substantial complexity is being discovered, identifying a composite of multiple diseases, rather than the few that were previously defined morphologically.[7] Emerging data from large sequencing initiatives encompassing various cancers[6,8] unveil an array of molecular aberrations in histologically indistinguishable cancers. As next-generation sequencing (NGS) and other omic technologies further advance, reclassification based on molecular criteria should provide sufficient granularity to define the distinctiveness of individual cancers.

Common malignancies are being segregated according to genomic analysis: colorectal cancer (*KRAS/BRAF/NRAS/PIK3CA* wild type and *KRAS*-mutated, *NRAS*-mutated, *BRAF*-mutated, *PIK3CA*-mutated tumors), malignant melanoma (*BRAF*, *NRAS*, or *KIT* mutated), and non–small cell lung cancer (NSCLC) (*EGFR*, *KRAS*, *BRAF* mutated; *ALK*-rearranged, *ROS1*-rearranged carcinomas). More recently, in colorectal cancer, genomic sequencing has established hypermutated and nonhypermutated subtypes. In the former, the genetic signature is marked by microsatellite instability (MSI); in the latter, differentiation is by *TP53* and *APC* mutations. In the nonhypermutated subtype, 60% of patients have a *TP53* mutation, whereas this mutation was present in only 20% of the hypermutated form.[6]

Pancreatic cancer (PC) specifically pancreatic ductal adenocarcinoma remains an unyielding adversary: it is the fourth leading cause of cancer death in western societies, with an overall 5-year survival rate of less than 5%, a figure that has remained unchanged for 50 years.[9] It is projected to be the second leading cause of cancer-related death by 2030.[10] Surgical resection remains the only chance of cure, with chemotherapy adding minimal benefit. With few exceptions, most clinical trials of systemic therapies have failed to affect survival in a statistically or clinically meaningful manner; however, noteworthy responses are sometimes observed in undefined subgroups.[11] Apart from the few common mutations that cannot be effectively targeted, most point mutations occur at a rate of less than 5%,[12,13] which hampers clinical testing because the responsive phenotype of a particular therapeutic regimen is likely to be below the detection threshold of conventional randomized controlled trial (RCT) designs.

The first PC genomics study, performed at Johns Hopkins University, used a combination of capillary-based exome sequencing and single-nucleotide polymorphism (SNP) microarrays to identify mutations and copy-number alterations in all protein coding genes for both cell lines and xenografts derived from primary and metastatic tumors of 24 patients.[9] This study uncovered the inherent genetic complexity of PC, reaffirming near-ubiquitous *KRAS* activation along with inactivation of *TP53*, *CDKN2A*, and *SMAD4* at rates of greater than 50%. The frequency of other genes harboring mutations with potential functional consequences decreased rapidly, with most less than 5%. The aberrations coalesced into 12 core signaling pathways contributing to fundamental processes underlying PC, including DNA damage repair and 11 other carcinogenic mechanisms. Therapeutic development is focused on negating the aberrant physiologic effects of many of these altered pathways and processes, a targeting strategy that may be preferable to targeting specific gene components. Somatic chromosomal structural rearrangement represents a common mutation class capable of disrupting gene sequences (eg, deletion, rearrangement), gene activation (eg, copy-number gain, amplification), and resulting in the formation of novel oncogenes (gene fusions). Often these occurrences promote carcinogenesis,[14,15] and may present therapeutic targets.[16,17] Karyotyping data have revealed such chromosomal rearrangements to be common in PC,[18] with subsequent assessment enabling characterization of structural rearrangements, suggesting that these variations contribute substantially to pancreatic carcinogenesis.[19,20] Significant intertumoral heterogeneity in the pattern of genomic instability was apparent, with variable prevalence (range, 3–558 per patient) and type of rearrangement. Analysis of clonal relationships among metastases in the same patients revealed that genomic instability frequently persists after cancer dissemination, resulting in ongoing, parallel, and even convergent genomic evolution.

Multinational collaborative efforts including the ICGC have accelerated the understanding of PC genes. Greater definition achieved by whole-exome sequencing delineated mutations along with DNA microarrays to survey copy-number alterations in 142 primary operable PCs characterizing novel mechanisms potentially central to PC carcinogenesis: axon guidance and chromatin modification.[12] Intense desmoplastic stroma characterizes PC, accounting for 70% or more of the tumor volume, and generates significant technical challenges for NGS across many cancer types.[21] Strategies for tumor epithelial content enrichment have included performing full-face frozen sectioning with macrodissection to improve epithelial cellularity and subsequently mutation detection sensitivity. An analysis tool (Qpure) allows estimation of tumor epithelial content using copy-number variation on SNP arrays to predict the relative sensitivity of mutation detection for a given sample before sequencing.[22] Resected samples with an epithelial cellularity of greater than 20% reveal significant heterogeneity of mutated PC genes, identifying 2016 genes with nonsilent mutations, and 1628 copy-number variations. There were on average 26 mutations per patient (range, 1–116). Significant mutated gene analysis identified 16 genes, including *KRAS*, *TP53*, *CDKN2A*, *SMAD4*, *MLL3*, *TGFBR2*, *ARID1A*, *SF3B1*, *PCDH15*, as well as novel genes implicated in chromatin modification (*EPC1* and *ARID2*) and *ATM*. In addition, 5 other previously unreported mutated genes were identified (*ZIM2*, *MAP2K4*, *NALCN*, *SLC16A4*, *MAGEA6*).[12] Copy-number alterations are common genomic events in PC; however, the degree of instability makes these events difficult to interpret, especially as epithelial cellularity decreases.

DRIVER VERSUS PASSENGER MUTATIONS

Although NGS has the power to uncover almost the full spectrum of mutations in a cancer genome, only a fraction of detected mutations are likely to be relevant contributors to tumorigenesis. Differentiating these candidate drivers from passenger mutations remains a substantial challenge in cancer genomics.[23] Such complexity suggests that innovative analytical approaches using large data sets are necessary to uncover further, unapparent mechanisms. Numerous computational tools assist in defining the probability of a given gene and/or mutation as a potential carcinogenic driver,[24] but they lack sensitivity and are inefficient when confronted with multiple infrequently mutated genes.

Further studies reinforced the molecular heterogeneity of PC and, although loss of function events predominated, a variety of secondary gain of function events seem to occur in genes that are known drivers in other cancer types.[12] This finding suggests that although *KRAS* is vital early in PC evolution, a second gain of function event (eg, *HER2*, *MET* amplification) may be essential for progression, which has implications for therapy because these are often targets of existing drugs. Integrating data from functional screens[25] and animal models may enrich for driver events.[26] Genetically engineered mouse models of PC are well developed.[27,28] In addition, *Sleeping Beauty* transposon–mediated mutagenesis screens in *KRAS* transgenic PC models[29,30] and in-vitro short hairpin RNA screens[31] provide a source of complementary data that can be used to inform human data. Such approaches have identified novel candidate genes in PC, including *USP9X*[29] and *MAP2K4*,[30] and pathway analysis supports important roles for pathways including G1/S checkpoint machinery, apoptosis, regulation of angiogenesis, transforming growth factor beta signaling, and novel pathways including chromatin modification and axon guidance, particularly SLIT/ROBO signaling.[12]

MUTATIONAL SIGNATURES IN CANCER

The accumulation of large-scale cohort-based cancer genome sequence data incorporating multiple cancer types has provided the opportunity to describe and classify mutational signatures distributed between them, and in some instances infer underlying mechanisms. Rather than being a random assortment of base changes spread across the genome, somatic tumor mutations reflect the sum of mutagenic exposures and mutational processes active during the evolution and progression of a cancer. Following the pioneering work that defined 5 common mutational signatures active in a breast cancer cohort,[32] a large Sanger Institute–led collaborative effort analyzed 4,942,984 mutations across 7042 tumors incorporating 30 cancer types, identifying more than 20 distinct mutational signatures.[32–34] Some signatures were associated with the age of the patient at diagnosis, established mutagenic exposures including smoking in lung cancer and ultraviolet light in malignant melanoma, or DNA damage repair defects, but approximately half were original signatures not previously described. Although some signatures are present in many cancer types, others are more restricted.

At present, data based on 100 whole-exome sequences in addition to 20 whole genomes indicate that there are 4 mutational signatures that correspond with known biological processes in PC. These signatures include, older age, BRCA-mediated defects in DNA damage repair, DNA mismatch repair deficiency, and a signature associated with the apolipoprotein B mRNA editing enzyme, catalytic polypeptide-like (APOBEC) family of cytidine deaminases.[33] This innovative approach to defining mutagenic processes vital in cancer evolution has the potential to inform strategies for cancer prevention, early diagnosis, and therapeutic development.

RATIONALE OF GENOTYPE-GUIDED MEDICINE

The ultimate goal of cancer research is a better understanding of underlying biological processes, enabling multidimensional components of patient care to be influenced, from time to diagnosis, to prognosis, to predictive markers of therapy. Despite the genetic complexity of cancer, a deeper understanding has led to a vast treatment armamentarium of therapies capable of selectively targeting putative molecular dependencies critical for cancer cell survival and proliferation. Clinical therapeutic benefit depends on the presence of specific cellular targets and is optimally directed by the presence of a robust, reproducible, companion biomarker of therapeutic responsiveness.[11]

Tamoxifen was the original targeted therapy, being an antagonist of the estrogen receptor in breast tissue and other tissues including the endometrium. Its use revolutionized the treatment of operable and metastatic breast cancer,[35] with further roles in prevention of contralateral breast cancer and disease prevention in high-risk individuals.[36] The availability of targeted therapies was extended only recently by the identification of HER2 amplification in breast cancer, in which genetic profiling and effective targeting by a monoclonal antibody, trastuzumab, improved survival in an aggressive tumor subtype.[37] Subsequent advancements, including imatinib in KIT-positive gastrointestinal stromal tumors[38] and the use of crizotinib in NSCLC with EML-ALK fusion gene, are shown in **Table 1**.[39] In triple-negative breast cancer, recurrent MAGI3-AKT3 fusion leading to constitutive AKT kinase activation, which is abolished by ATP-competitive AKT small-molecule inhibitors,[40] with genetic rearrangements leading to PTEN inactivation of gene fusions activating BRAF in prostate cancer subsets, provide rationale for clinical trials exploring phosphatidylinositol 3 kinase (PI3K) pathway BRAF/MEK inhibitors, respectively.[41,42] In-frame fusion transcripts of KIF5B and RET oncogenes are present in 1% to 2% of lung adenocarcinomas. In preclinical models, tyrosine kinase inhibitors (TKI) targeting RET suppress fusion-induced cell growth, introducing options for patients with NSCLC who possess this specific aberration.[43]

Table 1
Molecular targets for personalized cancer therapies

Cancer Type	Cellular Target	Targeted Agent	Class of Agent
Colorectal	KRAS	Cetuximab	EGFR mAb
Breast	HER2	Trastuzumab	HER2 mAb
Chronic myeloid leukemia	BCR-ABL fusion protein	Imatinib	TKI
Gastrointestinal stroma tumors	c-KIT	Imatinib	TKI
Non–small cell lung cancer	EGFR	Erlotinib and gefitinib	TKI
Non–small cell lung cancer	EML4-ALK fusion protein	Crizotinib	TKI
Malignant melanoma	BRAF^{V600E}	Vemurafenib	BRAF/MEK/ERK pathway inhibitor
Ovarian, breast, and prostate cancer	BRCA1, BRCA2	Olaparib	PARP inhibitor

Abbreviations: mAb, monoclonal antibody; PARP, poly(ADP-ribose) polymerase; TKI, tyrosine kinase inhibitor.

Successful translation of large-scale genomic data and other omic discoveries into improved patient care necessitate a paradigm shift in clinical oncology. Such a precision oncology approach incorporates a new molecular taxonomy, based on frequently mutated cancer genes largely not being specific for the tissue type of the tumor.[44,45] In addition to an organ-based and morphology-based classification, individual cancers are grouped and selected for optimal therapy according to their molecular signature or biotype, particularly for molecularly diverse cancers.[46] A lung cancer and a breast cancer with inappropriate activation of the same signaling pathways may share more genetic vulnerabilities than a lung or breast cancer lacking the same mutations. It remains unclear how best to identify and integrate these patients appropriately into clinical trials.

For a cancer with significant genomic heterogeneity and lacking a dominant phenotype such as PC, a genotype-guided stratified approach may be beneficial. Supportive examples of success include the activity of poly(ADP-ribose) polymerase (PARP) inhibitors in breast and ovarian cancers with BRCA1/2 mutations,[47] vemurafenib in BRAF^{V600E}-mutated melanoma and thyroid cancer,[48] and crizotinib in lung cancer and anaplastic large-cell lymphoma with ALK translocations.[49]

Strategies include an umbrella trial design, in which patients with a certain type of cancer are assigned a specific therapy according to the genetic characteristic of the cancer with many different arms under a single trial. It enables several targeted therapies and corresponding NGS-based profiling to test companion diagnostic assays that can be combined to treat either a single cancer or multiple cancer types.[50]

A further study design is the basket trial, which is a method to address the efficacy of companion biomarker (therapeutic target)–directed approaches to extend to low-prevalence actionable phenotypes, independent of tumor histology. Only those patients with a mutational profile suggestive of a therapeutic response are included. Genotyping individual cancers presents the opportunity to test the efficacy of targeted agents that are used in other cancers and other diseases, repurposing them to enable more rapid trial closure than studies focusing on a specific disease site, depending on patient response rates, and potentially enabling drug approval in multiple disease sites.[51] This hypothesis-driven strategy may be advantageous for mutations that are rare or difficult to study solely within a disease-specific context.

The key strengths of this approach are evident in the CUSTOM (Molecular Profiling and Targeted Therapies in Advanced Thoracic Malignancies) trial: namely the ability to identify a favorable response to targeted therapy with a small number of patients and the capacity to validate a clinical target. Only 15 patients with NSCLC and an epidermal growth factor receptor (EGFR) mutation were enrolled into the erlotinib treatment arm in this trial, and they had an overall response rate of 60%.[52] However, only 2 of the 15 treatment arms were successfully recruited as a result of feasibility issues stemming from the low incidence of certain mutations in specific histological subtypes. A true basket study that is independent of tumor histology may be more capable of addressing the efficacy of targeting specific genetic aberrations, as exemplified by the ongoing Vemurafenib basket trial (VE-BASKET) evaluating in multiple myeloma and solid malignancies with the BRAF V600 gene mutations (ClinicalTrials. gov identifier NCT01524978).

Whether common genetic events traversing different cancer lineages will translate into response to similar therapies remains unclear because specific genetic abnormalities often fail to confer sensitivity to targeted therapies across all tumor types, as exemplified by trastuzumab, which benefits patients with *HER2*-amplified breast cancer but failed to affect ovarian cancer outcome,[53] and by the poor response of *BRAF*^{V600E}-mutated colorectal cancer to vemurafenib.[54] It is likely that, if precision oncology strategies are to succeed, insights related to the underlying histology should not be entirely superseded by genetic aberrations.

MANAGING TUMOR HETEROGENEITY AND RESISTANCE TO TARGETED THERAPY

Despite advances in cancer genetics, intratumoral heterogeneity has yet to be fully understood and has significant implications for the development, interpretation, and translation of therapeutic strategies. Topographic differences in mutations, chromosome copy-number variations, and gene expression signatures reveal that multiple clonal subpopulations of tumor cells exist within a single neoplasm. Conventional pathology has previously described heterogeneity in common neoplasms as shown by regional separation of subclones harboring varying patterns of *HER2* amplification in breast cancer.[55] Notably, NGS techniques have revealed that the history of a tumor is encoded by its heterogeneity.[37] In renal cell carcinoma, common alterations in driver genes may be distinct across different tumoral regions.[56] As a consequence, biopsy samples may not adequately represent the cellular features and composition of the tumor bulk, with obvious implications for downstream biomarker utility and therapy selection. Clinical responses to targeted therapeutics are consistently negated by the development of drug resistance. Genomic analysis in relapsed tumor samples has revealed the emergence of secondary mutations, including *KIT*^{670I} for imatinib-resistant gastrointestinal stromal tumor (GIST),[57] and *EGFR*^{T790M} in gefitinib-resistant and erlotinib-resistant lung cancer.[58] These mechanisms affect response to TKIs either through alterations in drug targets (gatekeeper mutations) or change in the conformational state of the kinase, presumably representing positive selection of rare cell subpopulations already present in the primary.[59]

Tissue collected as part of clinical trials has the potential to enhance knowledge, identify new oncogenic mechanisms, define putative predictive and prognostic markers, as well as identify candidate drug resistance mechanisms. Specific rebiopsy protocols at the time of progression to molecular targeted therapy are becoming a standard of care for patients eligible for further treatment.[60] In *EGFR*-mutated NSCLC that has acquired resistance to erlotinib, secondary mutations have been identified in greater than 50% of patients.[61]

ADVANCING MOLECULAR PHENOTYPE–GUIDED THERAPY IN PANCREATIC CANCER

Overall response rates for PC have been disappointing when applied in an unselected fashion, with rapidly diminishing numbers eligible for second-line or third-line agents because of accumulating toxicity and cachexia. However, despite low overall response rates, palliative chemotherapy can be effective in undefined patient subgroups.[62,63]

Numerous prognostic and predictive biomarkers for PC have been explored, but few have been independently validated.[64] Despite the low mutation rates in PC, several actionable phenotypes of therapeutic responsiveness have been proposed (**Table 2**). Although individually small, cumulatively they account for up to 45% of PC, assuming minimal phenotype overlap. Mapping putative actionable molecular genotypes/phenotypes in PC using available tissue-based/genome-based assays and concentrating on repurposing or rescuing therapies potentially offers the opportunity to influence outcomes in a shorter timeframe than novel drug discovery and development.

Putative responsiveness biomarkers for gemcitabine include hENT1, hCNT1/3, and dCK,[65] with supportive preclinical evidence; however, clinical utility is not yet established.[66,67] SPARC (secreted protein acid and rich in cysteine) regulates extracellular

Table 2
Candidate actionable molecular phenotypes in pancreatic cancer

Actionable Phenotypes	Therapy	Rationale	Molecular Characterization Explored or Putative Biomarkers
Gemcitabine responsive	Gemcitabine	Phase 3 clinical trial data	High *hENT1, hCNT1, hCNT3* expression
DNA damage repair deficient	Platinum, MMC, PARP inhibitors	Case reports, clinical trials (FOLFIRINOX)	*BRCA2/ATM/PALB2* mutations Pangenomic instability
Nab-paclitaxel responsive	Nab-paclitaxel	Clinical trial; preclinical models	*SPARC* expression
Anti-EGFR responsive	Erlotinib	Phase 3 clinical trial (NCIC CTG PA.3)	*KRAS* wild type; epithelial signature
Fluoropyrimidine responsive	5-Fluorouracil; capecitabine	Phase 3 clinical trial data	Unknown
Irinotecan responsive	Irinotecan	Phase 3 clinical trial (FOLFIRINOX)	Topoisomerase 1 overexpression
HER2 amplified	Trastuzumab	Rescuing	*HER2* amplification
CSF1R mutation	Sunitinib	Repurposing	*CSF1R* mutation
STK11/LKB1 null	PI3K/mTOR/AKT inhibitors	Preclinical studies	*STK11/LKB1* mutation/loss
MET amplified	c-MET inhibitor	Preclinical studies	*MET* amplification
PTEN null/*PIK3CA* activated	PI3K/mTOR/AKT inhibitors	Preclinical studies	Loss of *PTEN* expression

Abbreviations: MMC, mitomycin C; mTOR, mammalian target of rapamycin.

matrix modeling and deposition.[68] With a prognostic biomarker role in PC[69,70] and because of its role as a so-called albumin sticker, it was developed as a therapeutic target for *nab*-paclitaxel (Abraxane). The phase III MPACT (Metastatic Pancreatic Adenocarcinoma Clinical Trial) RCT comparing gemcitabine versus gemcitabine plus Abraxane, showed that Abraxane conferred significant survival benefit in metastatic PC.[63] Although SPARC expression was potentially predictive in earlier phase studies,[71] the subsequent MPACT trial analysis did not validate a predictive role.[72] In the National Institute of Canada Clinical Trial Group (NCIC CTG) PA.3 study, the addition of erlotinib to gemcitabine showed a modest but significant survival advantage in advanced PC.[73] It remains unclear whether *KRAS* status can guide anti-EGFR therapy, which is akin to colorectal cancer in which activating mutations indicate therapy resistance. Preclinical data in normal pancreatic cell lines suggest an oncogenic role,[74] supporting efficacy for anti-HER2 therapy in *HER2*-overexpressing PC.[75,76] However, trastuzumab clinical trials have disappointed,[77,78] possibly as a consequence of nonstandardized assays leading to overestimation of *HER2* amplification, and hence underpowered studies.

A striking cellular hallmark of cancers with BRCA2-PALB2-Fanconi anemia DNA repair pathway defects is hypersensitivity to DNA damaging agents, including mitomycin C, platinum, and PARP inhibitors.[79,80] Platinum-based therapies in PC have mixed results in trials of unselected patients,[81] although a recent meta-analysis[82] and efficacy of FOLFIRINOX, a combination of 5-fluorouracil/leucovorin, irinotecan and oxaliplatin, shown by the PRODIGE (Partenariat de Recherche en Oncologie Digestive) 4/ACCORD (Actions Concertées dans les Cancers Colo-Rectaux et Digestifs) study suggests subgroup activity.[62] This combination can be associated with significant toxicity, so predicting responders would significantly improve outcomes. In addition, evidence suggests that oxaliplatin is the predominant active agent, implying that definition of tumors harboring DNA damage repair defects may diminish the need for this combination, and thus limit toxicity.

Both *BRCA1* and *BRCA2* proteins are integral to cross-linking DNA repair via homologous recombination,[83] therefore deficient cells accumulate DNA double-strand breaks, generating genomic instability with subsequent malignant transformation. Furthermore, they interact with Fanconi anemia pathways: *FANCC*, *FANCG*, and *PALB2*.[84] However, responsive phenotypes and corresponding biomarkers may extend beyond these. Trials are currently evaluating platinum agents and PARP inhibitors for breast and ovarian cancer treatment,[80,85] recruited according to germline or Fanconi anemia gene status.

Recently, genome-wide analysis of structural variation was used to classify PC into 4 subtypes according to genomic stability with potential clinical relevance: (1) stable, (2) locally rearranged, (3) scattered, and (4) unstable subtypes.[86] If those patients with an unstable genome, or the *BRCA*-mediated mutational signatures described earlier,[33] which have putative deficiencies in DNA damage repair, were included in addition to patients with traditional defects in DNA damage repair mechanisms such as detrimental somatic and germline point mutations in *BRCA1*, *BRCA2*, and *PALB2*, there is scope to capture a greater number of potential responders. It remains uncertain whether such surrogate biomarkers, in the absence of *BRCA* or *PALB2* mutations, will effectively predict therapeutic response. However, in that study,[86] 14% of tumors with an unstable genome had mutations in non-BRCA pathway targets known to be drivers of instability and chemosensitivity, suggesting that such a diagnostic whole-genome sequencing approach to detecting DNA maintenance defects may offer a potentially valuable method to predict platinum and PARP inhibitor therapy responsiveness in various cancer types.

INDIVIDUALIZED THERAPY INITIATIVES

Prospective clinical testing of actionable molecular phenotypes is challenging with novel, nimble, and adaptable approaches required. A collaborative effort including the Australian Pancreatic Cancer Genome Initiative (APCGI) has commenced an umbrella trial evaluating the feasibility of assessing a stratified approach for PC treatment using predefined actionable molecular phenotypes. Following screening for 3 molecular phenotypes, patients were recruited to the Individualised Molecular Pancreatic Cancer Therapy (IMPaCT) trial, a randomized phase II first-line study (Australian New Zealand Clinical Trial Registry ID: ACTRN12612000777897) that compares gemcitabine with a more stratified therapeutic approach. The initial molecular phenotypes and corresponding therapeutic agents include HER2 amplified (trastuzumab), germline BRCA1/2 or PALB2 mutations (DNA damaging agent or PARP inhibitor), and KRAS wild-type or KRAS G13D mutations (erlotinib). This adaptive trial enables inclusion of additional arms as emerging/novel actionable genotypes/phenotypes become defined. A much larger-scale example is the National Cancer Institute (NCI) Molecular Analysis for Therapy Choice (MATCH) trial, which in 2015 plans to screen more than 3000 patients, with enrollment of at least 1,000, for a targeted drug combination, independent of tumor histology, into a master protocol.[87] Similarly, to further evaluate the efficacy of treating tumors according targets, the NCI-MPACT (Molecular Profiling-Based Assignment of Cancer Therapy) trial is randomly assigning patients with a specific genetic mutation to either (1) pathway-targeted therapy or (2) treatment not known to be pathway specific (ClinicalTrials.gov identifier NCT01827384).

INHERITED SUSCEPTIBILITY OF CANCER IN THE ERA OF NEXT-GENERATION SEQUENCING

The traditional approach to understanding cancer predisposition emerged through the limitations associated with the sequencing of individual genes. At present there are 114 recognized cancer predisposition genes.[88] It is expected that the germline sequences that accompany collaborative genomic initiatives will provide insights into the prevalence of established predisposition loci, along with identification of novel loci, likely with small effect sizes.[89] Increasing availability of NGS will necessitate cautious interpretation of germline variations identified in the absence of traditionally identified high-risk kindreds. Unreliability of family history accounts for some misses; however, a higher than expected germline mutations prevalence in cancer predisposition genes is reported in other cancers, notably BRCA mutations in sporadic triple-negative breast cancer.[90]

At present only limited end points for cancer predisposition are recorded: young age of cancer onset and increased incidence, but further surrogates could potentially incorporate survival. Most genes investigated to date have well-known significant biological impact: TP53 in Li-Fraumeni syndrome, or KRAS mutations, which influence early carcinogenesis. An inherited deleterious gene variation may not substantially reduce the age of onset for a malignancy or dramatically influence the cancer incidence, because the founder mutation is still environmentally determined, but progressor mutations may be preexisting that then drive clonal evolution, resulting in the generation of a more aggressive tumor, with a worse prognosis. There is a need to define the clinical role of specific genomic variants, to better understand cancer predisposition using techniques including whole-genome sequencing and identify genetic defect surrogates including MSI and mutational signatures; for example, those associated with DNA maintenance defects.

EXCEPTIONAL RESPONDERS

The low prevalence of most molecular phenotypes may to an extent explain the failure of RCTs addressing heterogeneous cancers, including triple-negative breast cancer and PC, particularly when considering targeted agents. To overcome this, trials have been serially enlarged to increase the power to detect progressively smaller therapeutic benefits. In a simulation study, Stewart and Kurzrock[91] showed that addition of only 11 on-target patients was required to achieve significance and hence a positive, rather than a negative, outcome. However, many drugs are deemed ineffective and are quickly abandoned owing to limited overall efficacy, despite some patient subgroups having an exquisite sensitivity or an exceptional response to treatment.

Some eminently targetable mutations may be so rare that they are only discovered in the context of a negative trial. Recently, an inhibitor of the mTORC1 (mammalian target of rapamycin complex 1) complex, everolimus, traditionally an immunosuppressant, had extraordinary and durable efficacy for a single patient with metastatic bladder cancer despite failure of the phase II trial.[92] Whole-genome sequencing of the patient's tumor revealed coding mutations for *TSC1* and *NF2*, both previously associated with mTORC1 dependence in preclinical models, with partial responses to everolimus evident in 3 of 4 patients with a *TSC1* gene mutation present.[92] Subsequently, 2 further patients, one with metastatic urothelial cancer and another with metastatic anaplastic thyroid carcinoma, were noted to have experienced an exceptional response to everolimus and underwent whole-genome sequencing.[93,94] Experimental validation subsequently confirmed specific tumoral *mTOR* mutations that, if identified in further patients, may prompt off-label everolimus therapy irrespective of tumor histology. It is expected that the increased use of basket and umbrella clinical trial designs will identify more patients with an extreme or exceptional response to targeted therapies.

Study of the exceptional responses, particularly those in clinical trials, including those that failed to detect an overall benefit, enables genetics underlying cancer to inform future management strategies. Identifying molecular phenotypes that underlie exceptional responders will facilitate a stratified and rationalized approach to inform current clinical decision making, enabling research to focus on mechanisms of action and resistance, avoid ineffectual therapies, and unencumber the development of novel therapeutic strategies. The NCI has implemented an Exceptional Responders Initiative that is currently recruiting in an effort to improve patient selection and allow the development of more rational treatment strategies in the future (ClinicalTrials.gov identifier NCT02243592).

SUMMARY

The advent of NGS technologies along with a greater understanding of genomic data sets has brought some early promising signals that have potential to influence a profound transformation on the management of cancer through stratification and personalization of therapy. Such precision oncology strategies are designed to provide clinical management tailored toward the molecular characteristics of a patient's tumor, and this approach was outlined as a priority by the US government through the recently announced Precision Medicine Initiative.[95] However, numerous challenges remain and potentially the impact may prove substantive rather than transformative, with genomic profiling being relevant and important to many, but not necessarily all, cancer subtypes. Issues surrounding the impact of tumor heterogeneity along with challenges in optimal biospecimen acquisition will undoubtedly require development and refinement. Furthermore, educational issues remain and must be addressed if physicians are expected to order, understand, and act on diagnostic results generated from NGS genomic data. Resistance must be overcome with solid evidence that specific gene mutation stratified therapy combinations will provide clinical benefits, which may prove challenging to show in the current clinical trial framework. Integral to the success and impact of personalized cancer therapeutics is collaboration and alignment of the multiple stakeholders and health care systems.

REFERENCES

1. Boveri T. Concerning the origin of malignant tumours by Theodor Boveri. Translated and annotated by Henry Harris. J Cell Sci 2008;121(Suppl 1):1–84.
2. Sakurai M, Sandberg AA. Prognosis of acute myeloblastic leukemia: chromosomal correlation. Blood 1973;41(1):93–104.
3. Ma QC, Ennis CA, Aparicio S. Opening Pandora's Box–the new biology of driver mutations and clonal evolution in cancer as revealed by next generation sequencing. Curr Opin Genet Dev 2012;22(1):3–9.
4. Vucic EA, Thu KL, Robison K, et al. Translating cancer 'omics' to improved outcomes. Genome Res 2012;22(2):188–95.
5. International Cancer Genome Consortium, Hudson TJ, Anderson W, et al. International network of cancer genome projects. Nature 2010;464(7291):993–8.
6. Cancer Genome Atlas Network. Comprehensive molecular characterization of human colon and rectal cancer. Nature 2012;487(7407):330–7.
7. Watson IR, Takahashi K, Futreal PA, et al. Emerging patterns of somatic mutations in cancer. Nat Rev Genet 2013;14(10):703–18.
8. Cancer Genome Atlas Research Network. Comprehensive genomic characterization defines human glioblastoma genes and core pathways. Nature 2008; 455(7216):1061–8.
9. Siegel R, Naishadham D, Jemal A. Cancer statistics, 2013. CA Cancer J Clin 2013;63(1):11–30.
10. Rahib L, Smith BD, Aizenberg R, et al. Projecting cancer incidence and deaths to 2030: the unexpected burden of thyroid, liver, and pancreas cancers in the United States. Cancer Res 2014;74(11):2913–21.
11. Biankin AV, Hudson TJ. Somatic variation and cancer: therapies lost in the mix. Hum Genet 2011;130(1):79–91.
12. Biankin AV, Waddell N, Kassahn KS, et al. Pancreatic cancer genomes reveal aberrations in axon guidance pathway genes. Nature 2012;491(7424):399–405.
13. Jones S, Zhang X, Parsons DW, et al. Core signaling pathways in human pancreatic cancers revealed by global genomic analyses. Science 2008;321(5897):1801–6.
14. Stephens PJ, Greenman CD, Fu B, et al. Massive genomic rearrangement acquired in a single catastrophic event during cancer development. Cell 2011; 144(1):27–40.
15. Stephens PJ, Tarpey PS, Davies H, et al. The landscape of cancer genes and mutational processes in breast cancer. Nature 2012;486(7403):400–4.
16. Druker BJ, Sawyers CL, Kantarjian H, et al. Activity of a specific inhibitor of the BCR-ABL tyrosine kinase in the blast crisis of chronic myeloid leukemia and acute lymphoblastic leukemia with the Philadelphia chromosome. N Engl J Med 2001; 344(14):1038–42.
17. Gravalos C, Jimeno A. HER2 in gastric cancer: a new prognostic factor and a novel therapeutic target. Ann Oncol 2008;19(9):1523–9.
18. Griffin CA, Hruban RH, Morsberger LA, et al. Consistent chromosome abnormalities in adenocarcinoma of the pancreas. Cancer Res 1995;55(11):2394–9.

19. Campbell PJ, Yachida S, Mudie LJ, et al. The patterns and dynamics of genomic instability in metastatic pancreatic cancer. Nature 2010;467(7319):1109–13.

20. Yachida S, Jones S, Bozic I, et al. Distant metastasis occurs late during the genetic evolution of pancreatic cancer. Nature 2010;467(7319):1114–7.

21. Vogelstein B, Papadopoulos N, Velculescu VE, et al. Cancer genome landscapes. Science 2013;339(6127):1546–58.

22. Song S, Nones K, Miller D, et al. qpure: A tool to estimate tumor cellularity from genome-wide single-nucleotide polymorphism profiles. PLoS One 2012;7(9):e45835.

23. Stratton MR, Campbell PJ, Futreal PA. The cancer genome. Nature 2009; 458(7239):719–24.

24. Dees ND, Zhang Q, Kandoth C, et al. MuSiC: identifying mutational significance in cancer genomes. Genome Res 2012;22(8):1589–98.

25. Boehm JS, Hahn WC. Towards systematic functional characterization of cancer genomes. Nat Rev Genet 2011;12(7):487–98.

26. Chin L, Andersen JN, Futreal PA. Cancer genomics: from discovery science to personalized medicine. Nat Med 2011;17(3):297–303.

27. Hingorani SR, Wang L, Multani AS, et al. Trp53R172H and KrasG12D cooperate to promote chromosomal instability and widely metastatic pancreatic ductal adenocarcinoma in mice. Cancer Cell 2005;7(5):469–83.

28. Morton JP, Jamieson NB, Karim SA, et al. LKB1 haploinsufficiency cooperates with Kras to promote pancreatic cancer through suppression of p21-dependent growth arrest. Gastroenterology 2010;139(2):586–97, 597.e1–6.

29. Perez-Mancera PA, Rust AG, van der Weyden L, et al. The deubiquitinase USP9X suppresses pancreatic ductal adenocarcinoma. Nature 2012; 486(7402):266–70.

30. Mann KM, Ward JM, Yew CC, et al. Sleeping Beauty mutagenesis reveals cooperating mutations and pathways in pancreatic adenocarcinoma. Proc Natl Acad Sci U S A 2012;109(16):5934–41.

31. Cheung HW, Cowley GS, Weir BA, et al. Systematic investigation of genetic vulnerabilities across cancer cell lines reveals lineage-specific dependencies in ovarian cancer. Proc Natl Acad Sci U S A 2011;108(30):12372–7.

32. Nik-Zainal S, Alexandrov LB, Wedge DC, et al. Mutational processes molding the genomes of 21 breast cancers. Cell 2012;149(5):979–93.

33. Alexandrov LB, Nik-Zainal S, Wedge DC, et al. Signatures of mutational processes in human cancer. Nature 2013;500(7463):415–21.

34. Alexandrov LB, Nik-Zainal S, Wedge DC, et al. Deciphering signatures of mutational processes operative in human cancer. Cell Rep 2013;3(1):246–59.

35. Early Breast Cancer Trialists' Collaborative Group (EBCTCG). Effects of chemotherapy and hormonal therapy for early breast cancer on recurrence and 15-year survival: an overview of the randomised trials. Lancet 2005;365(9472): 1687–717.

36. Fisher B, Costantino JP. RESPONSE: re: tamoxifen for prevention of breast cancer: report of the National Surgical Adjuvant Breast and Bowel Project P-1 study. J Natl Cancer Inst 1999;91(21):1891A–1892.

37. Shibata D. Cancer. Heterogeneity and tumor history. Science 2012;336(6079): 304–5.

38. Tuveson DA, Willis NA, Jacks T, et al. STI571 inactivation of the gastrointestinal stromal tumor c-KIT oncoprotein: biological and clinical implications. Oncogene 2001;20(36):5054–8.

39. Kwak EL, Bang YJ, Camidge DR, et al. Anaplastic lymphoma kinase inhibition in non-small-cell lung cancer. N Engl J Med 2010;363(18):1693–703.

40. Banerji S, Cibulskis K, Rangel-Escareno C, et al. Sequence analysis of mutations and translocations across breast cancer subtypes. Nature 2012;486(7403): 405–9.

41. Berger MF, Lawrence MS, Demichelis F, et al. The genomic complexity of primary human prostate cancer. Nature 2011;470(7333):214–20.

42. Palanisamy N, Ateeq B, Kalyana-Sundaram S, et al. Rearrangements of the RAF kinase pathway in prostate cancer, gastric cancer and melanoma. Nat Med 2010; 16(7):793–8.

43. Kohno T, Ichikawa H, Totoki Y, et al. KIF5B-RET fusions in lung adenocarcinoma. Nat Med 2012;18(3):375–7.

44. Cancer Genome Atlas Research Network, Weinstein JN, Collisson EA, et al. The cancer genome atlas pan-cancer analysis project. Nat Genet 2013;45(10): 1113–20.

45. Kandoth C, McLellan MD, Vandin F, et al. Mutational landscape and significance across 12 major cancer types. Nature 2013;502(7471):333–9.

46. Accelerating progress against cancer: ASCO's blueprint for transforming clinical and translational cancer research. American Society of Clinical Oncology. 2011. Available at: http://www.asco.org/practice-research/ascos-research-blueprint. Accessed March 18, 2015.

47. Bryant HE, Schultz N, Thomas HD, et al. Specific killing of BRCA2-deficient tumours with inhibitors of poly(ADP-ribose) polymerase. Nature 2005;434(7035): 913–7.

48. Flaherty KT, Puzanov I, Kim KB, et al. Inhibition of mutated, activated BRAF in metastatic melanoma. N Engl J Med 2010;363(9):809–19.

49. Gambacorti-Passerini C, Messa C, Pogliani EM. Crizotinib in anaplastic large-cell lymphoma. N Engl J Med 2011;364(8):775–6.

50. Ledford H. 'Master protocol' aims to revamp cancer trials. Nature 2013; 498(7453):146–7.

51. Willyard C. 'Basket studies' will hold intricate data for cancer drug approvals. Nat Med 2013;19(6):655.

52. Lopez-Chavez A, Thomas A, Rajan A, et al. Molecular profiling and targeted therapy for advanced thoracic malignancies: a biomarker-derived, multiarm, multihistology phase II basket trial. J Clin Oncol 2015;33(9):1000–7.

53. Bookman MA, Darcy KM, Clarke-Pearson D, et al. Evaluation of monoclonal humanized anti-HER2 antibody, trastuzumab, in patients with recurrent or refractory ovarian or primary peritoneal carcinoma with overexpression of HER2: a phase II trial of the Gynecologic Oncology Group. J Clin Oncol 2003;21(2):283–90.

54. Prahallad A, Sun C, Huang S, et al. Unresponsiveness of colon cancer to BRAF(V600E) inhibition through feedback activation of EGFR. Nature 2012; 483(7387):100–3.

55. Cottu PH, Asselah J, Lae M, et al. Intratumoral heterogeneity of HER2/neu expression and its consequences for the management of advanced breast cancer. Ann Oncol 2008;19(3):595–7.

56. Gerlinger M, Rowan AJ, Horswell S, et al. Intratumor heterogeneity and branched evolution revealed by multiregion sequencing. N Engl J Med 2012;366(10): 883–92.

57. Gajiwala KS, Wu JC, Christensen J, et al. KIT kinase mutants show unique mechanisms of drug resistance to imatinib and sunitinib in gastrointestinal stromal tumor patients. Proc Natl Acad Sci U S A 2009;106(5):1542–7.

58. Choi YL, Soda M, Yamashita Y, et al. EML4-ALK mutations in lung cancer that confer resistance to ALK inhibitors. N Engl J Med 2010;363(18):1734–9.

59. Garraway LA, Janne PA. Circumventing cancer drug resistance in the era of personalized medicine. Cancer Discov 2012;2(3):214–26.
60. Arcila ME, Oxnard GR, Nafa K, et al. Rebiopsy of lung cancer patients with acquired resistance to EGFR inhibitors and enhanced detection of the T790M mutation using a locked nucleic acid-based assay. Clin Cancer Res 2011;17(5): 1169–80.
61. Sequist LV, Waltman BA, Dias-Santagata D, et al. Genotypic and histological evolution of lung cancers acquiring resistance to EGFR inhibitors. Sci Transl Med 2011;3(75):75ra26.
62. Conroy T, Desseigne F, Ychou M, et al. FOLFIRINOX versus gemcitabine for metastatic pancreatic cancer. N Engl J Med 2011;364(19):1817–25.
63. Von Hoff D, Ervin T, Arena F, et al. Results of a randomized phase III trial (MPACT) of weekly nab-paclitaxel plus gemcitabine versus gemcitabine alone for patients with metastatic adenocarcinoma of the pancreas with PET and CA19-9 correlates. J Clin Oncol 2013;(Suppl 31):abstr 4005.
64. Jamieson NB, Carter CR, McKay CJ, et al. Tissue biomarkers for prognosis in pancreatic ductal adenocarcinoma: a systematic review and meta-analysis. Clin Cancer Res 2011;17(10):3316–31.
65. Marechal R, Bachet JB, Mackey JR, et al. Levels of gemcitabine transport and metabolism proteins predict survival times of patients treated with gemcitabine for pancreatic adenocarcinoma. Gastroenterology 2012;143(3):664–74.e1-6.
66. Farrell JJ, Elsaleh H, Garcia M, et al. Human equilibrative nucleoside transporter 1 levels predict response to gemcitabine in patients with pancreatic cancer. Gastroenterology 2009;136(1):187–95.
67. Poplin EA, Wasan H, Rolfe L, et al. Randomized, multicenter, phase II study of CO-101 versus gemcitabine in patients with metastatic pancreatic ductal adenocarcinoma: including a prospective evaluation of the role of hENT1 in gemcitabine or CO-101 sensitivity. J Clin Oncol 2013;31(35):4453–61.
68. Neuzillet C, Tijeras-Raballand A, Cros J, et al. Stromal expression of SPARC in pancreatic adenocarcinoma. Cancer Metastasis Rev 2013;32(3–4):585–602.
69. Infante JR, Matsubayashi H, Sato N, et al. Peritumoral fibroblast SPARC expression and patient outcome with resectable pancreatic adenocarcinoma. J Clin Oncol 2007;25(3):319–25.
70. Mantoni TS, Schendel RR, Rodel F, et al. Stromal SPARC expression and patient survival after chemoradiation for non-resectable pancreatic adenocarcinoma. Cancer Biol Ther 2008;7(11):1806–15.
71. Von Hoff DD, Ramanathan RK, Borad MJ, et al. Gemcitabine plus nab-paclitaxel is an active regimen in patients with advanced pancreatic cancer: a phase I/II trial. J Clin Oncol 2011;29(34):4548–54.
72. Hidalgo M, Plaza C, Illei P, et al. SPARC analysis in the phase III MPACT trial of nab-paclitaxel (nab-p) plus gemcitabine (gem) vs gem alone for patients with metastatic pancreatic cancer (PC). Ann Oncol 2014;25:ii106.
73. Moore MJ, Goldstein D, Hamm J, et al. Erlotinib plus gemcitabine compared with gemcitabine alone in patients with advanced pancreatic cancer: a phase III trial of the National Cancer Institute of Canada Clinical Trials Group. J Clin Oncol 2007;25(15):1960–6.
74. Chang Z, Li Z, Wang X, et al. Deciphering the mechanisms of tumorigenesis in human pancreatic ductal epithelial cells. Clin Cancer Res 2013;19(3):549–59.
75. Kimura K, Sawada T, Komatsu M, et al. Antitumor effect of trastuzumab for pancreatic cancer with high HER-2 expression and enhancement of effect by combined therapy with gemcitabine. Clin Cancer Res 2006;12(16):4925–32.

76. Buchler P, Reber HA, Eibl G, et al. Combination therapy for advanced pancreatic cancer using Herceptin plus chemotherapy. Int J Oncol 2005;27(4):1125–30.

77. Safran H, Iannitti D, Ramanathan R, et al. Herceptin and gemcitabine for metastatic pancreatic cancers that overexpress HER-2/neu. Cancer Invest 2004;22(5): 706–12.

78. Harder J, Ihorst G, Heinemann V, et al. Multicentre phase II trial of trastuzumab and capecitabine in patients with HER2 overexpressing metastatic pancreatic cancer. Br J Cancer 2012;106(6):1033–8.

79. Xia B, Dorsman JC, Ameziane N, et al. Fanconi anemia is associated with a defect in the BRCA2 partner PALB2. Nat Genet 2007;39(2):159–61.

80. Byrski T, Huzarski T, Dent R, et al. Response to neoadjuvant therapy with cisplatin in BRCA1-positive breast cancer patients. Breast Cancer Res Treat 2009;115(2): 359–63.

81. Tabernero J, Macarulla T. Changing the paradigm in conducting randomized clinical studies in advanced pancreatic cancer: an opportunity for better clinical development. J Clin Oncol 2009;27(33):5487–91.

82. Ciliberto D, Botta C, Correale P, et al. Role of gemcitabine-based combination therapy in the management of advanced pancreatic cancer: a meta-analysis of randomised trials. Eur J Cancer 2013;49(3):593–603.

83. Schutte M, da Costa LT, Hahn SA, et al. Identification by representational difference analysis of a homozygous deletion in pancreatic carcinoma that lies within the BRCA2 region. Proc Natl Acad Sci U S A 1995;92(13):5950–4.

84. Slater EP, Langer P, Niemczyk E, et al. PALB2 mutations in European familial pancreatic cancer families. Clin Genet 2010;78(5):490–4.

85. Clark-Knowles K, O'Brien A, Weberpals J. BRCA1 as a therapeutic target in sporadic epithelial ovarian cancer. J Oncol 2010;2010:891059.

86. Waddell N, Pajic M, Patch AM, et al. Whole genomes redefine the mutational landscape of pancreatic cancer. Nature 2015;518(7540):495–501.

87. National Cancer Institute - Molecular Analysis for Therapy Choice Program (NCI-MATCH). 2014. Available at: http://deainfo.nci.nih.gov/advisory/ncab/164_1213/Conley.pdf. Accessed March 18, 2015.

88. Rahman N. Realizing the promise of cancer predisposition genes. Nature 2014; 505(7483):302–8.

89. Stadler ZK, Schrader KA, Vijai J, et al. Cancer genomics and inherited risk. J Clin Oncol 2014;32(7):687–98.

90. Couch FJ, Hart SN, Sharma P, et al. Inherited mutations in 17 breast cancer susceptibility genes among a large triple-negative breast cancer cohort unselected for family history of breast cancer. J Clin Oncol 2015;33(4):304–11.

91. Stewart DJ, Kurzrock R. Fool's gold, lost treasures, and the randomized clinical trial. BMC Cancer 2013;13:193.

92. Iyer G, Hanrahan AJ, Milowsky MI, et al. Genome sequencing identifies a basis for everolimus sensitivity. Science 2012;338(6104):221.

93. Wagle N, Grabiner BC, Van Allen EM, et al. Response and acquired resistance to everolimus in anaplastic thyroid cancer. N Engl J Med 2014;371(15):1426–33.

94. Wagle N, Grabiner BC, Van Allen EM, et al. Activating mTOR mutations in a patient with an extraordinary response on a phase I trial of everolimus and pazopanib. Cancer Discov 2014;4(5):546–53.

95. Collins FS, Varmus H. A new initiative on precision medicine. N Engl J Med 2015; 372(9):793–5.

The Triple-Code Model for Pancreatic Cancer

Cross Talk Among Genetics, Epigenetics, and Nuclear Structure

Gwen A. Lomberk, PhD[a],*, Raul Urrutia, MD[b,c,d],*

KEYWORDS

- Pancreatic adenocarcinoma • Epigenetics • Triple-code hypothesis

KEY POINTS

- Many researchers and practitioners still see pancreatic cancer exclusively as a disease of epithelial exocrine cells, which become transformed by the accumulation of genetic alterations.
- Genetic alterations cross talk with epigenetic and nuclear structure changes to give rise to not only neoplastic transformation but also to determine most features of the cancer phenotype and its symptoms.
- This updated paradigm for the progression of pancreatic cancer integrates the concept that the patterns of gene expression networks to define the pancreatic cancer phenotype are dictated by the combination of genetic, epigenetic, and nuclear structure instructions according to the triple-code hypothesis, which considers that all of these codes contribute to the development and progression of this disease.
- Many epigenetic alterations are significantly ameliorated by a new type of therapeutics that targets the epigenome. Promising epigenetics-based therapies are currently being evaluated through different types of trials.

Work in the authors' laboratories is supported by funding from the National Institutes of Health R01 DK52913 (R. Urrutia) and R01 CA178627 (G.A. Lomberk), as well as the Mayo Clinic Center for Cell Signaling in Gastroenterology (P30DK084567) and the Mayo Clinic SPORE in Pancreatic Cancer (P50 CA102701).
Conflicts of Interest: The authors declare that they have no competing interests.
[a] Laboratory of Epigenetics and Chromatin Dynamics, Gastroenterology Research Unit, Division of Gastroenterology and Hepatology, Department of Medicine, Mayo Clinic, 200 First Street Southwest, Guggenheim 10-24A, Rochester, MN 55905, USA; [b] Laboratory of Epigenetics and Chromatin Dynamics, Gastroenterology Research Unit, Department of Biochemistry and Molecular Biology, Mayo Clinic, Guggenheim 10-42C, Rochester, MN 55905, USA; [c] Laboratory of Epigenetics and Chromatin Dynamics, Gastroenterology Research Unit, Department of Biophysics, Mayo Clinic, Guggenheim 10-42C, Rochester, MN 55905, USA; [d] Laboratory of Epigenetics and Chromatin Dynamics, Gastroenterology Research Unit, Department of Medicine, Mayo Clinic, Guggenheim 10-42C, Rochester, MN 55905, USA
* Corresponding author.
E-mail addresses: lomberk.gwen@mayo.edu; urrutia.raul@mayo.edu

Surg Clin N Am 95 (2015) 935–952
http://dx.doi.org/10.1016/j.suc.2015.05.011
0039-6109/15/$ – see front matter © 2015 Elsevier Inc. All rights reserved.

Pancreatic adenocarcinoma (PDAC) remains a national health priority and significant therapeutic challenge. This dismal disease ranks fourth as a leading cause of cancer-related deaths in the United States, with a median survival of 6 months and a 5-year survival of 3% to 5%.[1] The bleak prognosis of PDAC is due to an aggressive biology, its immediate dissemination, and late diagnosis, rapidly leading to an incurable stage for which therapeutic intervention is a challenge. Surgical resection is the only curative modality; however, this only applies to 10% of patients, with their 5-year survival barely 20%.[2] Notably, these aggressive neoplasms are highly resistant to conventional chemotherapy and radiation.[3] Gemcitabine, a nucleoside analog, remains the standard chemotherapy option for metastatic PDAC.[4,5] Numerous trials have attempted to improve gemcitabine clinical benefit through alternative schedules or combination with other agents, to no avail.[6–8] Thus, there is an urgent need to develop novel therapies in PDAC, in particular, targeting pathways highly relevant to its pathobiology.

The genetics revolution has significantly advanced pancreatic cancer research. Searching for genetic mechanisms, many laboratories discovered oncogenes and tumor suppressor genes for PDAC.[9] These discoveries led to the seminal working model from the John Hopkins group[9] that expanded the understanding that PDAC arises from epithelial cells through accumulation of genetic alterations, driving transitions through increasingly aggressive lesions known as pancreatic intraepithelial neoplasias (PanINs). In particular, mutation of the KRAS oncogene is almost universally found in most PDAC cases.[10] Preneoplastic diseases, such as chronic pancreatitis, also harbor initiating KRAS mutations,[11] which seem to contribute to its evolution into cancer. This work prompted the development of animal models and tools to study, diagnose, and treat PDAC.[12,13] Thus, genetic concepts and tools have advanced the understanding of pancreatic diseases. Moreover, this work has led to the characterization of oncogenic signals that, for instance, in the case of kinases have allowed the development of novel therapeutics tools for this disease. However, despite these remarkable achievements, pancreatic cancer remains incurable.

The emergence of a new scientific revolution, epigenetics, has further advanced the study of pancreatic cancer by generating new tools for management and treatment. In 1942, Waddington[14] coined the term epigenetics to refer to inheritance that occurs independently of the coding capacity of DNA. Epigenetic mechanisms confer pluripotent progenitor cells that possess identical genomic DNA, the ability to differentiate into distinct populations. This wide range of differentiation originates from modulating genome expression in manners that are inheritable during cell division. Unlike genetics, epigenetics deals with the inheritance not of the genome but of the mechanisms that regulate the expression of entire gene networks at the right time, right time, level, and place to define and maintain the integrity of phenotypes. Since Waddington, it has been known that a cell has the potential to follow paths of distinct differentiation programs, similar to a ball rolling through different landscapes. Today, it is understood that these landscapes are defined by gene expression patterns. Recent Nobel Prize-winning discoveries have revealed that cells can be induced to undergo incredible phenotypic changes by manipulating gene expression in a manner that promotes rapid transit though these landscapes.[15] The generation of induced pluripotent stem cells, which promise to be key for cell-based therapies, involve the manipulation of the epigenetics of the cell, for example, in a manner that leads a fibroblast to convert into an adult pancreatic cell. More importantly, once they divide, these cells give rise to identical adult pancreatic cells. This fundamental stepping-stone will lead to the potential manipulation of the expressed genome for therapeutic purposes in a manner that will revolutionize biology and medicine. However, epigenetics promises much more. For instance, it is now known that, similar to genetic aberrations, epigenetic changes are inherited, giving rise to disease.[16] In addition, environmental insults induce epigenetic modifications to influence health and disease.[17] Thus, through genetics, humans inherit the potential to be who we are. However, epigenetics transforms this into the reality of who we are in health and in disease. In contrast to genetic alterations, epigenetic mechanisms are amenable to reversal by small molecule drugs, giving rise to the new area of epigenetic therapeutics, with many agents being tested in clinical trials. Thus, epigenetics is promising to provide deeper mechanistic insight into diseases, as well as provide new diagnostic and therapeutic tools for their management.

CROSS TALK BETWEEN GENETICS AND EPIGENETICS AS A PROMISING PARADIGM IN PANCREATOLOGY

Since its inception 25 years ago, the authors' laboratory has helped to promulgate that DNA methylation, histone modification, nucleosome remodeling, and regulatory noncoding RNAs regulate most biological processes that associate to neoplastic transformation in the pancreas. A significant amount of evidence suggests that epigenetic deregulation is involved in pancreatic cancer development, spreading, and some signs and symptoms such as thrombosis and cachexia. Epigenetics studies the activation and inactivation of gene networks independent of mutations, therefore, this article considers how these mechanisms fit within the genetic-centric paradigm. This exercise has previously led to the proposal that cross talk between genetics and epigenetics is critical for carcinogenesis.[18] This article reviews and updates this model.

The overarching concept of cancer genetics is that if a gene is over-amplified in cancer, it might have been selected to provide cells with an advantage to grow and survive during neoplastic transformation. On the other hand, similar advantages can be gained by cells via the downregulation of other genes, known as tumor suppressors. Following this premise along with the knowledge available from sequencing, Hruban and colleagues proposed a model in which PDAC arises from epithelial cells through an accumulation of genetic alterations in oncogenes and tumor suppressors, which promotes the development of precursor PanIN lesions.[19] Although over time this model increasingly materializes as incomplete, it is still highly valuable because it establishes the types of mutations that associate to a particular type of progressive preneoplastic lesion. For instance, the most universal mutation found in pancreatic cancer, oncogenic activation of KRAS, is necessary for initiation, but must be complemented later by genetic disruption of tumor suppressor pathways (eg, p16, p53, SMAD4) to give rise to frank invasive cancer.[9] The validity of this model has been shown in an elegant manner using genetically engineered models, which have been primarily supported by the National Institutes of Health via the Mouse Model Consortium funded by the National Cancer Institute.[20] However, this model does not explain epigenetic changes, which occur between landmark mutations and are responsible for either activating or repressing entire gene expression networks that drive cancer progression. Therefore, this article will give examples of these epigenetic mechanisms, namely DNA methylation, histone-based epigenetics, and noncoding RNA epigenetic molecules. In summary, this updated paradigm for the progression of pancreatic cancer integrates the concept of the triple-code hypothesis to include 2 additional types of processes besides genetics: epigenetic changes and alterations in nuclear architecture (**Fig. 1**). The intention in proposing this new paradigm is for investigators to dive into pancreatic cancer research with a more in-depth mechanistic approach than using only the tools of molecular pathology.

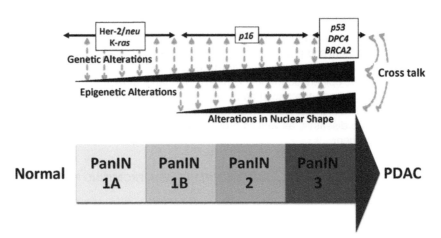

Fig. 1. Cross talk between genetics, epigenetics, and nuclear structure in a revised comprehensive progression model for pancreatic cancer. This model incorporates the genetic events described in the previous model as well as epigenetic changes and other alterations caused by changes in nuclear shape. Importantly, this model integrates the concept that these alterations do not occur in isolation, rather genetic alterations cross talk with epigenetic and nuclear structure changes to give rise to neoplastic transformation as well as most features of the cancer phenotype and its symptoms.

MECHANISTIC BASIS OF EPIGENETICS: THE NUCLEOSOME

Chromatin, which is composed of genomic DNA, histones, nonhistone regulatory proteins, and both small and long noncoding RNAs, are at the mechanistic core of epigenetics. These molecules are packed inside cells in the unit of the nucleosome, which can be viewed as the key nanomachine that senses both environmental and cell-autonomous signals to convert them into a gene-regulatory response that ultimately defines distinct phenotypes. It is at the level of the nucleosome that the processes of environment-gene interactions that have been robustly documented by genetic epidemiologists take place.[21] The nucleosome is composed of approximately 150 base pairs of nuclear DNA wrapped around a histone octamer built from 2 molecules of each core histone protein: H2A, H2B, H3, and H4. In addition, a linker histone, H1, attaches to the external face of the DNA-histone octamer complex to facilitate further compaction, a process that has vital biological importance. The N-terminal domain of histones, commonly referred to as histone tails, extend out from the nucleosome particle, and thereby become easily accessible to epigenetic regulator complexes and serve as the platform on which epigenetic signals are written, read, and erased to codify for the expression of distinct gene expression networks. The body of each core histone, which locates inside of the DNA, is thus less accessible but, in certain circumstances, becomes exposed to receive fewer, yet similarly critical, signals. A plethora of studies, originally pioneered independently by Strahl and Allis[22] as well as Turner,[23] revealed that these epigenetic signals, known as histone marks, are made by covalent chemical modifications. Today, it is known that histones receive many marks, including acetylation of lysines, methylation of lysines and arginines, phosphorylation of serines and threonines, adenosine diphosphate–ribosylation of glutamic acids, and ubiquitination and sumoylation of lysine residues, among others. More importantly, it is understood that it is the type and combination of these marks that serves as the instruction for cells to regulate gene expression in an inheritable manner. This concept is fundamental because it points to the existence of an epigenetic code (histone code) that is used to read the instruction provided by ancestors and cell progenitors to subsequent generations in the form of the genetic code. Aberrant patterns of histone marks are increasingly being associated to clinical phenotype and/or outcome in various cancers.[24–26] In pancreatic cancer, low cellular levels of distinct marks on histone H3, such as dimethyl lysine 4 (H3K4me2), dimethyl lysine 9, or acetyl lysine 18 (H3K18ac), were found to be significant and independent predictors of poor survival, with the most significant predictor of overall survival resulting from combined low levels of H3K4me2 and/or H3K18ac.[27] Histone marks alone, however, are not sufficient for the associated regulatory mechanism. To better understand epigenetics, the molecular machinery involved in the deposition, reading, and erasing necessary to give these instructions must be considered. Consequently, insight into these phenomena, which are critical for cells to gain and maintain their normal phenotype, is provided.

Sequence Specific Transcription Factors Function as Adaptor Proteins to Link DNA to Epigenetic Regulators

The first types of molecules above the layer of nucleosomes to consider in epigenetics are called sequence specific transcription factors. These proteins are most often modular molecules, which contain specialized domains that mediate their nuclear localization, binding to specific regions of DNA, and coupling to epigenetic regulators.[28] Most epigenetic regulators are armed with a specialized enzymatic activity that allows them to deposit, read, or erase posttranslational modifications in DNA and associated proteins. These marks function, therefore, as the signaling cascades of epigenetics and are interpreted as instructions for turning on and off extensive networks of genes. This article focuses on a selective group of transcription factor proteins that assist the RNA polymerase type II, the enzyme that copies most protein-coding genes as well as many, though not all, noncoding RNAs. An example of this type of transcription factor is the tumor suppressor p53, which contains a DNA-binding domain to recognize specific DNA sequences in promoters and other important regulatory regions, including enhancers of target genes (eg, p21).[29] The most frequent hot spot for mutation of this protein in cancer, including 50% to 75% of pancreatic cancers,[30] is within this DNA-binding domain.[31] In addition, this protein also contains a cluster of basic amino acids that function as a nuclear localization signal and a transcriptional regulatory domain that binds to epigenetic regulators that, in turn, will mark either the regulatory DNA domains or proteins associated with them. Depending on the chemical nature of these marks, they serve as the initial epigenetic signal to dictate whether the target gene will be expressed or silenced. Thus, it is important to describe how DNA is stored within the cell nucleus and is eventually sequestered away or accessed by transcription factors, marked, and regulated.

Nucleosome Remodeling Machines and Histone-Modifying Enzymes Work in Concert to Regulate Histone Marks

As mentioned previously, genomic DNA is highly packed into chromatin within the nucleus of eukaryotic cells. It is thought that this sequestration of the genome by a cover of proteins and RNA help to protect it from chemical and physical insults, as well as maintain many genes in a state of dormancy until necessary for access by the messenger RNA (mRNA) synthesis machinery to convert them into messages, which are then translated into proteins that help to define phenotypes. However, these associated proteins and RNA have the ability to regulate the genome by directing the expression of genes at the right level, right time, and right place to give rise to particular structures and functions. Among the genome-associated molecular machines that turn on and off genes (epigenetic regulatory complexes) are 2 major groups: nucleosome remodeling machines and histone-modifying enzymes. Nucleosome remodeling machines are multisubunit protein complexes that use energy from adenosine triphosphate (ATP) to move nucleosomes along the DNA template, thereby exposing or sequestering binding sites that function to specifically recruit other complexes (eg, histone-modifying enzymes) to specific regions of the genome. There are 4 families of nucleosome remodeling machines, which are typically identified by the type of ATPase subunits.[32] These complexes have different subunits of various types and sizes, including members of the switching defective/sucrose non-fermenting (SWI/SNF); imitation SWI (ISWI); inositol-requiring 80 (INO80); and nucleosome remodeling and deacetylation/Mi-2/chromodomain, helicase, DNA-binding (NuRD/Mi2/CHD) families. It has been long known that nucleosome remodeling machines are mutated in many cancers. Because these complexes consist of numerous subunits that perform a single net function, the sum of mutations in individual subunits must be considered to evaluate the prevalence in cancer similar to a single gene, such as *TP53*. For example, the average incidence of SWI/SNF mutations across all cancer types is nearly 20%, with a frequency of 26% in pancreatic cancer.[33]

Histone-modifying enzymes are currently considered among the most critical parts of the epigenome, other than noncoding RNAs. However, in contrast to noncoding RNAs, more is now known about the structures, functions, pathobiologic roles, and pharmacologic manipulation of the histone-modifying enzymes. Collectively, they possess enzymatic activities that allow them to deposit epigenomic marks (mark writers) and reverse these reactions when needed (mark erasers), as well as interpret these marks in context (mark readers). Among these proteins, histone methylases, acetylases, and ubiquitin ligases are among the most known and studied histone mark writers. The reactions catalyzed by these enzymes are then reversed by histone code erasers, including deacetylases, demethylases, and deubiquinases. Several histone-modifying enzymes are dysregulated in pancreatic cancer. For instance, in a recent study by Mazur and colleagues,[34] SMYD3, MLL5, EZH2, SETD5, and WHSC1L1 were found to be consistently upregulated in pancreatic cancer samples in a screen of 54 known and candidate human lysine methyltransferases, which are histone code writers. Several studies had previously found EZH2 overexpression in pancreatic cancer.[35–37] Interestingly, the oncogenic mutant KRAS signal was found to increase the expression of EZH2.[38] Furthermore, EZH2 suppresses the p16INK4 tumor suppressor gene, which is critical during injury-induced regeneration during pancreatitis and, therefore, contributes to the progression to pancreatic cancer.[39] In addition, EZH2 has been characterized as directly affecting the maintenance of the pancreatic cancer stem cell phenotype, which is also associated with its H3K27me3 catalytic activity.[40] Overexpression of some histone code erasers, such as the histone demethylases KDM2B[41] and LSD1,[42] enhance pancreatic cancer growth, whereas loss of the KDM6B histone demethylase associates with PDAC aggressiveness.[43] Probably the first class of histone-modifying enzymes identified to be dysregulated in PDAC was the histone deacetylase (HDAC). For instance, class I HDACs were strongly expressed in a subset of PDACs from a larger cohort of 82 samples. Strong nuclear immunoreactivity for HDAC1, 2, and 3 was observed for 32%, 63%, and 79% of PDAC cases, respectively.[44] In another expression profile of class I HDACs, HDAC1, HDAC2, HDAC3, and HDAC8 were positive in 17 (85%), 18 (90%), 20 (100%), and 18 (90%) of 20 pancreatic cancer cases, respectively, as observed with immunohistochemistry.[45] Further studies in PDAC have linked elevated HDAC1 and HDAC2 levels with poor tumor differentiation and overall survival.[46–48] Ouaïssi and colleagues[49] reported that approximately 80% of examined PDAC samples had a significant increase of HDAC7 at the RNA and protein levels. Notably, HDAC7 levels were reduced in chronic pancreatitis, serous cystadenoma, and intraductal papillary mucinous tumor of the pancreas samples, suggesting that HDAC7 overexpression can discriminate PDAC from other pancreatic diseases. Therefore, the histone marks and the type of instruction that each provides, as well as the associated histone-modifying enzymes, which are responsible of their regulation, should be carefully studied.[50–53] This suggestion is of particular importance because many drugs that are used to manipulate these pathways are being developed and tested at an unprecedented rate.[54–56] Many other compounds, such as neuroepileptic and other psychotropic drugs, that have been used for several decades, have potent epigenetic effects, which further supports the need for the medical community to become familiarized with this important family of epigenetic regulators. Similarly, there are writers, readers, and erasers of marks on DNA in addition to histones, which contribute to the instructions dictated to entire gene expression networks (see later discussion). In summary, the final outcome of these cascades is codified by the type and combination of marks controlled in context by writer, reader, and eraser enzymes in response to either cell-autonomous clues or environmental signals.

MARKING THE GENOME BY METHYLATION

The methylation of DNA was the first epigenetic modification to be discovered. Indeed, for decades, the methylation of CpG dinucleotides has been known to play a key role in X-chromosome inactivation, silencing of transposable DNA elements, and imprinting.[57] Methylation occurs in promoters and along gene bodies,[58] although the functional role of the latter remains poorly understood. Today, there are several types DNA methylation marks are identified, including the best known, which occurs by the covalent addition of a methyl (CH_3) group at the 5-carbon of the cytosine ring resulting in 5-methylcytosine (5 mC), as well as its oxidized forms, 5-hydroxymethyl-cytosine (5hmC), 5-formylcytosine, and 5-carboxylcytosine.[59] Sterically, when present in promoters and similar regulatory elements, the 5 mC mark protrudes into the major groove of DNA, which is the main region recognized by the molecular machinery that regulates gene expression and, thereby, inhibits transcription. For instance, methylation of the E-box (CACGTG) prevents n-Myc from binding to the EGFR promoter.[60] In addition, a significant amount of information exists on the type of writers, readers, and erasers of these marks.[59,61,62] Methylated CpG islands form a docking site for a family of methyl binding proteins, which read these marks to interfere with RNA synthesis to result in gene silencing. In the gene body, however, DNA methylation correlates with active transcription, splicing, and elongation,[63] though the detailed molecular mechanisms for this phenomenon are undefined. Similarly important, in contrast to the widely assumed notion that DNA methylation is a stable epigenetic mark, active methylation-demethylation cycles also occur. Dynamic regulation of DNA methylation is mainly achieved through a cyclical enzymatic cascade comprised of cytosine methylation by a group of writer enzymes called DNMTs; demethylation by ten-eleven translocation (TET) dioxygenases (TET1, TET2, and TET3), which act as erasers of these marks; and reconstitution of unmethylated cytosines by replication-dependent dilution and base excision during DNA repair. DNMT1 functions as a maintenance methyltransferase responsible for faithfully reproducing the level and pattern of methylation during somatic cell division.[61] DNMT3a and DNMT3b are involved in adding de novo methyl groups to DNA, in particular during development.[61] The methyltransferase 3-like protein (DNMT3L) does not have enzymatic activity but works as a necessary partner for the other DNMTs to perform their function. Interestingly, although Dnmt1 has up to a 50-fold preference for hemimethylated CpG sites present at the replication fork, it also seems to promote de novo methylation at non-CpG cytosines.[61] For performing the methylation reaction, all these enzymes use a derivative of the amino acid methionine, namely S-adenosylmethionine, as a methyl donor. The product of this reaction gives S-adenosylhomocysteine, which later becomes homocysteine to be catabolized or remethylated to methionine. Notably, because of the use of these cofactors, epigenetically driven methylation reactions are influenced by metabolism and nutritional intake.[64] Thus, besides signaling cascades, these 2 processes can influence DNA methylation and affect gene expression.

The effects of DNA methylation on pancreatic cancer have been extensively studied, both in experimental models and in human tissues. The results of these studies have revealed an increase in promoter-associated CpG island methylation, which often results in the silencing of tumor suppressor genes.[20,61,65] This phenomenon has led to the development and utilization of several drugs that function as DNMT inhibitors and, partially due to their effects on reactivating tumor suppressor genes, can slow down the progression of pancreatic cancer in both mice and humans.[66,67] However, promoter hypermethylation is accompanied by the concomitant hypomethylation of repetitive sequences corresponding to dormant retrotransposons, which can become activated. Hypomethylation of these sequences also becomes more pronounced by treatment with demethylating drugs.[68] However, the effect of these processes on the pathobiology of cancer is not completely clear. Interestingly, levels of 5hmC have been found reduced in pancreatic cancer and other cancer types along with a concomitant reduction in the expression of all 3 TET genes.[69] Besides its mechanistic importance and its relevance for cancer treatment, DNA methylation has been studied as a marker for the early detection of cancer. Cancer-specific DNA methylation patterns can be measured in DNA from detached tumor cells that are released to the blood, in pancreatic juice, or feces.[70–73] Unfortunately, despite its promise, there is not yet a clinically applicable assay for this purpose.

EPIGENETIC REGULATION BY NONCODING RNAs

Recent advances in sequencing technologies have revealed that the genome is extensively transcribed, yielding a large repertoire of noncoding RNAs. These include long noncoding RNAs (lncRNAs) and many small noncoding RNAs, such as microRNAs (miRNAs), small interfering RNAs, and Piwi-interacting RNAs (piRNAs). These mRNA-like molecules do not code for proteins but instead play key regulatory roles in a variety of cellular processes by modulating the levels and translation of other RNAs, including those coding for proteins.[74] Thus, it is important to briefly describe the biochemical constitution and function of these molecules. The most common among these molecules, miRNAs are small single-stranded molecules (20–25 nucleotides [nt]) that arise from pre-miRNAs, which are characterized by the presence of a hairpin structure.[75,76] This hairpin is processed to give rise to a mature miRNA, which is used to assemble an RNA-induced silencing complex (RISC), containing key regulatory proteins such as Dicer. Once released, the miRNA hybridizes in a complementary manner to target mRNAs via their 3′ untranslated region to subsequently induce cleavage by Argonaute, the catalytic component of RISC, and cause its silencing.

Distinct from miRNAs in size, lack of sequence conservation, and increased complexity, small 24 to 30 nt-long piRNAs interact in an RNA-protein complex with Piwi proteins, thus imparting their name.[76] These small RNAs are characterized by the presence of a uridine base at the 5′ end and a 2′-O-methyl modification at the 3′ end. Piwi proteins are a subclass of Argonaute protein family and are key to the biogenesis of these molecules.[77] The function of these molecules has been ascribed to epigenetic and posttranscriptional silencing of transposable elements during germline development.[78] Perhaps one of the most rapidly advancing fields within RNA research is the study of lncRNAs. These non–protein-coding transcripts are longer than 200 nt in length, which, like protein-coding RNAs, undergo splicing and polyadenylation.[79] A subgroup of lncRNAs, large intergenic noncoding RNAs (lincRNAs), have long been known by their role in epigenetic gene silencing, such as X-inactive specific transcript. However, different than miRNAs, lncRNAs seem to regulate gene expression and translation in various ways without a common mode of action. Thus far, lncRNA function has been categorized into 4 types of molecular mechanisms: signal, decoy, guide, and scaffold.[79] The lncRNAs assigned to the signal type function as molecular signals of transcriptional activity. For the decoy type, the lncRNAs bind to and titrate away other regulatory RNAs or proteins. As a guide, the lncRNAs serve to localize ribonucleoprotein complexes to specific targets, whereas the scaffold lncRNAs provide a structural platform for the assembly of relevant proteins and/or RNA components. Finally, enhancer RNAs and promoter-associated RNAs are the most recent types of noncoding RNA to be described.[80] The role of these molecules in epigenetics is just beginning to be uncovered. Enhancer RNAs are 800 nt in length on average, which up to now have been shown to be only transcriptional activators. Promoter-associated RNAs are noncoding transcripts that range from 16 nt to 200 nt, and they are expressed near the vicinity of promoters. Most of these molecules seem to associate with highly expressed genes and have short half-lives. Though investigations on the functional significance of these molecules have just started, thus far they are believed to mediate transcriptional activation and repression.

As a result of numerous studies, PDAC cell lines, tissues, and blood samples have been extensively profiled for miRNA expression levels and compared with normal and chronic pancreatitis samples to determine a miRNA expression signature that is associated with PDAC. Recently, however, Ma and colleagues[81] performed a comprehensive metareview of published studies in PDAC to evaluate a total of 538 tumor and 206 noncancerous control samples. This analysis revealed a meta-signature of 7 upregulated and 3 downregulated miRNAs, namely miR-155, miR-100, miR-21, miR-221, miR-31, miR-143, and miR-23a with increased expression and miR-217, miR-148a and miR-375 with decreased expression. In addition, alterations in miRNA levels are able to modulate chemosensitivity or radiosensitivity of PDAC cells in a variety of settings, with certain miRNAs serving as indicators of chemotherapy efficacy.[82] Therefore, miRNAs continue to be an active area of investigation for diagnostic biomarkers and therapeutic targets in PDAC. During the past 2 to 3 years, a few studies in pancreatic cancer on lncRNAs have emerged. For instance, expression of HOTAIR, a lincRNA that associates with Polycomb repressive complex 2 and its overexpression correlates with poor survival in several cancers, was found increased in pancreatic tumors, in particular more aggressive tumors, compared with control tissue.[83] Furthermore, knockdown of HOTAIR in PDAC cell lines resulted in decreased cell proliferation, altered cell cycle progression, induced apoptosis, reduced cell invasion, and inhibited tumor growth in xenografts. Similarly, overexpression of the lncRNAs MALAT1, HULC, and PVT1 have been associated with poor outcome in PDAC subjects.[84–86] Another study that evaluated lncRNAs by microarray found that subjects with high expression levels of the lncRNA BC008363 had significantly improved survival rates compared with those with lower levels.[87] Another lncRNA frequently downregulated in PDAC, ENST00000480739, was found to suppress tumor invasion and metastasis through regulation of hypoxia-inducible factor 1α on reexpression,[88] suggesting that lncRNAs may serve as a focus of future therapies.

SHAPING GENE EXPRESSION THROUGH NUCLEAR ARCHITECTURE

One of the most universal hallmarks of cancer cells is visible morphologic alteration of the nuclei detectable by light microscopy on routine staining and this is often used by pathologists to grade and specify cancer type and stage, such as the transition of PanIN 1B to PanIN 2.[89] Changes in nuclear structure include increased size, distortions in shape, and alterations in the internal organization of the nucleus.[90,91] The spatial arrangement of chromosomes and other nuclear components, which defines the nuclear architecture, imparts a scaffold to organize the regulation of distinct functional processes. Any observed alterations in nuclear architecture may result from changes in the nuclear matrix, higher order chromatin folding, and/or the spatial arrangement of nucleic acid metabolism. Therefore, these changes, as seen in cancer, have the potential to affect the fidelity of genome replication, chromatin organization, and gene expression. Studies have indicated that nuclear morphometry may serve as a prognostic indicator in nonresectable pancreatic cancer,[92] as well as provide important preoperative information in assessing pancreas resectability.[93] Another report demonstrated that there is significant deformation of the chromosome 8 territory in a small cohort of PDAC samples compared with histologically normal ductal epithelium.[94] However, the detailed evaluation of common alterations in nuclear architecture in PDAC along with the mechanistic links and its specific impact on nuclear functions remains in its infancy. Nevertheless, it is the authors opinion that this field is perhaps the most promising for future advances in epigenetics and pancreatic cancer. Therefore, it is important to underscore its importance in an attempt to stimulate future research.

EPIGENETICS OPENS A NEW ERA FOR PANCREATIC CANCER MARKERS AND NOVEL THERAPEUTIC MODALITIES

Working primarily with pancreatic cells, the authors' laboratory has contributed to the better understanding of some key aspects of the current paradigm for epigenetics. Working with transcription factors, for instance, we cloned and characterized several members of the KLF family of epigenetic regulators from the human pancreas. We subsequently found that these proteins work at the intersection of metabolism and cancer. More importantly, thus far, the work performed on these proteins has provided a comprehensive model of epigenetic pathways in the human pancreas leading to the characterization of several histone acetylase, deacetylase, methylase, and reader proteins, among others. For this purpose, we underscore the importance of KLF11 and KLF14. Although we identified these proteins in the context of their ability to suppress pancreatic cancer cell growth,[95–97] it was later discovered through our own and other work that these sequence-specific transcription factors function primarily through the regulation of metabolic gene networks.[98–101] This is important owing to the key relationship between metabolism and cancer uniquely found in pancreatic cancer (the diabetes–pancreatic cancer connection). Interestingly, the tumor suppression function of KLF11 is inactivated in PDAC by methylation-mediated gene silencing.[102] On the other hand, mutations in the protein impair certain distinct functions of KLF11 to give rise to type 1diabetes (MODY VII).[103] More importantly, alterations in a KLF11 binding site within the insulin promoter are responsible for neonatal diabetes.[104] A highly related member of the family, KLF14, is associated with obesity and diabetes, as well as basal cell carcinoma.[101,105] Studies on these proteins led us to define that they function as a link between the DNA sequence they recognize and histone-modifying enzymes. They are modular proteins, which contain small domains that serve as docking platforms for the Sin3-HDAC complex, HATs, WW- and WD40 domain proteins, histone methyl-transferase, and chromodomain reader molecules.[100,104,106–109] In addition, these proteins also heterodimerize with NFκB and PPARγ, which bring additional complexes along for regulatory purposes.[99,110,111] For instance, by coupling to the HP1-SUV39H1 as well as to the Sin3-HDAC pathway, these proteins are able to mark the promoters of metabolic gene networks to affect cell survival and growth.[98] In this regard, it is impor-tant to take into consideration that oncogenic activation, for instance of KRAS, in the pancreas leads to distinct metabolic changes.[112] KLF proteins are necessary for antagonizing KRAS.[95] Thus, it is likely that these proteins act early during the PDAC initiation process to change metabolic profiles of transforming cells. Noteworthy, how-ever, significant efforts have been devoted to directly characterizing some of the his-tone code readers, writers, and erasers, whether in the context of functioning with or without recruitment by a specific transcription factor. In 2001, a widely known domain for the recruitment of HDACs was described.[109] This mechanism, which was discov-ered in the exocrine pancreas, is also used by many tumor suppressor genes, including Mad1, an antagonist of the Myc oncogene.[113] Subsequently, how histone code readers work to mediate growth stimuli downstream of growth factor receptor pathways was characterized.[114] Next, new Polycomb-type writer complexes from the pancreas were isolated and their growth-promoting role in pancreatic cells was defined.[115] Together, it is now known that these molecular cascades are essential to define the cancer phenotype, thereby becoming attractive targets for develop-mental therapeutics.

SUMMARY

This article seeks to promote a change in the conceptual bias, which currently affects the pancreatic cancer field. For instance, many researchers and practitioners still see pancreatic cancer exclusively as a disease of epithelial exocrine cells, which become transformed by the accumulation of genetic alterations. This view, combined with solid observations from the authors' laboratory and others, reveals that genetic alterations cross talk with epigenetic and nuclear structure changes to give rise to neoplastic transformation as well as determines most features of the cancer phenotype and its symptoms (see **Fig. 1**). This new framework has significant mechanistic value in com-prehending how this disease originates and evolves. This updated paradigm for the progression of pancreatic cancer integrates the concept that the patterns of gene expression networks to define the pancreatic cancer phenotype are dictated by the combination of genetic, epigenetic, and nuclear structure instructions according to the triple-code hypothesis, which considers that all 3 of these codes contribute to the development and progression of this disease (**Fig. 2**). More importantly, however, many epigenetic alterations are significantly ameliorated by a new type of therapeu-tics, which target the epigenome. Promising epigenetics-based therapies are currently being evaluated through different types of trials. Thus, the concepts discussed here should fuel a new era of studies that promise to provide the medical community with new tools to diagnose and treat this dismal disease.

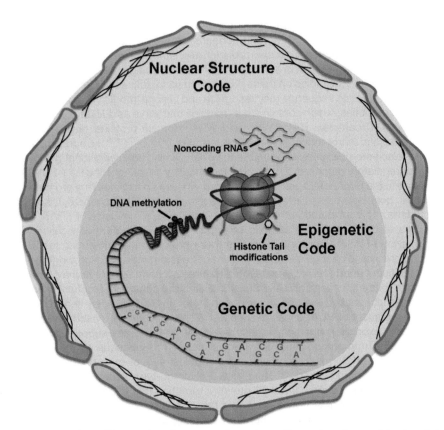

Fig. 2. Integration of instructions from genetics, epigenetics, and nuclear architecture into the triple-code hypothesis. This comprehensive model for the development and progression of PDAC is based on the understanding that gene expression networks are regulated by the combination of instructions dictated by genetics, epigenetics, and nuclear architecture, which the authors have coined the triple-code hypothesis. Alterations in the genetic code form the foundation of the well-known DNA-centric hypothesis for the establishment and maintenance of the cancer phenotype, which includes mutations and deletions. The epigenetic code takes into account changes in DNA methylation, noncoding RNA molecules, and chromatin via histone modifications and the writers, readers, and erasers of the histone code. Finally, the nuclear structure code, which includes the nuclear matrix and higher-order chromatin organization, affects the fidelity of genome replication, chromatin organization, and gene expression.

REFERENCES

1. Iovanna J, Mallmann M, Goncalves A, et al. Current knowledge on pancreatic cancer. Front Oncol 2012;2:6.
2. Sharma C, Eltawil K, Renfrew P, et al. Advances in diagnosis, treatment and palliation of pancreatic carcinoma: 1990-2010. World J Gastroenterol 2011;17:867–97.
3. Yu X, Zhang Y, Chen C, et al. Targeted drug delivery in pancreatic cancer. Biochim Biophys Acta 2010;1805:97–104.
4. Burris H, Moore M, Andersen J, et al. Improvements in survival and clinical benefit with gemcitabine as first-line therapy for patients with advanced pancreas cancer: a randomized trial. J Clin Oncol 1997;15:2403–13.

5. Heinemann V. Gemcitabine: progress in the treatment of pancreatic cancer. Oncology 2001;60:8–18.
6. Rocha Lima C, Green M, Rotche R, et al. Irinotecan plus gemcitabine results in no survival advantage compared with gemcitabine monotherapy in patients with locally advanced or metastatic pancreatic cancer despite increased tumor response rate. J Clin Oncol 2004;22:3776–83.
7. Louvet C, Labianca R, Hammel P, et al. Gemcitabine in combination with oxaliplatin compared with gemcitabine alone in locally advanced or metastatic pancreatic cancer: results of a GERCOR and GISCAD phase III trial. J Clin Oncol 2005;23:3509–16.
8. Scheithauer W, Schull B, Ulrich-Pur H, et al. Biweekly high-dose gemcitabine alone or in combination with capecitabine in patients with metastatic pancreatic adenocarcinoma: a randomized phase II trial. Ann Oncol 2003;14:97–104.
9. Hruban RH, Goggins M, Parsons J, et al. Progression model for pancreatic cancer. Clin Cancer Res 2000;6:2969–72.
10. Kanda M, Matthaei H, Wu J, et al. Presence of somatic mutations in most early-stage pancreatic intraepithelial neoplasia. Gastroenterology 2012;142:730–3.e739.
11. Rivera JA, Rall CJN, Graeme-Cook F, et al. Analysis of K-ras oncogene mutations in chronic pancreatitis with ductal hyperplasia. Surgery 1997;121: 42–9.
12. Herreros-Villanueva M, Hijona E, Cosme A, et al. Mouse models of pancreatic cancer. World J Gastroenterol 2012;18:1286–94.
13. Perez-Mancera PA, Guerra C, Barbacid M, et al. What we have learned about pancreatic cancer from mouse models. Gastroenterology 2012;142:1079–92.
14. Waddington CH. The epigenotype. 1942. Int J Epidemiol 2012;41:10–3.
15. Colman A. Profile of John Gurdon and Shinya Yamanaka, 2012 nobel laureates in medicine or physiology. Proc Natl Acad Sci U S A 2013;110:5740–1.
16. Egger G, Liang G, Aparicio A, et al. Epigenetics in human disease and prospects for epigenetic therapy. Nature 2004;429:457–63.
17. Ho S-M, Johnson A, Tarapore P, et al. Environmental epigenetics and its implication on disease risk and health outcomes. ILAR J 2012;53:289–305.
18. Lomberk G, Urrutia R. Epigenetics and its applications to a revised progression model of pancreatic cancer. In: Neoptolemos JP, Urrutia R, Abbruzzese JL, et al, editors. Pancreatic cancer. New York: Springer; 2010. p. 143–69.
19. Maitra A, Fukushima N, Takaori K, et al. Precursors to invasive pancreatic cancer. Adv Anat Pathol 2005;12:81–91.
20. Frese KK, Tuveson DA. Maximizing mouse cancer models. Nat Rev Cancer 2007;7:654–8.
21. Mazzio EA, Soliman KFA. Basic concepts of epigenetics: impact of environmental signals on gene expression. Epigenetics 2012;7:119–30.
22. Strahl BD, Allis CD. The language of covalent histone modifications. Nature 2000;403:41–5.
23. Turner BM. Histone acetylation and an epigenetic code. Bioessays 2000;22: 836–45.
24. Seligson DB, Horvath S, McBrian MA, et al. Global levels of histone modifications predict prognosis in different cancers. Am J Pathol 2009;174:1619–28.
25. Esteller M. The necessity of a human epigenome project. Carcinogenesis 2006; 27:1121–5.
26. Kanai Y, Arai E. Multilayer-omics analyses of human cancers: exploration of biomarkers and drug targets based on the activities of the International Human Epigenome Consortium. Front Genet 2014;5:24.

27. Manuyakorn A, Paulus R, Farrell J, et al. Cellular histone modification patterns predict prognosis and treatment response in resectable pancreatic adenocarcinoma: results from RTOG 9704. J Clin Oncol 2010;28:1358–65.

28. Lomberk G, Urrutia R. The family feud: turning off Sp1 by Sp1-like KLF proteins. Biochem J 2005;392:1–11.

29. Freeman JA, Espinosa JM. The impact of post-transcriptional regulation in the p53 network. Brief Funct Genomics 2013;12:46–57.

30. Koorstra J-BM, Hustinx SR, Offerhaus GJA, et al. Pancreatic carcinogenesis. Pancreatology 2008;8:110–25.

31. Rivlin N, Brosh R, Oren M, et al. Mutations in the p53 tumor suppressor gene: important milestones at the various steps of tumorigenesis. Genes Cancer 2011;2:466–74.

32. Lusser A, Kadonaga JT. Chromatin remodeling by ATP-dependent molecular machines. Bioessays 2003;25:1192–200.

33. Shain AH, Pollack JR. The spectrum of SWI/SNF mutations, ubiquitous in human cancers. PLoS One 2013;8:e55119.

34. Mazur PK, Reynoird N, Khatri P, et al. SMYD3 links lysine methylation of MAP3K2 to Ras-driven cancer. Nature 2014;510:283–7.

35. Ougolkov AV, Bilim VN, Billadeau DD. Regulation of pancreatic tumor cell proliferation and chemoresistance by the histone methyltransferase enhancer of zeste homologue 2. Clin Cancer Res 2008;14:6790–6.

36. Qazi AM, Aggarwal S, Steffer CS, et al. Laser capture microdissection of pancreatic ductal adeno-carcinoma cells to analyze EzH2 by Western Blot analysis. Methods Mol Biol 2011;755:245–56.

37. Toll AD, Dasgupta A, Potoczek M, et al. Implications of enhancer of zeste homologue 2 expression in pancreatic ductal adenocarcinoma. Hum Pathol 2010;41:1205–9.

38. Fujii S, Fukamachi K, Tsuda H, et al. RAS oncogenic signal upregulates EZH2 in pancreatic cancer. Biochem Biophys Res Commun 2012;417:1074–9.

39. Lasfargues C, Pyronnet S. EZH2 links pancreatitis to tissue regeneration and pancreatic cancer. Clin Res Hepatol Gastroenterol 2012;36:323–4.

40. van Vlerken LE, Kiefer CM, Morehouse C, et al. EZH2 Is required for breast and pancreatic cancer stem cell maintenance and can be used as a functional cancer stem cell reporter. Stem Cells Translational Med 2013;2:43–52.

41. Tzatsos A, Paskaleva P, Ferrari F, et al. KDM2B promotes pancreatic cancer via Polycomb-dependent and -independent transcriptional programs. J Clin Invest 2013;123:727–39.

42. Qin Y, Zhu W, Xu W, et al. LSD1 sustains pancreatic cancer growth via maintaining HIF1α-dependent glycolytic process. Cancer Lett 2014;347:225–32.

43. Yamamoto K, Tateishi K, Kudo Y, et al. Loss of histone demethylase KDM6B enhances aggressiveness of pancreatic cancer through downregulation of C/EBPα. Carcinogenesis 2014;35:2404–14.

44. Lehmann A, Denkert C, Budczies J, et al. High class I HDAC activity and expression are associated with RelA/p65 activation in pancreatic cancer in vitro and in vivo. BMC Cancer 2009;9:395.

45. Nakagawa M, Oda Y, Eguchi T, et al. Expression profile of class I histone deacetylases in human cancer tissues. Oncol Rep 2007;18:769–74.

46. Miyake K, Yoshizumi T, Imura S, et al. Expression of hypoxia-inducible factor-1alpha, histone deacetylase 1, and metastasis-associated protein 1 in pancreatic carcinoma: correlation with poor prognosis with possible regulation. Pancreas 2008;36:e1–9.

47. Wang W, Gao J, Man XH, et al. Significance of DNA methyltransferase-1 and histone deacetylase-1 in pancreatic cancer. Oncol Rep 2009;21:1439–47.
48. Fritsche P, Seidler B, Schüler S, et al. HDAC2 mediates therapeutic resistance of pancreatic cancer cells via the BH3-only protein NOXA. Gut 2009;58:1399–409.
49. Ouaïssi M, Sielezneff I, Silvestre R, et al. High histone deacetylase 7 (HDAC7) expression is significantly associated with adenocarcinomas of the pancreas. Ann Surg Oncol 2008;15:2318–28.
50. Yun M, Wu J, Workman JL, et al. Readers of histone modifications. Cell Res 2011;21:564–78.
51. Kouzarides T. Chromatin modifications and their function. Cell 2007;128:693–705.
52. Izzo A, Schneider R. Chatting histone modifications in mammals. Brief Funct Genomics 2010;9:429–43.
53. Kim YZ. Altered histone modifications in gliomas. Brain Tumor Res Treat 2014;2:7–21.
54. Ivanov M, Barragan I, Ingelman-Sundberg M. Epigenetic mechanisms of importance for drug treatment. Trends Pharmacol Sci 2014;35:384–96.
55. Rotili D, Mai A. Targeting histone demethylases: a new avenue for the fight against cancer. Genes Cancer 2011;2:663–79.
56. Arrowsmith CH, Bountra C, Fish PV, et al. Epigenetic protein families: a new frontier for drug discovery. Nat Rev Drug Discov 2012;11:384–400.
57. Bird AP, Wolffe AP. Methylation-induced repression—belts, braces, and chromatin. Cell 1999;99:451–4.
58. Jones PA. Functions of DNA methylation: islands, start sites, gene bodies and beyond. Nat Rev Genet 2012;13:484–92.
59. Kohli RM, Zhang Y. TET enzymes, TDG and the dynamics of DNA demethylation. Nature 2013;502:472–9.
60. Perini G, Diolaiti D, Porro A, et al. In vivo transcriptional regulation of N-Myc target genes is controlled by E-box methylation. Proc Natl Acad Sci U S A 2005;102:12117–22.
61. Subramaniam D, Thombre R, Dhar A, et al. DNA methyltransferases: a novel target for prevention and therapy. Front Oncol 2014;4:80.
62. Parry L, Clarke AR. The roles of the Methyl-CpG binding proteins in cancer. Genes Cancer 2011;2:618–30.
63. Liyanage VRB, Jarmasz JS, Murugeshan N, et al. DNA modifications: function and applications in normal and disease states. Biology (Basel) 2014;3:670–723.
64. Kaelin WG, McKnight SL. Influence of metabolism on epigenetics and disease. Cell 2013;153:56–69.
65. Ueki T, Toyota M, Sohn T, et al. Hypermethylation of multiple genes in pancreatic adenocarcinoma. Cancer Res 2000;60:1835–9.
66. Shakya R, Gonda T, Quante M, et al. Hypomethylating therapy in an aggressive stroma-rich model of pancreatic carcinoma. Cancer Res 2013;73:885–96.
67. Missiaglia E, Donadelli M, Palmieri M, et al. Growth delay of human pancreatic cancer cells by methylase inhibitor 5-aza-2'-deoxycytidine treatment is associated with activation of the interferon signalling pathway. Oncogene 2005;24:199–211.
68. Ehrlich M. DNA hypomethylation in cancer cells. Epigenomics 2009;1:239–59.
69. Yang H, Liu Y, Bai F, et al. Tumor development is associated with decrease of TET gene expression and 5-methylcytosine hydroxylation. Oncogene 2013;32:663–9.
70. Matsubayashi H, Canto M, Sato N, et al. DNA methylation alterations in the pancreatic juice of patients with suspected pancreatic disease. Cancer Res 2006;66:1208–17.

71. Fukushima N, Walter KM, Uek T, et al. Diagnosing pancreatic cancer using methylation specific PCR analysis of pancreatic juice. Cancer Biol Ther 2003;2:78–83.

72. Dauksa A, Gulbinas A, Barauskas G, et al. Whole blood DNA aberrant methylation in pancreatic adenocarcinoma shows association with the course of the disease: a pilot study. PLoS One 2012;7:e37509.

73. Kisiel JB, Yab TC, Taylor WR, et al. Stool DNA testing for the detection of pancreatic cancer: assessment of methylation marker candidates. Cancer 2012;118: 2623–31.

74. Santosh B, Varshney A, Yadava PK. Non-coding RNAs: biological functions and applications. Cell Biochem Funct 2015;33:14–22.

75. Taft RJ, Pang KC, Mercer TR, et al. Non-coding RNAs: regulators of disease. J Pathol 2010;220:126–39.

76. Ghildiyal M, Zamore PD. Small silencing RNAs: an expanding universe. Nat Rev Genet 2009;10:94–108.

77. Seto AG, Kingston RE, Lau NC. The coming of age for Piwi proteins. Mol Cell 2007;26:603–9.

78. Malone CD, Hannon GJ. Small RNAs as guardians of the genome. Cell 2009; 136:656–68.

79. Li X, Wu Z, Fu X, et al. lncRNAs: insights into their function and mechanics in underlying disorders. Mutat Res Rev Mutat Res 2014;762:1–21.

80. Kaikkonen MU, Lam MTY, Glass CK. Non-coding RNAs as regulators of gene expression and epigenetics. Cardiovasc Res 2011;90:430–40.

81. Ma M-Z, Kong X, Weng M-Z, et al. Candidate microRNA biomarkers of pancreatic ductal adenocarcinoma: meta-analysis, experimental validation and clinical significance. J Exp Clin Cancer Res 2013;32:71.

82. Sun T, Kong X, Du Y, et al. Aberrant MicroRNAs in Pancreatic Cancer: Researches and Clinical Implications. Gastroenterol Res Pract 2014;2014:386561.

83. Kim K, Jutooru I, Chadalapaka G, et al. HOTAIR is a negative prognostic factor and exhibits pro-oncogenic activity in pancreatic cancer. Oncogene 2013;32: 1616–25.

84. Huang CS, Yu W, Cui H, et al. Increased expression of the lncRNA PVT1 is associated with poor prognosis in pancreatic cancer patients. Minerva Med 2015; 106(3):143–9.

85. Pang EJ, Yang R, Fu XB, et al. Overexpression of long non-coding RNA MALAT1 is correlated with clinical progression and unfavorable prognosis in pancreatic cancer. Tumour Biol 2015;36(4):2403–7.

86. Peng W, Gao W, Feng J. Long noncoding RNA HULC is a novel biomarker of poor prognosis in patients with pancreatic cancer. Med Oncol 2014;31:346.

87. Li J, Liu D, Hua R, et al. Long non-coding RNAs expressed in pancreatic ductal adenocarcinoma and lncRNA BC008363 an independent prognostic factor in PDAC. Pancreatology 2014;14:385–90.

88. Sun YW, Chen YF, Li J, et al. A novel long non-coding RNA ENST00000480739 suppresses tumour cell invasion by regulating OS-9 and HIF-1[alpha] in pancreatic ductal adenocarcinoma. Br J Cancer 2014;111:2131–41.

89. Hruban RH, Adsay NV, Albores–Saavedra J, et al. Pancreatic intraepithelial neoplasia: a new nomenclature and classification system for pancreatic duct lesions. Am J Surg Pathol 2001;25:579–86.

90. Reddy KL, Feinberg AP. Higher order chromatin organization in cancer. Semin Cancer Biol 2013;23:109–15.

91. Chow K-H, Factor RE, Ullman KS. The nuclear envelope environment and its cancer connections. Nat Rev Cancer 2012;12:196–209.

92. Linder S, Lindholm J, Falkmer U, et al. Combined use of nuclear morphometry and DNA ploidy as prognostic indicators in nonresectable adenocarcinoma of the pancreas. Int J Pancreatol 1995;18:241–8.
93. Vasilescu C, Giza DE, Petrisor P, et al. Morphometrical differences between resectable and non-resectable pancreatic cancer: a fractal analysis. Hepato-gastroenterology 2012;59:284–8.
94. Timme S, Schmitt E, Stein S, et al. Nuclear position and shape deformation of chromosome 8 territories in pancreatic ductal adenocarcinoma. Anal Cell Pathol (Amst) 2011;34:21–33.
95. Fernandez-Zapico ME, Lomberk GA, Tsuji S, et al. A functional family-wide screening of SP/KLF proteins identifies a subset of suppressors of KRAS-mediated cell growth. Biochem J 2011;435:529–37.
96. Fernandez-Zapico ME, Mladek A, Ellenrieder V, et al. An mSin3A interaction domain links the transcriptional activity of KLF11 with its role in growth regulation. EMBO J 2003;22:4748–58.
97. Truty MJ, Lomberk G, Fernandez-Zapico ME, et al. Silencing of the transforming growth factor-beta (TGFbeta) receptor II by Kruppel-like factor 14 underscores the importance of a negative feedback mechanism in TGFbeta signaling. J Biol Chem 2009;284:6291–300.
98. Calvo E, Grzenda A, Lomberk G, et al. Single and combinatorial chromatin coupling events underlies the function of transcript factor Krüppel-like factor 11 in the regulation of gene networks. BMC Mol Biol 2014;15:10.
99. Loft A, Forss I, Siersbaek MS, et al. Browning of human adipocytes requires KLF11 and reprogramming of PPARgamma superenhancers. Genes Dev 2015;29:7–22.
100. Lomberk G, Grzenda A, Mathison A, et al. Kruppel-like factor 11 regulates the expression of metabolic genes via an evolutionarily conserved protein interaction domain functionally disrupted in maturity onset diabetes of the young. J Biol Chem 2013;288:17745–58.
101. Civelek M, Lusis AJ. Conducting the metabolic syndrome orchestra. Nat Genet 2011;43:506–8.
102. Fernandez-Zapico M, Molina J, Ahlquist D, et al. Functional characterization of KLF11, a novel TGFb-regulated tumor suppressor for pancreatic cancer. Pancreatology 2003;3:436.
103. Neve B, Fernandez-Zapico ME, Ashkenazi-Katalan V, et al. Role of transcription factor KLF11 and its diabetes-associated gene variants in pancreatic beta cell function. Proc Natl Acad Sci U S A 2005;102:4807–12.
104. Bonnefond A, Lomberk G, Buttar N, et al. Disruption of a novel Kruppel-like transcription factor p300-regulated pathway for insulin biosynthesis revealed by studies of the c.-331 INS mutation found in neonatal diabetes mellitus. J Biol Chem 2011;286:28414–24.
105. Stacey SN, Sulem P, Masson G, et al. New common variants affecting susceptibility to basal cell carcinoma. Nat Genet 2009;41:909–14.
106. Seo S, Lomberk G, Mathison A, et al. Krüppel-like factor 11 differentially couples to histone acetyltransferase and histone methyltransferase chromatin remodeling pathways to transcriptionally regulate dopamine D2 receptor in neuronal cells. J Biol Chem 2012;287:12723–35.
107. Lomberk G, Mathison AJ, Grzenda A, et al. Sequence-specific recruitment of heterochromatin protein 1 via interaction with Krüppel-like factor 11, a human transcription factor involved in tumor suppression and metabolic diseases. J Biol Chem 2012;287:13026–39.

108. Fernandez-Zapico ME, van Velkinburgh JC, Gutierrez-Aguilar R, et al. MODY7 gene, KLF11, is a novel p300-dependent regulator of Pdx-1 (MODY4) transcription in pancreatic islet beta cells. J Biol Chem 2009;284:36482–90.

109. Zhang J-S, Moncrieffe MC, Kaczynski J, et al. A conserved α-helical motif mediates the interaction of Sp1-like transcriptional repressors with the corepressor mSin3A. Mol Cell Biol 2001;21:5041–9.

110. Yin KJ, Fan Y, Hamblin M, et al. KLF11 mediates PPARgamma cerebrovascular protection in ischaemic stroke. Brain 2013;136:1274–87.

111. Fan Y, Guo Y, Zhang J, et al. Krüppel-like factor-11, a transcription factor involved in diabetes mellitus, suppresses endothelial cell activation via the nuclear factor-kappaB signaling pathway. Arterioscler Thromb Vasc Biol 2012; 32:2981–8.

112. Pylayeva-Gupta Y, Grabocka E, Bar-Sagi D. RAS oncogenes: weaving a tumorigenic web. Nat Rev Cancer 2011;11:761–74.

113. Ayer DE, Lawrence QA, Eisenman RN. Mad-Max transcriptional repression is mediated by ternary complex formation with mammalian homologs of yeast repressor Sin3. Cell 1995;80:767–76.

114. Lomberk G, Bensi D, Fernandez-Zapico ME, et al. Evidence for the existence of an HP1-mediated subcode within the histone code. Nat Cell Biol 2006;8:407–15.

115. Grzenda A, Lomberk G, Svingen P, et al. Functional characterization of EZH2β reveals the increased complexity of EZH2 isoforms involved in the regulation of mammalian gene expression. Epigenetics Chromatin 2013;6:3.

Principles of Cancer Screening

Paul F. Pinsky, PhD

KEYWORDS

- Cancer screening • Overdiagnosis • Lead time • Targeted screening
- Number needed to screen • Performance characteristics

KEY POINTS

- Early detection of cancer through screening can reduce cancer mortality; detection of pre-cancerous lesions, achievable currently with colorectal and cervical cancer screening, also reduces cancer incidence.
- Sensitivity and specificity are critical metrics for researchers assessing the predictive ability of a screening modality; positive predictive value (probability of cancer given a positive test) is more relevant for clinicians.
- The gold standard for evaluating cancer screening tests is the randomized controlled trial (RCT). Caution must be taken when using observational data, and especially survival statistics, to assess cancer screening.
- Harms from screening include false-positive tests and their downstream sequellae, including invasive diagnostic tests and complications thereof, and overdiagnosed and overtreated cancers.
- Targeting screening to high-risk subjects is a strategy to make screening more efficient, in terms of optimizing the benefits to harms tradeoff and the cost-effectiveness of screening.

INTRODUCTION

For more than a half century, cancer screening has been an important component of the struggle to reduce the burden of morbidity and mortality from cancer. In certain cases, such as with cervical cancer, the effects have been dramatic, with mortality decreasing more than 80% in the United States after implementation of widespread screening with Pap smears.[1] For most other cancers, however, the effects of screening have been substantially less pronounced. Benefits of screening have generally been on the modest side, and there has been increasing recognition of screening-related harms. The promise of cancer screening still beckons, however, and many new

Disclosures: None.
Division of Cancer Prevention, National Cancer Institute, 9609 Medical Center Drive, Room 5E108, Bethesda, MD 20910, USA
E-mail address: pp4f@nih.gov

Surg Clin N Am 95 (2015) 953–966
http://dx.doi.org/10.1016/j.suc.2015.05.009
0039-6109/15/$ – see front matter Published by Elsevier Inc.
surgical.theclinics.com

technologies continue to be evaluated for their potential to generate new screening modalities.

A standard introduction for a scientific paper concerning cancer screening proceeds as follows: the 5-year survival rate for cancer X is very low. Among stage I cases, however, 5-year survival is much higher; however, few cases are diagnosed in this stage. Therefore, if cancer X could only be detected earlier, the prognosis for subjects diagnosed with cancer X can be much improved.

In a nutshell, this is the basic, and very intuitive, rationale behind cancer screening. Although intuitively appealing, some caveats are in order. First, cancers diagnosed in early stages have a (relatively) good prognosis, but that does not necessarily mean that if those cancers currently diagnosed in late stage were detected earlier they would also have the same favorable prognosis. It is possible, for some cancer types, that inherent properties of late-stage tumors, such as their potential for early metastasis, and not the time of initial treatment, determine their eventual clinical outcome. Second, as a preventive intervention, screening tests are applied to asymptomatic and apparently healthy populations where, because of the relatively low prevalence of any given cancer type, most of those being screened cannot benefit from the screening but can be harmed because of either the screening test itself or of downstream consequences of it.

On the more favorable side for screening, there is the concept of detection through screening of precancerous lesions. Although standard screening programs are an example of secondary prevention, whereby cancer incidence is not reduced but mortality from the cancer is, screening modalities, such as those for colorectal and cervical cancer, that detect early cancers and precancerous lesions provide primary prevention (ie, incidence reduction) and secondary prevention. In addition to incidence reduction being a substantial benefit in itself, in terms of patient well-being and societal costs, screening modalities that reduce cancer incidence have greater magnitude reductions in cancer mortality than those that only provide secondary prevention.

This article provides an overview of some basic concepts and principles in cancer screening. Discussed are performance characteristics of screening tests (related to test accuracy), measures of screening benefit, some potential biases associated with evaluating screening benefits, harms of screening, the concept of cost-effectiveness of screening, and the related concept of targeting screening to high-risk groups. Finally, current recommendations for cancer screening in North America are summarized.

PERFORMANCE CHARACTERISTICS OF SCREENING TESTS

The performance characteristics of a screening test refer to its ability to accurately predict disease state. **Table 1** shows some common test performance characteristics. Sensitivity and specificity, and more generally the receiver-operating characteristic curve of sensitivity at varying levels of specificity for continuous or ordinal valued tests, are critical in the research setting for evaluating the potential of new screening modalities. Positive predictive value (PPV) is more relevant in the clinical setting, in that it assesses the probability that a patient with a positive test has the cancer of interest. Importantly, PPV depends not only on sensitivity and specificity, but also critically on the prevalence of the cancer being screened for (technically, this is the prevalence of underlying, undiagnosed cancer). With fixed sensitivity and specificity, PPV decreases as prevalence decreases. Because cancer prevalence in a screened population is low, even high specificity values can lead to very low values of PPV, regardless of sensitivity. For example, for a prevalence of 0.6% (eg, breast cancer in women

Table 1
Common performance characteristics of screening tests

Performance Characteristic	Definition
Sensitivity	Proportion of subjects with cancer who test positive
Specificity	Proportion of subjects without cancer who test negative
ROC curve	Curve of sensitivity at varying levels of 1-specificity
Area under the ROC curve	Area below the ROC curve; 1 = perfect prediction, 0.5 = no predictive ability
Positive predictive value	Proportion of subjects who test positive that have cancer
Negative predictive value	Proportion of subjects who test negative that do not have cancer

Abbreviation: ROC, receiver-operating characteristic.
From U.S. Preventive Services Task Force, Rockville, MD.

recommended for mammography screening) and sensitivity and specificity of 90%, PPV is only 5%; PPV increases to 10% and 21%, respectively, as specificity increases to 95% and 98%. This highlights the general requirement in cancer screening that specificity should be quite high. Negative predictive value (NPV) can be useful in a diagnostic context for a rule-out; however, in a screening context it is generally not informative because the pretest probability that the disease is absent is already so high.

The term "false-positive rate" in a screening context usually refers to 1-Specificity (or 100-Specificity when specificity is expressed as a percent). However, it may be used also to refer to 100-PPV, so use of the term may be confusing. Because specificity is generally well higher than 50% in a cancer screening context and PPV lower than 50%, the value of the false-positive rate usually gives a hint as to which definition is being used (a false-positive rate higher than 50% usually refers to 100-PPV and lower than 50% to 100-Specificity).

A cancer screening test may produce a continuous measure (eg, a blood concentration, such as prostate-specific antigen [PSA]) or a binary (Yes/No) result of whether a suspicious lesion is present. With some imaging modalities, such as low-dose computed tomography (CT) for lung cancer screening, the size of the largest nodule may essentially provide a continuous-valued result among positive screens. With continuous or ordinal-valued tests, a standardized cutoff generally determines whether the test is considered positive (eg, >4 ng/mL for PSA). Additionally, for continuous or ordinal-valued tests, PPV can be reported per positive test category or range and overall. For example, in the National Lung Screening Trial (NLST), overall PPV at baseline for low-dose CT was 3.8%, but PPV ranged from 0.5% for positive screens with nodule size of 4 to 6 mm to 41% for positive screens with nodule size greater than 30 mm.[2]

Note that a common error is to attempt to estimate PPV directly from a 2 × 2 table from a case-control study. Because the case to control ratio is arbitrary in such a design, it is erroneous to compute PPV as the number of cases with a positive test divided by the number of all study subjects with a positive test. In a prospective (cohort) study such a method is legitimate, but in a case-control design an outside estimate of prevalence is needed to compute PPV.

A standard assumption is that a cancer screening test must have a high level of sensitivity for it to be effective. However, high sensitivity alone for a screening modality does not necessarily imply that the modality will have any mortality benefit, and a sensitivity level sufficient for one screening modality and cancer type may not be sufficient for another. For example, a recent large study demonstrated sensitivity for film screen mammography, a screening modality with a demonstrated mortality benefit, of 66%.[3] In the Prostate, Lung, Colorectal and Ovarian (PLCO) Cancer Screening Trial, the combined modality of CA125 and transvaginal ultrasound for ovarian cancer screening had a similar 66% sensitivity; however, there was no observed mortality benefit of screening (the screened arm actually had slightly higher mortality from ovarian cancer).[4]

With screening tests where precancerous lesions may be detected, with a proved resultant decrease in cancer incidence, such as those for colorectal cancer (CRC), it is important to also consider sensitivity for such lesions. The fecal immunochemical test (FIT) has shown relatively high sensitivity for CRC, 61% to 91% compared with 90% to 95% for colonoscopy.[5] However, for the important cancer precursor of advanced adenoma, the relative sensitivity of FIT compared with colonoscopy is much lower.

This example of FIT and colonoscopy brings up the concept of program sensitivity. Program sensitivity measures the ability of a periodic screening regimen (eg, annual screening) to detect cancer early, or to detect cancer precursors. Because FIT is recommended for annual use, whereas colonoscopy is recommended only every 10 years, FIT could have several opportunities to detect a preclinical cancer, or an advanced adenoma, whereas colonoscopy would (generally) only have one. Therefore, examined as an overall screening program, the sensitivity of FIT for cancer or advanced adenoma is closer to that of colonoscopy than the values at a single time point might imply.

Analogous to program sensitivity is the concept of the cumulative false-positive rate. With periodic screening, the chance of experiencing at least one false-positive test obviously increases over time. The choice of a specific screening program, in terms of testing frequency, does not affect the false-positive rate at any given screen but does influence the cumulative false-positive rate. For example, biennial instead of annual screening over a fixed age range would clearly lead to a reduced cumulative false-positive rate over subjects' lifetimes; note it could also reduce program sensitivity.

MEASURES OF SCREENING BENEFIT

In a randomized controlled trial (RCT) of cancer screening, the primary outcome is typically cancer-specific mortality, defined as the rate of death from the cancer of interest.[6] A metric of screening efficacy is the cancer-specific mortality rate ratio (RR), or the ratio of cancer-specific death rates in the screening versus control arm. Overall mortality is not used as the primary end point in cancer screening trials; because deaths from the cancer of interest are a small fraction of all deaths, there is too much "noise" from nonrelevant deaths and the trial would require enormous sample size to be adequately statistically powered.[6]

Meta-analyses of randomized trials of mammography showed pooled RR estimates for breast cancer mortality of 0.85 for women aged 40 to 49, 0.86 for women 50 to 59, and 0.68 for women 60 to 69.[7] In the NLST comparing low-dose CT with chest radiograph, the updated lung cancer mortality RR was 0.84.[8] For PSA-based prostate cancer screening, the European Randomised Study of Screening for Prostate Cancer (ERSPC) showed a mortality RR of 0.79; however, the US PLCO trial did not show any mortality benefit (RR = 1.09).[9,10] Four randomized trials of flexible sigmoidoscopy screening showed a mean (range) of RR for CRC mortality of 0.75 (0.69–0.80).[11–14] Several trials are ongoing for colonoscopy screening but none have reported primary outcomes to date. Because colonoscopy covers the entire colorectum and flexible sigmoidoscopy only the distal colorectum, the RR would be expected to be lower for colonoscopy. Mortality RRs for distal CRC with flexible sigmoidoscopy were lower than those for overall CRC (mean, 0.67; range, 0.50–0.87).[11–14]

For screening modalities that also prevent cancer, such as flexible sigmoidoscopy and colonoscopy, the cancer incidence RR from an RCT is a measure of efficacy for primary cancer prevention. RRs for CRC incidence in the previously mentioned four flexible sigmoidoscopy trials averaged 0.81 (range, 0.77–0.87).[11–14]

Another metric commonly used is the number needed to screen (NNS), which is calculated as the reciprocal of the difference in cancer-specific mortality rates between arms.[15] For example, in NLST, which enrolled high-risk ever-smokers, the NNS was 320, meaning 320 (NLST-eligible) subjects would have to be screened with low-dose CT according to the NLST protocol (a total of three annual screens) to prevent one lung cancer death.[8] The NNS measure is more appropriate from a public health and cost-effectiveness perspective because it measures how many deaths will be prevented per number of subjects undergoing screening. The NNS takes into account the mortality RR and the background death rate of the cancer of interest. For the same RR, NNS increases (meaning screening becomes less efficient) as the background death rate decreases. For example, comparing low-dose CT in high-risk smokers with mammography, the mortality RRs are roughly the same but the death rate from lung cancer in high-risk ever-smokers is approximately five times the death rate from breast cancer in the population recommended for mammography. Therefore, the NNS is roughly five times higher for mammography in its recommended population than for low-dose CT in its recommended population of high-risk ever-smokers.

Population Measures

A screening modality only has true benefit when it disseminates outside of research settings to the general population. The ultimate metric of benefit of a cancer screening test is the overall population reduction in deaths from the cancer of interest that is attributable to screening. This is a function of the degree of dissemination of screening and the effectiveness of screening in reducing cancer-specific mortality. For screening modalities that prevent cancer incidence (eg, screening for CRC and cervical cancer), reduction in population incidence is also a critical metric.

The reduction in mortality that is attributable to screening is often difficult to assess unless there is a dramatic effect, such as with cervical cancer, where the screening modality reduced incidence and very sharply reduced mortality. Mortality rates from cervical cancer in the United States were 12 to 13 (per 100,000 women) in the 1950s before the common use of Pap smears, versus around two currently, and cervical cancer incidence decreased by about 60% from before to after the introduction of Pap smears.[1] CRC screening also reduces cancer incidence, although the effects to date have not been as dramatic as for cervical cancer screening. CRC incidence rates (age adjusted) in the United States were about 65 per 100,000 from 1975 to 1985 (prescreening), with corresponding mortality rates of around 28 per 100,000.[16] In 2011, incidence was 39 per 100,000 and mortality 15 per 100,000.[16]

For those screening modalities that do not prevent cancer, analyzing secular trends in mortality is a starting point to evaluating the effect of screening. However, because the mortality benefits of such screening are generally modest at best, it is often difficult to tease apart the effect of screening from that of improvement in treatment or other factors. For example, a high-profile modeling analysis of mammography by seven independent groups (incorporating breast cancer natural history, mammography sensitivity, RCT results, population incidence and mortality trends, and mammography usage rates) estimated the effect of the introduction of mammography on breast cancer mortality. The estimates across the seven models ranged from 7.5% to 22.7% for the mortality decrease because of mammography.[17]

COMMON BIASES IN ASSESSING THE BENEFITS OF SCREENING

The RCT is the gold standard for assessing the effectiveness of a cancer screening modality. However, screening may be implemented in the absence of an RCT, or before results from an RCT are reported. For example, prostate cancer screening with PSA began to be implemented in the United States in the early 1990s, before an RCT was initiated.[18] No RCTs reported until 2009, when the European trial (ERSPC) reported a positive result and the US PLCO trial reported a negative result, making the question of PSA benefit still uncertain.[9,10] In addition, with changes in screening technology or improvements in treatment, prior RCT results may have become out of date and more recent data may be needed to evaluate screening as currently practiced.

Researchers thus must often rely on observational or population-level studies to help assess screening benefit. This is problematic, however, because of several important potential biases that tend to affect studies of screening.

Two common related biases in nonrandomized studies of screening are lead time bias and overdiagnosis bias.[6] Early detection through screening implies advancement in the time of diagnosis of the cancer from what would have otherwise occurred in the absence of screening. The concept of lead time refers to the length of this period of time advancement. Because diagnosis is advanced and before any symptoms, it is possible that, in the absence of screening, clinical diagnosis would never have occurred, either because of the inherent indolence of the cancer or of competing causes of death. This phenomenon of screening detecting a cancer that never would have otherwise become clinically apparent is known as overdiagnosis. Overdiagnosis and lead time are theoretic concepts, in that they can generally not be observed in a given individual but can be estimated statistically in populations. **Fig. 1** shows hypothetical examples of individual time courses of screened subjects, illustrating lead time and overdiagnosis, and a true benefit of screening. Lead time and overdiagnosis can lead to scenarios in observational studies where screening seems to be beneficial even though the modality may actually have no effectiveness in reducing mortality from the cancer.

A common approach in observational studies of screening is to compare cancer survival among screened and nonscreened populations. Note that in the cancer screening context, "survival" refers to death rates following cancer diagnosis, whereas "mortality" refers to the death rate in an entire population cohort, whether or not diagnosed with cancer. Survival is a notoriously misleading statistic for evaluating screening effectiveness because of the effects of lead time and overdiagnosis bias, which tend to make survival rates more favorable in screened populations. By definition, there are no deaths from the cancer of interest among overdiagnosed cases or during screen-detected cases' lead time (except for deaths caused by the cancer treatment itself). Therefore, even in the absence of any mortality benefit of screening, survival metrics can be greatly improved on implementation of screening. For prostate cancer in the United States, 5-year relative survival increased from around 70% in the late 1970s to 99.3% by 2005.[16] In terms of death rates (ie, 100-survival), this corresponds to a 97% decrease (30%–0.7%). Yet mortality rates decreased much more modestly, from 31 per 100,000 in the late 1970s to 24 per 100,000 in 2005 (only a 23% decrease). Whether (or how much of) this 23% decrease was caused by

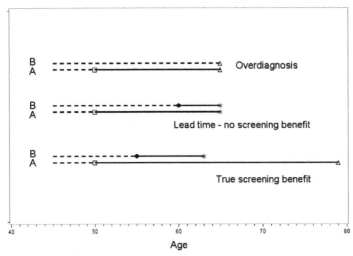

Fig. 1. Schematic of screening scenarios. In each panel, *A* represents the scenario with screening at age 50 and *B* represents the hypothetical scenario if there had been no screening. *Square* and *circle* represent screen-detected and clinical diagnosis, respectively; *dotted line* and *solid line* represent preclinical cancer and postdiagnosis cancer, respectively. *Star* and *triangle* denote death from the cancer of interest and death from other causes, respectively. In the "lead time - no screening benefit" scenario, "survival" increases from 5 to 15 years on screening, but time and cause of death are unchanged.

screening, as compared with improvements in treatment, is not totally clear; however, even with no mortality benefit a large survival improvement would still have been observed because of lead time and overdiagnosis bias. When examining survival specifically in subjects with screen-detected cancers, as opposed to analyzing survival in population registries, the potential for bias is even greater because it is not diluted by cancers in subjects not undergoing screening.

For comparison, for Hodgkin disease, a cancer with no screening but improvements in treatment, 5-year survival improved from 1975 to 2006 from 71.4% to 88.3%, corresponding to a change in 5-year case-fatality rates (ie, 100-survival rate) from 28.6% to 11.7%, a 59% decrease. In that same period, death rates from the disease decreased by a similar 66%.[16]

Using survival statistics to make a case for screening benefit is thus extremely problematic, although it is still commonly used. The case of prostate cancer also highlights how misleading improvements in 5-year survival rates over time can be when there has been a corresponding increase in the use of screening.

Another bias in evaluating the effect of screening is selection bias.[6] This issue arises when one examines the (cancer-specific) mortality rate among a group undergoing screening to that in a group not undergoing screening or to population-wide statistics. Because those who choose to be screened may be different with respect to the incidence of and survival from the cancer of interest, these underlying factors, and not the screening itself, may be contributing to any observed differences in mortality rates between the screened and nonscreened (or population-wide) group. Other studies examine the same geographic population over different time periods or different geographic populations at the same time with different exposures to screening; again, differences other than the screening per se may be operating across the populations.

HARMS OF SCREENING

In general, there are few medical harms of the actual cancer screening tests themselves. Modalities that rely on x-ray radiation (low-dose CT, mammography) do convey some added cancer risk; however, that excess risk is generally acknowledged to be quite small.[19,20] Colonoscopy carries some risks, including for perforation, which is estimated in the range of 2 to 4 per 10,000.[21,22] There is minor discomfort with some screening tests, and some reported short-term anxiety associated with false-positive test results.[23]

However, the primary medical harms of cancer screening come from downstream events, from the diagnostic work-up of false-positive screens, and from diagnosis and treatment of cancers that may never have become clinically apparent without screening (overdiagnosed and overtreated cases). With respect to harms from the diagnostic work-up of false-positives, the overall harm is a function of the false-positive rate (defined as 100-Specificity) and the nature of the diagnostic work-up. For example, in the NLST, the false-positive rate was high (average of 24% over all screening rounds); however, only a small fraction of false-positives, 2.6%, were followed up by invasive diagnostic procedures (thoracotomy, thoracoscopy, bronchoscopy, or needle biopsy).[24] Of these, 2.4% were associated with a major complication (9.6% with any complication). Thus, as a proportion of all low-dose CT screens (without a cancer diagnosis), the major complication rate was very low, 1.5 per 10,000 (6.0 per 10,000 for any complication). For another example, with screening for prostate cancer with PSA and digital rectal examination, the PLCO trial found a postbiopsy complication rate of 2.0%.[25] Based on the false-positive rate (12%–14% across screening rounds), the frequency of follow-up biopsy, and this complication rate, the frequency of complications from biopsy was about 7 per 10,000 screens. Although these rates per screen are low, for many screening programs persons may undergo 20 to 30 screens over their lifetime, so the lifetime risk of experiencing a complication is substantially greater than the one-time risk. Also, with mass screening of healthy populations, the absolute number of people with complications as a result of screening-induced diagnostic work-up is considerable.

Overdiagnosis

Overdiagnosis and overtreatment are harms of screening that are being increasingly recognized. The harms of overdiagnosis depend not only on the magnitude of overdiagnosis, but also on the costs and harms, and likelihood, of treatment. Overdiagnosis is the critical issue in PSA-based screening for prostate cancer because there is an elevated level of overdiagnosis and a high rate of serious quality of life harms (eg, urinary incontinence, impotence) associated with the standard curative treatments of radiation and radical prostatectomy. Overdiagnosis is also a serious issue in mammography screening for breast cancer, and has even been recognized in low-dose CT lung cancer screening.

Quantitative definitions of overdiagnosis rates vary considerably; therefore, care must be taken when comparing estimates from different sources or across cancer types. For example, the "overdiagnosis rate" may be defined as the percentage of screen-detected cancers that are overdiagnosed; the percentage of all cancers that are overdiagnosed in a population attending screening or in a population invited to attend screening; and finally, as the percentage of overdiagnosed cases among an entire population, only a fraction of which is actually undergoing screening.

Perhaps the most straightforward method for estimating the overdiagnosis rate is from a randomized screening trial of screening versus no screening; here the excess of screened arm (vs control arm) cancers following a long enough observation period without further screening, to allow the control arm to "catch up" to the screened arm in diagnosed cases, can be used to estimate overdiagnosis rates. In the ERSPC, prostate cancer incidence was 63% higher in the screened than the control arm; assuming no further control arm catch-up, this leads to an estimate of about 50% of the screen-detected prostate cancers in ERSPC being overdiagnosed.[9] However, because of variations in data sources and methods, and definitions, estimates of overdiagnosis rates vary greatly. A meta-analysis showed a range of estimated overdiagnosis rates for invasive breast cancer associated with mammography of 1% to 54%.[26]

A method of indirectly assessing overdiagnosis is to examine the change in incidence rates after the introduction of screening, assuming there has been no observed change in any known major risk factors for the cancer, as is true for prostate cancer in the United States. Annual prostate cancer incidence rates in the United States ranged from 105 to 115 (per 100,000 men) in the period from 1980 to 1985, before the start of the PSA era.[16] In the middle of the PSA era (1995–2005), the average prostate cancer incidence rate was 173, almost a 60% increase.

COST-EFFECTIVENESS AND TARGETED SCREENING

Even if a cancer screening modality has been shown in RCTs, or with other solid evidence, to reduce mortality from the cancer of interest, and if the benefits of the screening clearly outweigh the (medical) harms, there is still the question of cost-effectiveness. Cost-effectiveness analysis (CEA) is an approach to assessing the benefits and harms of a medical intervention that also takes into account resource use and/or cost issues.

CEAs often use the metric of cost per quality-adjusted life-year (QALY) gained from screening, where the QALY attempts to incorporate quality of life effects and longevity. In a cancer screening context, the harms of screening contribute to lower QALYs. For example, with PSA screening, the side effects of treatment decrease the QALYs in those treated cases that are estimated to have been overdiagnosed. Note that if the case were not overdiagnosed, then presumably the side effects and QALY decrement would have occurred even without screening, so such side effects would not impact the CEA. The costs of screening include those of the screening test itself, the diagnostic follow-up and treatment of any complications thereof, and costs of overtreated cases. It may also include such factors as time lost from work for the screening visit, and other associated costs.

A standard benchmark for interventions that are cost-effective is $100,000 per QALY. Several analyses of colorectal screening have shown that at least some modalities (including annual screening with FIT and flexible sigmoidoscopy) can actually reduce health care costs while increasing QALYs (ie, their cost per QALY is actually negative).[27] This is because CRC screening can reduce the incidence of CRC, CRC is a relatively common cancer, and the cost of treating CRC can be very high. For other modalities where the screening does not reduce cancer incidence, the estimated cost per QALY has always been positive, meaning that the introduction of these modalities into the health care system does not reduce health care costs. Although some costs associated with treatment of late-stage cancers may be reduced, this effect is overwhelmed by the cost of screening and diagnostic follow-up.

Cost effectiveness and cost per QALY estimates for the same screening modality and scenarios often vary widely, because of not only the underlying data sources and/or models that quantify the various harms and benefits, but also because of variability in numerical cost values, differences in what types of costs are included (eg, lost productivity), and the choice of perspective (provider/patient vs societal). Assessing quality of life effects to estimate QALYs is also inherently subjective and variable. A study using five breast cancer natural history models with costs and some other factors standardized across models showed a cost per QALY mean (range) for biennial screening with digital mammography for women 50 to 74 of $36,000 ($23,000–$72,000).[28]

Targeted Screening

A general principle of cancer screening is that the net benefit (benefits minus harms) of screening generally increases as the incidence rate of the cancer of interest in the screened population increases. This follows because only those who have the cancer of interest can benefit from screening, whereas the harms of screening and diagnostic follow-up apply to all screened persons. Likewise, the relative cost-effectiveness of screening also increases with incidence, because costs and harms accrue from all screened persons.

Therefore, a strategy to maximize the net benefit of screening, and its cost-effectiveness, is to target screening to an identifiable subset of the population that

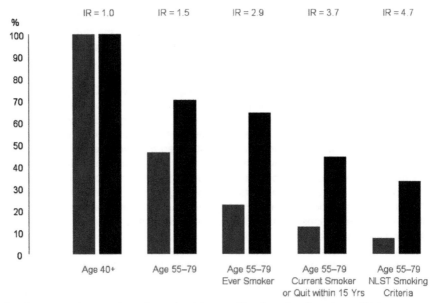

Fig. 2. Targeted screening through risk stratification for low-dose CT lung cancer screening. *Blue bars* represent overall population (older than age 40), *black bars* represent incident lung cancers. For the scenario of screening everyone older than age 40 (left-most column), 100% of the population and 100% of lung cancers (in the 40+ population) are covered. With increasing age and/or smoking history requirements, the percentage of incident lung cancers covered decreases, but the percentage of the population screened decreases more sharply. The incidence ratio (IR) represents the ratio of incidence rates in the restricted population over that in the overall population; it is also the ratio of the height of the *black bar* versus *blue bar*. NLST smoking criteria is 30+ pack-years and current smoking or quit within 15 years. (*Data from* Pinsky PF, Berg C. Applying the National Lung Screening Trial eligibility criteria to the US population: what percent of the population and of incident lung cancers would be covered. J Med Screen 2012;19:154–6.)

is at above average risk for the cancer of interest; this is sometimes denoted as risk stratification or targeted screening.

For most cancer screening programs in the United States, the primary criteria for who is recommended for screening is age and sex. The minimum age requirement is used because cancer incidence generally increases with age, and screening in a setting where the incidence of the cancer of interest is too low may lead to an unfavorable benefits to harms tradeoff and cost-effectiveness ratio. Some screening recommendations also incorporate family history. For example, with colonoscopy screening for CRC, an earlier start age and more frequent colonoscopy is recommended for those with a first-degree relative diagnosed with CRC younger than age 60, or two or more first-degree relatives diagnosed with CRC.[29]

The primary exception to only using age, sex, and family history for choosing who should be screened is lung cancer screening with low-dose CT, where most guidelines recommend screening only for those at high risk because of heavy smoking history (30+ pack years and current smoker or recent quitter).[30,31] **Fig. 2** illustrates the power

Table 2
USPSTF cancer screening guidelines

Cancer	Screening Modality	Updated	Population	Recommendation
Colorectal	Colonoscopy/fecal occult blood test/flexible sigmoidoscopy	2008	Age 50–75 Age 75–85 Age >85	A C D
Breast	Mammography	2009	Women age 40–49 Women age 50–74 Women age 75+	C B I
Prostate	Prostate-specific antigen	2012	Men any age	D
Lung	Low-dose computed tomography	2013	Age 55–80, 30+ pack-years current smoker or quit within 15 y	B
Cervical	Pap smear, human papillomavirus testing	2012	Women age 21–65 Women younger than 21 or older than 65 (with prior screens)	A D
Ovarian	CA125, transvaginal ultrasound	2012	Any age	D
Skin	Whole-body skin examination	2009	Any age	I
Oral cavity	Clinical examination	2013	Any age	I
Bladder	Urinalysis for hematuria; urine cytology	2011	Any age	I
Pancreatic	Ultrasound, abdominal palpation, serology	2004	Any age	D
Testicular	Self or clinical examination	2011	Adolescent/adult men	D

Recommendation Code: A, recommends the service—high certainty of substantial net benefit; B, recommends the service—high certainty of moderate benefit/moderate certainty of moderate-substantial net benefit; C, recommends selective offering or providing service based on professional judgment/patient preference; D, recommends against the service; I, insufficient evidence; balance of benefits and harms cannot be determined.

From U.S. Preventive Services Task Force. Available at: http://www.uspreventiveservicestaskforce.org/. Accessed November 10, 2014; with permission.

of targeted screening in this setting to increase the efficiency of screening by selecting for higher-risk subjects. Although screening is more efficient in the targeted population, the reach of screening in the overall population is diminished with targeting, as is the overall proportional reduction in cancer mortality achievable.

Several studies examined targeting for bladder cancer screening based on age, sex, and smoking history. Because smoking is less strong a risk factor for bladder than for lung cancer, the degree of risk concentration achievable with bladder cancer is less than that for lung cancer.[32,33]

CURRENT RECOMMENDED CANCER SCREENING TESTS IN NORTH AMERICA

Table 2 displays all of the recommendations for cancer screening modalities from the US Preventive Services Task Force.[34] There are only two cancers for which screening received the top A recommendation; not coincidentally, these are the two cancers where screening reduces incidence and mortality, namely cervical cancer and CRC. An additional two cancers received a B recommendation for screening, breast cancer with mammography and lung cancer with low-dose CT. Screening for several cancers received an I rating, meaning there is insufficient evidence to judge whether screening is beneficial. The recommendation for PSA-based screening for prostate cancer was changed to a D (from a C) in 2012. Screening for ovarian, pancreatic, and testicular cancer also received a D recommendation.

In Canada, the Canadian Task Force on Preventive Health Care issues recommendations for cancer screening.[35] Cervical cancer screening with Pap smears is recommended for age 30 to 69 (strong recommendation) and 25 to 29 (weak recommendation). Mammography is recommended every 2 to 3 years for women 50 to 74 (weak recommendation). For CRC, there is a recommendation from 2001 for fecal occult blood testing (strong) and flexible sigmoidoscopy (weak); new guidelines are expected soon that will cover colonoscopy. For prostate cancer, there is a recommendation not to undergo screening. Lung cancer screening guidelines with low-dose CT are also forthcoming.

REFERENCES

1. Habbema D, de Kok I, Brown ML. Cervical cancer screening in the United States and the Netherlands: a tale of two countries. Milbank Q 2012;90:5–37.
2. National Lung Screening Trial Research Team. Results of initial low-dose computed tomographic screening for lung cancer. N Engl J Med 2013;368: 1980–91.
3. Pisano ED, Gatsonis G, Hendrick E, et al. Diagnostic performance of digital versus film mammography for breast-cancer screening. N Engl J Med 2005; 353:1773–83.
4. Buys SS, Partridge E, Black A, et al. Effect of screening on ovarian cancer mortality: the Prostate, Lung, Colorectal and Ovarian (PLCO) cancer screening randomized controlled trial. JAMA 2011;305:2295–302.
5. Whitlock EP, Lin JS, Liles E, et al. Screening for colorectal cancer: a targeted, updated systematic review for the U.S. Preventive Services Task Force. Ann Intern Med 2008;149:638–58.
6. Croswell JM, Ransohoff DF, Kramer BS. Principles of cancer screening: lessons from history and study design issues. Semin Oncol 2010;37:202–15.
7. U.S. Preventive Services Task Force. Screening for breast cancer: U.S. Preventive Services Task Force Recommendation Statement. Ann Intern Med 2009; 151:1716–26.

8. Pinsky PF, Church T, Izmirlian G, et al. The National Lung Screening Trial: results stratified by demographics, smoking history and lung cancer histology. Cancer 2013;119:3976–83.

9. Schroder FH, Hugosson H, Roobol MJ, et al. Screening and prostate cancer mortality: results of the European Randomised Study of Screening for Prostate Cancer (ERSPC) at 13 years of follow-up. Lancet 2014;384:2027–35.

10. Andriole GL, Crawford ED, Grubb R, et al. Prostate cancer screening in the randomized Prostate, Lung, Colorectal and Ovarian Screening Trial: mortality results after 13 years of follow-up. J Natl Cancer Inst 2012;104:125–32.

11. Schoen RE, Pinsky PF, Weissfeld JL, et al. Colorectal-cancer incidence and mortality with screening flexible sigmoidoscopy. N Engl J Med 2011;366(25): 2345–57.

12. Atkin WS, Edwards R, Kralj-Hans I, et al. Once-only flexible sigmoidoscopy screening in prevention of colorectal cancer: a multicentre randomised controlled trial. Lancet 2010;375:1624–33.

13. Segnan N, Armaroli P, Bonelli L, et al. Once-only sigmoidoscopy in colorectal cancer screening: follow-up findings of the Italian Randomized Controlled Trial – SCORE. J Natl Cancer Inst 2011;103:1310–22.

14. Holme O, Loberg M, Kalager M, et al. Effect of flexible sigmoidoscopy screening on colorectal cancer incidence and mortality: a randomized trial. JAMA 2014;312: 606–15.

15. Rembold CM. Number needed to screen: development of a statistic for disease screening. BMJ 1998;317:307–12.

16. SEER – National Cancer Institute. SEER statistical summaries. Available at: www. seer.cancer.gov. Accessed January 15, 2015.

17. Berry DA, Cronin KA, Plevritis SK, et al. Effect of screening and adjuvant therapy on mortality from breast cancer. N Engl J Med 2005;353:1784–92.

18. Etzioni R, Legler JM, Feuer EJ, et al. Cancer surveillance series: interpreting trends in prostate cancer. Part III: quantifying the link between population prostate-specific antigen testing and recent declines in prostate cancer mortality. J Natl Cancer Inst 1999;16:1033–9.

19. De Gelder R, Draisma G, Heijnsdijk E, et al. Population-based mammography screening below age 50: balancing radiation-induced vs prevented breast cancer deaths. Br J Cancer 2011;104:1214–20.

20. Brenner DJ. Radiation risks potentially associated with low-dose CT screening of adult smokers for lung cancer. Radiology 2004;231:440–5.

21. Bielawska B, Day AG, Lieberman DA, et al. Risk factors for early colonoscopic perforation include non-gastroenterologist endoscopists: a multivariable analysis. Clin Gastroenterol Hepatol 2014;12:85–92.

22. Rutter CM, Johnson E, Miglioretti DL, et al. Adverse events after screening and follow-up colonoscopy. Cancer Causes Control 2012;23:289–96.

23. Byrne MM, Weissfeld J, Roberts MS. Anxiety, fear of cancer, and perceived risk of cancer following lung cancer screening. Med Decis Making 2008;28:917–25.

24. National Lung Screening Trial Research Team. Reduced lung-cancer mortality with low-dose computed tomographic screening. N Engl J Med 2011;365: 395–409.

25. Pinsky PF, Parnes HL, Andriole G. Mortality and complications following prostate biopsy in the PLCO cancer Screening Trial. Br J Urol Int 2014;113:254–9.

26. Biesheuvel C, Barratt A, Howard K, et al. Effects of study methods and biases on estimates of invasive breast cancer over-detection with mammography screening. Lancet Oncol 2007;8:1129–38.

27. Sharaf RN, Ladabaum U. Comparative effectiveness and cost-effectiveness of screening colonoscopy vs. sigmoidoscopy and alternative strategies. Am J Gastroenterol 2013;108:120–32.

28. Stout NK, Lee SJ, Schechter CB, et al. Benefits, harms and costs for breast cancer screening after US implementation of digital mammography. J Natl Cancer Inst 2014;106:dju092.

29. Rex DK, Johnson DA, Anderson JC, et al. American College of Gastroenterology guidelines for colorectal cancer screening 2008. Am J Gastroenterol 2009;104: 739–50.

30. U.S. Preventive Services Task Force. Screening for lung cancer: U.S. Preventive Services Task Force Recommendation Statement. Ann Intern Med 2014;160: 330–8.

31. Pinsky PF, Berg C. Applying the National Lung Screening Trial eligibility criteria to the US population: what percent of the population and of incident lung cancers would be covered. J Med Screen 2012;19:154–6.

32. Krabbe LM, Svatek RS, Shariat SF, et al. Bladder cancer risk: use of the PLCO and NLST to identify a suitable screening cohort. Urol Oncol 2015;33(2): 65.e19–25.

33. Mir MC, Stephenson AJ, Grubb R, et al. Predicting risk of bladder cancer using clinical and demographic information from prostate, lung colorectal and ovarian cancer screening trial participants. Cancer Epidemiol Biomarkers Prev 2013;22: 2241–9.

34. United States Preventive Services Task Force. Recommendations for primary care practice. Available at: http://www.uspreventiveservicestaskforce.org. Accessed January 12, 2015.

35. Canadian Task Force on Preventive Health Care. Canadian Task Force on Preventive Health Care guidelines. Available at: http://canadiantaskforce.ca/ctfphc-guidelines. Accessed January 12, 2015.

Lung Cancer Screening

Mark E. Deffebach, MD[a,b,*], Linda Humphrey, MD, MPH[b,c]

KEYWORDS

- Low Dose CT • Smoking • Screening • Multidisciplinary program

KEY POINTS

- Screening for lung cancer in high-risk individuals with annual low-dose computed tomography (LDCT) has been shown to reduce lung cancer mortality by 20% and is recommended by multiple health care organizations.
- Screening for lung cancer by chest radiography (CXR) or in low-risk individuals is not recommended.
- Lung cancer screening is not a specific test; it is a process that involves appropriate selection of high-risk individuals, careful interpretation and follow-up of imaging, and annual testing.
- Screening should be performed in the context of a multidisciplinary program experienced in the diagnosis and management of lung nodules and early-stage lung cancer.

INTRODUCTION

The burden of lung cancer is immense. It is the leading cause of cancer-related death in the United States and worldwide, and was estimated to account for almost 160,000 cancer deaths in the United States in 2013[1] and 1.4 million deaths worldwide in 2008. Some of the major risks for developing lung cancer are easily identified, most notably cigarette smoking, and there is evidence that the reduced rates of smoking in the United States are resulting in reduced incidence of lung cancer. Even if trends in smoking cessation continue, the substantial burden of lung cancer will continue for many years. Smoking cessation is the most important public health measure for reducing this burden. However, early detection through screening asymptomatic at-risk individuals also holds promise for decreasing the morbidity and mortality of lung cancer.

The rationale for lung cancer screening is strong. The disease has a long preclinical phase, the clinical outcomes in early disease are substantially better than when

[a] Division of Hospital and Specialty Medicine, Pulmonary and Critical Care Medicine, Portland VA Health Care System, P3PULM, 3710 Southwest US Veterans Hospital Road, Portland, OR 97201, USA; [b] Department of Medicine, Oregon Health and Science University, Portland, OR 97239, USA; [c] Division of Hospital and Specialty Medicine, Portland VA Health Care System, P3PULM, 3710 Southwest US Veterans Hospital Road, Portland, OR 97201, USA
* Corresponding author. Division of Hospital and Specialty Medicine, Pulmonary and Critical Care Medicine, Portland VA Health Care System, P3PULM, 3710 Southwest US Veterans Hospital Road, Portland, OR 97201.
E-mail address: Mark.Deffebach@va.gov

Surg Clin N Am 95 (2015) 967–978
http://dx.doi.org/10.1016/j.suc.2015.05.006
0039-6109/15/$ – see front matter Published by Elsevier Inc.

surgical.theclinics.com

detected as advanced disease, and currently, most lung cancer presents at an advanced stage. In addition, more so than with most cancers, a substantial portion of at-risk individuals can be readily identified and targeted for screening.

Imaging has been the focus of lung cancer screening since the early 1960s. The use of CXR for lung cancer screening was the focus of several large-scale clinical trials, including 6 randomized controlled trials.[2–5] One of these, the Mayo Lung Project, included a 20-year follow-up.[6] None demonstrated a mortality benefit. In the Prostate, Lung, Colorectal, and Ovarian Cancer (PLCO) Screening trial, 154,942 subjects from the general population, including nonsmokers, were randomized to annual CXR compared with a baseline CXR and usual care in the control group. After 13 years of follow-up, only 20% of lung cancers in the screening group were detected by screening, and no mortality benefit was seen in either the general population or the subset at higher risk of lung cancer based on smoking history and age.[7] The Mayo Clinic also conducted a randomized trial of CXR and sputum analysis versus usual care for lung cancer screening. In a long-term follow-up of the Mayo Lung Project, although significantly more cancers were detected in the screening group, there was a higher overall lung cancer death rate.[8] These studies, along with others, led to recommending against using CXR for screening.[9] With the failure of CXR-based lung cancer screening, computed tomography (CT)-based screening with LDCT began to be explored.

The initial studies of LDCT screening were observational, including the Early Lung Cancer Project (ELCAP),[10] the International ELCAP,[11] the Mayo Clinic CT study,[12] and the Continuous Observation of Smoking (COSMOS) study in Italy.[13] These studies demonstrated the ability of CT to detect lung cancer at an early stage. However, none were randomized and all subject to several forms of bias, most notably lead-time and overdiagnosis bias (see later discussion). The observational studies are important because they confirmed that most lung cancer detected through screening is early stage and can inform the practice of lung cancer screening. Despite demonstrating the ability to detect early-stage lung cancers, analysis of the observational studies did not result in a recommendation for CT-based lung cancer screening.[9] Only a randomized clinical trial could determine the true efficacy of CT-based lung cancer screening.

The most important trial to date, the National Lung Screening Trial (NLST), is a large randomized trial conducted by the National Cancer Institute of LDCT for lung cancer screening.[14,15] The NLST had its origins in the PLCO screening trial, and because of the background with accumulated data from the PLCO screening trial and the demonstration that CXR was ineffective compared with no screening,[7] the NLST was designed to compare CXR with LDCT. To date it is the only published large-scale randomized trial of LDCT lung cancer screening. There are other ongoing randomized trials, but it is not clear if they are adequately powered to detect a mortality benefit.

The NLST is one of the largest and most expensive clinical trials ever conducted, and it is possible that it will be the only North American randomized controlled trial of LDCT lung cancer screening. A total of 53,454 high-risk persons at 33 medical centers across the United States were enrolled. Age and smoking history were the main determinates of risk: individuals enrolled had to be between 55 and 74 years of age with at least 30 pack-years of smoking. Subjects could not have quit smoking greater than 15 years before enrollment. Exclusions included any prior history of lung cancer, other cancer within the past 5 years (other than a nonmelanoma skin cancer), a chest CT scan in the past 18 months, unexplained weight loss or symptoms suggestive of lung cancer, or a medical condition that posed a significant risk of mortality during the trial period. Enrollment first began in 2002, with subjects randomized to either an annual CXR or annual LDCT during 3 consecutive years. Imaging was completed in 2007, with continued follow-up until the trial was stopped in November 2010 when an interim analysis showed a significant benefit for LDCT screening. At a median follow-up of 6.5 years, there were 1060 lung cancers and 247 lung cancer deaths in the LDCT group compared with 941 lung cancers and 309 lung cancer deaths in the CXR group, a 20% reduction in lung cancer mortality and a 6.7% reduction in all-cause mortality.[14]

The NLST included careful monitoring of image quality and clear definitions of negative and positive scan results.[15] Evaluation of positive findings was left to the discretion of individual providers but generally occurred in the study-associated academic center. Positive findings were defined as any noncalcified nodule seen on CXR and any nodule 4 mm or more seen on LDCT. During all 3 rounds of screening, 24% of subjects in the LDCT arm had a positive result, with 96.4% of all positive results not shown to be lung cancer and considered false positive. Most false-positive results were evaluated and resolved with additional imaging but included surgery in 297 subjects. Overall, the rate of complications from the evaluation of true or false-positive findings was low, 1.4% in the LDCT group.

Based largely on the strength of the results of the NLST, multiple organizations involved in lung cancer and cancer screening now recommend annual lung cancer screening with LDCT for high-risk individuals. These organizations include the American Cancer Society,[16] the American Association of Thoracic Surgeons (AATS),[17] the American College of Chest Physicians (ACCP),[18] the American Society of Clinical Oncology and the American Thoracic Society (ATS),[19] and the US Preventative Services Task Force.[20,21] The Centers for Medicare and Medicaid Services has proposed coverage for LDCT and visits for counseling and shared decision making (http://www.cms.gov/medicare-coverage-database/details/nca-proposed-decision-memo.aspx?NCAId=274) (**Table 1**).

In the NLST, 70% of the lung cancers detected by LDCT were stage I or II, mostly adenocarcinoma. The rate of cancer detection was similar during the 3 years of screening, and there were fewer advanced cancers in the LDCT group. The predictive

Table 1		
Potential Benefits and Harms from LDCT Screening		
	Events/1000 Screened	**Reference**
Benefits		
Diagnosis of Stage I or II lung cancer	16	14
Prevented Lung Cancer Death	3	14
Harms		
False positive CT		
Nodule size considered abnormal		
>4 mm	263	14
>5 mm	155	39
>6 mm	93	45
>7 mm	61	45
Invasive biopsy for benign lesion	41	14
Surgery for benign lesion	10	14
Major complication during evaluation of a benign lesion	3	14
Overdiagnosis of lung cancer	0.6–1.2	45

value of LDCT improved during the 3 rounds of screening, probably because positive findings in round 1 that were shown to be stable were then considered to be negative.[22]

The cost-effectiveness of the NLST has been assessed, linking all costs for the time horizon of the study and predicted lifetime of the subjects.[23] The cost per quality-adjusted life year gained was estimated to be $81,000, within a commonly held threshold of $100,000 used to evaluate other prevention strategies. Cost-effectiveness was greater in women and individuals at higher lung cancer risk and can be significantly affected by screening protocol details such as the cost of the screening study, definitions of a positive result, and evaluation of findings.

Post hoc analysis of the NLST has included an application of a more complete lung cancer risk assessment model.[24,25] Using a model based on the PLCO screening trial cohort that included smoking history and age, as in the NLST, along with race or ethnicity, education, obesity, chronic obstructive pulmonary disease, and personal or family history of cancer, the NLST cohort was divided into quintiles of risk for death from lung cancer over 6 years. Although the 20% reduction in lung cancer deaths was observed in all quintiles, only 1% of the prevented lung cancer deaths occurred in the lowest-risk quintile. The number needed to screen to prevent 1 lung cancer death varied greatly with lung cancer risk; the lowest-risk quintile required 5276 enrollees to prevent 1 lung cancer death, whereas in the highest-risk quintile, only 161 enrollees were required (**Fig. 1**). In addition, the proportion of false-positive results decreased with increasing risk of lung cancer. This result suggests that further application of lung cancer risk models to lung cancer screening can improve the cost-effectiveness and efficiency of screening.

There are several ongoing studies of lung cancer screening that, although under-powered for determining the effect of LDCT on lung cancer screening mortality, are able to inform on the practice of lung cancer screening. NELSON (Dutch-Belgian Lung Cancer Screening Trial) is a randomized trial of LDCT versus usual care (no screening) being conducted in Europe with 7557 subjects undergoing LDCT screening with a baseline CT followed by repeat LDCT at years 1 and 3.[26–30] Positive scan results were defined based on nodule volume and change in volume.[31] Unlike the NLST, 5-year lung cancer survivors were eligible for inclusion. NELSON investigators have published data on the screening group, and analysis that includes comparison to the control group is anticipated in 2015–16.

Using a volumetric approach to classifying and following lung nodules found through screening, NELSON, compared with the NLST, has a shown a lower false-

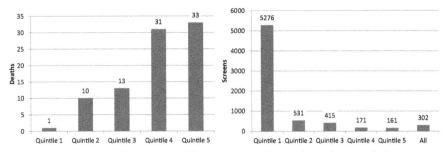

Fig. 1. Lung cancer deaths prevented by LDCT screening and number needed to treat to prevent 1 lung cancer death in NLST. Screened subjects were divided into quintiles of risk for lung cancer death over 5 years. (*Data from* Kovalchik SA, Tammemagi M, Berg CD, et al. Targeting of low-dose CT screening according to the risk of lung-cancer death. N Engl J Med 2013;369(3):245–54.)

positive rate and a higher true-positive rate with a comparable overall yield for screening.[26] The study has also shown that interval cancers, those diagnosed outside of screening and between rounds of screening, and cancers detected at later rounds of screening tend to be more aggressive.[32]

RISKS AND HARMS OF LUNG CANCER SCREENING
Radiation

LDCT screening for lung cancer exposes individuals to radiation, which may include repeated exposure over 20 years. The risks of radiation are often extrapolated from environmental exposures, including atomic bomb survivors.[33] Analyses have suggested that serial imaging may independently add to the risk of developing a malignancy,[34] and consideration of the risks of radiation need to include not only the LDCT screening CT but also the radiation exposure from studies of positive, mostly false-positive, findings. Restricting screening to the appropriate (older) age group, close attention to adherence and monitoring of a LDCT protocol, and judicious use of follow-up imaging are required to minimize the risks of radiation. The reported radiation dose for LDCT in screening studies ranges from 0.61 to 1.5 mSv, with 1 study documenting cumulative doses up to 7 mSv for the screening and follow-up studies.[35]

Invasive Procedures

In the NLST, more than 90% of all positive findings were false-positive findings and required some evaluation, and 11% led to an invasive procedure. Many of the procedures that might be used carry substantial risks, such as image-guided biopsies, bronchoscopies, and surgery. Judicious use of these tests and expertise in their conduct are required to minimize associated risks.

Anxiety and Stress

Any abnormal finding that might indicate malignancy can cause anxiety, and this has been demonstrated in the context of lung cancer screening. Assessing the definition of abnormal and carefully crafted communication are important to reducing stress and anxiety associated with screening for lung cancer.[36]

Overdiagnosis

Overdiagnosis occurs when there is a diagnosis of a cancer or other disease that would otherwise not go on to cause symptoms or death.[37] This result is not a false-positive diagnosis, as these are individuals diagnosed with cancer with tumors that meet pathologic criteria for cancer. The challenge is that one currently cannot determine which cancers will progress and which will not, and therefore evaluation and treatment typically occurs for all of them. However, when a patient is exposed to the harms of evaluation and treatment of disease that would not have become symptomatic during their lifetime, overdiagnosis has occurred with no benefit and only harm is incurred to the patient. Although overdiagnosis is sometimes questioned, there is no doubt that it occurs with most cancers, including lung cancer, and is a major risk in patients screened for any type of cancer. Only randomized studies with long-term follow-up can determine the actual rate of overdiagnosis. Determinates of overdiagnosis include the aggressiveness of the cancer and the competing comorbidities in patients being diagnosed with cancer. Although lung cancer is generally an aggressive malignancy, it is heterogeneous with many cancers, including some of those detected through screening, being very indolent. Studies have found that very indolent lung cancer, defined as having a doubling time greater than 400 days make up anywhere from 3% to 31% of detected cancers.[38] Furthermore, with smoking and age being the major lung cancer risks, patients at risk for developing lung cancer often have significant comorbidities, some of which result in death before development of symptoms from a screen-detected cancer.

Estimates of the Rate of Overdiagnosis in Lung Cancer Screening

In the Mayo Lung project, a randomized trial of CXR-based screening study in the 1970s that included more than 9000 subjects, 17% more lung cancers were detected in the screening group without any reduction in lung cancer mortality.[12] This observation was seen during the initial 6 years of the study and during an additional 16 years of follow-up.[6,8] However, this study had several significant flaws, including a substantial amount of screening in the control group. In the larger PLCO study comparing CXR screening to usual care, the lung cancer incidence rates, lung cancer mortality, and fraction of late-stage diagnoses were the same in the 2 groups, demonstrating that CXR screening was ineffective and without evidence for overdiagnosis.[7] This result was true for the general population as well as a subset selected for increased lung cancer risk using the NLST criteria.

Estimates of overdiagnosis in the NLST have been made. Comparing cancer detection rates in the LDCT- and CXR-screened groups during the 6 years of observation, 1089 lung cancers were found in the LDCT group and 969 lung cancers in the CXR (control) group, indicating a maximum overdiagnosis rate of 18%.[39] Because this analysis only includes short-term follow-up, the true rate of overdiagnosis of LDCT screening is probably lower. Using a model of extended lifetime follow-up after LDCT screening, the overdiagnosis rate of LDCT for non–small cell lung cancer was estimated to decrease to less than 4%. It has been suggested that lesions presenting as pure ground-glass nodules and typically associated with bronchoalveolar cell carcinoma or minimally invasive adenocarcinoma, although pathologically classified as cancers, may be candidates for overdiagnosis.[39] Whether these lesions, when detected by screening, can be managed as truly indolent lesions, avoiding invasive procedures, is not known.[40]

PRACTICE OF LUNG CANCER SCREENING
Multidisciplinary Lung Cancer Screening Program

Lung cancer screening is not simply obtaining an LDCT and reacting to what is found. It is a multidisciplinary process that should be conducted in the context of a multidisciplinary program that includes all the relevant specialties. The goals and elements of such a program have been outlined by the ACCP and the ATS.[41] A lung cancer screening program should include specialists experienced in nodule management and diagnosis and treatment of lung cancer, and ideally include pulmonary medicine, thoracic imaging, thoracic surgery, medical oncology, and radiation oncology. Lung cancer screening programs should develop policies and collect data related to all aspects of lung cancer screening, along with monitoring adherence to those policies.

Eligibility for Lung Cancer Screening

Several different, but closely related, eligibility criteria can be applied to lung cancer screening. The NLST enrolled subjects considered at risk for developing lung cancer based on smoking and age, with the major criteria being age 55 to 74 years with at least 30 pack-years smoking history and having smoked within the last 15 years. Current recommendations for screen eligibility are based on this, with some organizations including some minor variations (see **Table 1**). The NLST also excluded subjects with symptoms suggestive of lung cancer, a prior history of a significant cancer, and significant comorbidities that would preclude lung cancer treatment, generally considered to mean surgical resection. Adherence to eligibility criteria is key to effective lung cancer screening; enrolling low-risk individuals results in inefficient screening and enrolling individuals with significant comorbidities may increase overdiagnosis and complications from procedures associated with evaluation of positive results and the treatment of detected lung cancer. One analysis illustrated this by assessing a wide range of lung cancer risks that were within the range being offered by lung cancer screening in some institutions; the number of persons needed to screen during 3 years to prevent 1 lung cancer death ranged from a low of 82 in high-risk subjects to a high of 35,186 in very-low-risk subjects still considered candidates for screening.[42] Basing eligibility on individual risk models may improve lung cancer screening efficiency. For example, Kovalchik and colleagues[24] found that application of a validated lung cancer risk model to the NLST population could reduce the number screened by 8% and increase the lung cancer diagnosis rate by 12%, with the number needed to screen to prevent 1 lung cancer death reduced from 320 to 255 (see **Fig. 1**). Risk assessment tools are available online (http://www.brocku.ca/lung-cancer-risk-calculator), but how to operationalize individual risk assessment has not been studied. The same investigators developed a risk model for never smokers and concluded that a sufficient risk to support screening in never smokers could not be identified.[43] Lung cancer screening programs should incorporate methods to adhere to accepted eligibility criteria and mechanisms to adapt to new developments in eligibility criteria, such as individualized risk assessments.

Computed Tomography Protocol

The detection of lung nodules that are possibly malignant is the goal of LDCT screening for lung cancer. Screening is currently recommended annually and may occur for more than 20 years; therefore, LDCT has been optimized to provide quality images with the lowest delivered radiation dose. In the NLST, the delivered dose ranged from 2 to 5 mGy.[44] New methods of acquisition and processing may be able to substantially reduce this exposure. The American College of Radiology has published guidelines for LDCT image acquisition, reporting, and quality control, along with criteria for designation as a lung cancer screening center with an emphasis on the imaging components.[45]

Definition of Abnormal Results on Low-Dose Computed Tomography

The definition of a nodule determines the number of screening studies in need of further evaluation. In the NLST, greater than 4 mm was the threshold for considering a nodule abnormal. This criterion resulted in 27% of all baseline scan results considered abnormal.[14] Raising the threshold results in fewer studies in need of evaluation (**Table 2**) but can reduce the sensitivity for detection of lung cancer. Yip and colleagues[46] analyzed the NLST data using abnormal thresholds from 5 to 9 mm and found that the rate of abnormal results decreased from 16% to 4%, as a larger nodule size was used to define an abnormal result. No lung cancer diagnoses were missed going from 4 to 5 mm, and only 6 of 232 cancers were missed with a 7-mm threshold. These data suggest that modifying the definition of a positive LDCT result might preserve the mortality benefit while substantially reducing the number of false-positive LDCT results and the subsequent evaluations. The National Cancer Care Network currently recommends a 5-mm threshold. Several guidelines are available that include definitions and recommendations, including the American College of Radiology[47,48] (http://www.acr.org/Quality-Safety/Resources/LungRADS). For efficient lung cancer screening, it is key that each lung cancer program apply specific definitions of abnormal that are applied uniformly. Geographic variation in the number and types of lung nodules may also need to be taken into account.

Table 2 Studies on nodule threshold		
Organization	Recommendation	Year
US Preventative Services Task Force	Recommends annual LDCT screening for high-risk individuals (ages 55–80 y with a 30 pk-y history of smoking and current smoker or quit within past 15 y). Discontinue when person has not smoked for 15 y or if limited life expectancy	2013
American Cancer Society	Recommends annual LDCT screening for high-risk individuals (ages 55–74 y with a 30 pk-y history of smoking and current smoker or quit within past 15 y). Informed individual decision making before testing	2013
American College of Chest Physicians	Recommends annual LDCT screening for high-risk individuals (ages 55–74 y with a 30 pk-y history of smoking and current smoker or quit within past 15 y)	2012
American Academy of Thoracic Surgeons	Recommends annual LDCT screening for high-risk individuals (ages 55–74 y with a 30 pk-y history of smoking and current smoker or quit within past 15 y) or age $\geq$50 y with cumulative risk >5% over next 5 y	2012
National Comprehensive Cancer Network	Recommends annual LDCT screening for high-risk individuals (ages 55–74 y with a 30 pk-y history of smoking and current smoker or quit within past 15 y) or age $\geq$50 y and $\geq$20 pk-y smoking history with 1 additional risk factor	2015
American Academy of Family Physicians	Concludes there is insufficient evidence to recommend for or against screening for lung cancer with LDCT in persons at high risk for lung cancer based on age and smoking history	2013
Canadian Task Force on the Periodic Health Examination	Recommends against the use of CXR in asymptomatic persons. Evidence is insufficient for or against screening with CT in asymptomatic persons	2003 (under review)
Centers for Medicare and Medicaid Services	Recommends annual LDCT screening for high-risk individuals (ages 55–77 y with a 30 pk-y history of smoking and current smoker or quit within past 15 y) and initiate only after visit for screening counseling with shared decision making	2014

Reporting and Communication

Most of the findings on lung cancer screening LDCT are indeterminate small lung nodules that eventually prove to be benign, and a consistent approach to measurement and description is key to ensuring that follow-up is appropriate and that patients and referring providers do not experience unnecessary stress[49]; this is particularly important in an era of direct patient access to medical records. The language used can be important. As part of Radiology Lung Imaging Reporting and Data System (LungRADS), the ACR offers one approach to consistent reporting.[47]

Evaluation of Abnormal Findings

Several guidelines are available for the management of pulmonary nodules, including guidelines for solid and subsolid nodules from the Fleischner Society,[50,51] ACCP,[52] AATS,[17] and the National Comprehensive Cancer Network (http://www.nccn.org/professionals/physician_gls/pdf/lung_screening.pdf). Volumetric measurement of nodules and changes in nodule volume may improve both sensitivity and specificity of LDCT for correctly characterizing smaller nodules[26,31,53] but was not used by NSLT and is not currently in wide use. Appropriate management of nodules detected should be multidisciplinary and can reduce the number of diagnostic procedures and improve the efficiency of the screening process.[48]

Smoking Cessation

Despite the mortality benefit of lung cancer screening in at-risk individuals, smoking cessation is the most important public health measure for the prevention of lung cancer. A systematic review of smoking cessation and lung cancer screening showed that screening for lung cancer in and of itself does not seem to influence smoking cessation rates,[54] but receipt of a positive result may[55] and therefore be an opportunity for an effective smoking cessation intervention. Lung cancer screening should integrate smoking cessation, either as part of the multidisciplinary program or by referral to a smoking cessation program.

Education

Subjects undergoing lung cancer screening should be fully informed of both the potential benefits and risks of lung cancer screening and the importance of compliance with annual or follow-up scans. There are several printed and online resources available, including excellent patient education materials from the following:

1. The National Cancer Care Network (NCCN) (http://www.nccn.org/patients/guidelines/lung_screening/index.html#)
2. The National Cancer Institute (NCI) (http://www.cancer.gov/cancertopics/pdq/screening/lung/Patient/page3)
3. The US Department of Veteran Affairs (VA) (http://www.prevention.va.gov/Lung_Cancer_Screening.asp)

The ACCP and ATS also recommend that lung cancer screening programs become active in provider education, and this is especially important as criteria for screening and technology evolve.

SUMMARY

Screening for early lung cancer with LDCT in at-risk individuals has the potential to significantly reduce the burden of lung cancer. To be safe and efficient it requires a multidisciplinary approach with careful adherence to eligibility criteria and experienced management of detected findings. Lung cancer screening programs should be designed to adapt to changes in eligibility criteria, definitions of abnormal nodules, and evolving approaches to monitoring detected nodules. Lastly, every individual undergoing screening while still smoking should also be referred for smoking cessation.

REFERENCES

1. American Cancer Society. Cancer facts and figures 2013. Atlanta (GA); 2013. p. 1–64.

2. Kubík A, Parkin DM, Khlat M, et al. Lack of benefit from semi-annual screening for cancer of the lung: follow-up report of a randomized controlled trial on a population of high-risk males in Czechoslovakia. Int J Cancer 1990;45(1):26–33.
3. Friedman GD, Collen MF, Fireman BH. Multiphasic health checkup evaluation: a 16-year follow-up. J Chronic Dis 1986;39(6):453–63.
4. Melamed MR. Lung cancer screening results in the National Cancer Institute New York study. Cancer 2000;89(11 Suppl):2356–62.
5. Berlin NI, Buncher CR, Fontana RS, et al. The National Cancer Institute Cooperative Early Lung Cancer Detection Program. Results of the initial screen (prevalence). Early lung cancer detection: introduction. Am Rev Respir Dis 1984; 130(4):545–9.
6. Marcus PM, Bergstralh EJ. Lung cancer mortality in the Mayo Lung Project: impact of extended follow-up. J Natl Cancer Inst 2000;92(16):1308–16. Available at: http://eutils.ncbi.nlm.nih.gov/entrez/eutils/elink.fcgi?dbfrom=pubmed&id=10944552&retmode=ref&cmd=prlinks.
7. Oken MM, Hocking WG, Kvale PA, et al. Screening by chest radiograph and lung cancer mortality: the Prostate, Lung, Colorectal, and Ovarian (PLCO) randomized trial. JAMA 2011;306(17):1865–73.
8. Marcus PM, Bergstralh EJ, Zweig MH, et al. Extended lung cancer incidence follow-up in the Mayo Lung Project and overdiagnosis. J Natl Cancer Inst 2006; 98(11):748–56.
9. U.S. Preventive Services Task Force. Lung cancer screening: recommendation statement. Ann Intern Med 2004;140(9):738–9.
10. Henschke CI, McCauley DI, Yankelevitz DF, et al. Early lung cancer action project: overall design and findings from baseline screening. Lancet 1999; 354(9173):99–105.
11. International Early Lung Cancer Action Program Investigators, Henschke CI, Yankelevitz DF, et al. Survival of patients with stage I lung cancer detected on CT screening. N Engl J Med 2006;355(17):1763–71.
12. Swensen SJ, Jett JR, Hartman TE, et al. Lung cancer screening with CT: Mayo Clinic experience. Radiology 2003;226(3):756–61.
13. Veronesi G, Maisonneuve P, Spaggiari L, et al. Diagnostic performance of low-dose computed tomography screening for lung cancer over five years. J Thorac Oncol 2014;9(7):935–9.
14. National Lung Screening Trial Research Team, Aberle DR, Adams AM, et al. Reduced lung-cancer mortality with low-dose computed tomographic screening. N Engl J Med 2011;365(5):395–409.
15. National Lung Screening Trial Research Team. The National Lung Screening Trial: overview and study design. Radiology 2011;258(1):243–53.
16. Wender R, Fontham ET, Barrera E Jr, et al. American Cancer Society lung cancer screening guidelines. CA Cancer J Clin 2013;63(2):106–17.
17. Jaklitsch MT, Jacobson FL, Austin JH, et al. The American Association for Thoracic Surgery guidelines for lung cancer screening using low-dose computed tomography scans for lung cancer survivors and other high-risk groups. J Thorac Cardiovasc Surg 2012;144(1):33–8.
18. Detterbeck FC, Mazzone PJ, Naidich DP, et al. Screening for lung cancer: diagnosis and management of lung cancer, 3rd ed: American College of Chest Physicians evidence-based clinical practice guidelines. Chest 2013;143(5 Suppl): e78S–92S.
19. Bach PB, Mirkin JN, Oliver TK, et al. Benefits and harms of CT screening for lung cancer: a systematic review. JAMA 2012;307(22):2418–29.

20. Moyer VA. Screening for lung cancer: U.S. preventive services task force recommendation statement. Ann Intern Med 2014;160(5):330–8.
21. Humphrey LL, Deffebach M, Pappas M, et al. Screening for lung cancer with low-dose computed tomography. Ann Intern Med 2014;160(3):212.
22. Aberle DR, DeMello S, Berg CD, et al. Results of the two incidence screenings in the National Lung Screening Trial. N Engl J Med 2013;369(10):920–31.
23. Black WC, Gareen IF, Soneji SS, et al. Cost-effectiveness of CT screening in the National Lung Screening Trial. N Engl J Med 2014;371(19):1793–802.
24. Kovalchik SA, Tammemagi M, Berg CD, et al. Targeting of low-dose CT screening according to the risk of lung-cancer death. N Engl J Med 2013; 369(3):245–54.
25. Tammemägi MC, Katki HA, Hocking WG, et al. Selection criteria for lung-cancer screening. N Engl J Med 2013;368(8):728–36.
26. Horeweg N, van der Aalst CM, Vliegenthart R, et al. Volumetric computed tomography screening for lung cancer: three rounds of the NELSON trial. Eur Respir J 2013;42(6):1659–67.
27. Horeweg N, van der Aalst CM, Thunnissen E, et al. Characteristics of lung cancers detected by computer tomography screening in the randomized NELSON trial. Am J Respir Crit Care Med 2013;187(8):848–54.
28. van den Bergh KA, Essink Bot ML, Bunge EM, et al. Impact of computed tomography screening for lung cancer on participants in a randomized controlled trial (NELSON trial). Cancer 2008;113(2):396–404.
29. Xu DM, Gietema H, de Koning H, et al. Nodule management protocol of the NELSON randomised lung cancer screening trial. Lung Cancer 2006;54(2):177–84.
30. van Iersel CA, de Koning HJ, Draisma G, et al. Risk-based selection from the general population in a screening trial: selection criteria, recruitment and power for the Dutch-Belgian randomised lung cancer multi-slice CT screening trial (NELSON). Int J Cancer 2006;120(4):868–74.
31. van Klaveren RJ, Oudkerk M, Prokop M, et al. Management of lung nodules detected by volume CT scanning. N Engl J Med 2009;361(23):2221–9.
32. Horeweg N, Scholten ET, de Jong PA, et al. Detection of lung cancer through low-dose CT screening (NELSON): a prespecified analysis of screening test performance and interval cancers. Lancet Oncol 2014;15:1342–50.
33. Brenner DJ. Radiation risks potentially associated with low-dose CT screening of adult smokers for lung cancer. Radiology 2004;231(2):440–5.
34. Berrington de Gonzalez A, Kim KP, Berg CD. Low-dose lung computed tomography screening before age 55: estimates of the mortality reduction required to outweigh the radiation-induced cancer risk. J Med Screen 2008; 15(3):153–8.
35. Mascalchi M, Mazzoni LN, Falchini M, et al. Dose exposure in the ITALUNG trial of lung cancer screening with low-dose CT. Br J Radiol 2012;85(1016):1134–9.
36. Slatore CG, Sullivan DR, Pappas M, et al. Patient-centered outcomes among lung cancer screening recipients with computed tomography: a systematic review. J Thorac Oncol 2014;9(7):927–34.
37. Welch HG, Black WC. Overdiagnosis in Cancer. J Natl Cancer Inst 2010;102(9): 605–13.
38. Infante M, Berghmans T, Heuvelmans MA, et al. Slow-growing lung cancer as an emerging entity: from screening to clinical management. Eur Respir J 2013;42(6): 1706–22.
39. Patz EF, Pinsky P, Gatsonis C, et al. Overdiagnosis in low-dose computed tomography screening for lung cancer. JAMA Intern Med 2014;174(2):269–74.

40. Revel MP. Avoiding overdiagnosis in lung cancer screening: the volume doubling time strategy. Eur Respir J 2013;42(6):1459–63.

41. Mazzone P, Powell CA, Arenberg D, et al. Components necessary for high quality lung cancer screening: American College of Chest Physicians and American Thoracic Society Policy Statement. Chest 2015;147(2):295–303.

42. Bach PB, Gould MK. When the average applies to no one: personalized decision making about potential benefits of lung cancer screening. Ann Intern Med 2012; 157(8):571–3.

43. Tammemägi MC, Church TR, Hocking WG, et al. Evaluation of the lung cancer risks at which to screen ever- and never-smokers: screening rules applied to the PLCO and NLST cohorts. PLoS Med 2014;11(12):e1001764.

44. Cody DD, Kim HJ, Cagnon CH, et al. Normalized CT dose index of the CT scanners used in the National Lung Screening Trial. Am J Roentgenol 2010;194(6):1539–46.

45. Kazerooni EA, Armstrong MR, Amorosa JK, et al. ACR CT Accreditation Program and the Lung Cancer Screening Program Designation. J Am Coll Radiol 2015; 12(1):38–42.

46. Yip R, Henschke CI, Yankelevitz DF, et al. CT screening for lung cancer: alternative definitions of positive test result based on the National Lung Screening Trial and International Early Lung Cancer Action Program databases. Radiology 2014; 273(2):591–6.

47. Manos D, Seely JM, Taylor J, et al. The Lung Reporting and Data System (LU-R-ADS): a proposal for computed tomography screening. Can Assoc Radiol J 2014; 65(2):121–34.

48. McKee BJ, Regis SM, McKee AB, et al. Performance of ACR Lung-RADS in a Clinical CT Lung Screening Program. J Am Coll Radiol 2015;12(3):273–6.

49. Harris RP, Sheridan SL, Lewis CL, et al. The harms of screening. JAMA Intern Med 2014;174(2):281–6.

50. Naidich DP, Bankier AA, MacMahon H, et al. Recommendations for the management of subsolid pulmonary nodules detected at CT: a statement from the Fleischner Society. Radiology 2013;266(1):304–17.

51. MacMahon H, Austin JH, Gamsu G, et al. Guidelines for management of small pulmonary nodules detected on CT scans: a statement from the Fleischner Society. Radiology 2005;237(2):395–400.

52. Gould MK, Donington J, Lynch WR, et al. Evaluation of individuals with pulmonary nodules: when is it lung cancer? Diagnosis and management of lung cancer, 3rd ed: American College of Chest Physicians evidence-based clinical practice guidelines. Chest 2013;143(5 Suppl):e93S–120S.

53. Mehta HJ, Ravenel JG, Shaftman SR, et al. The utility of nodule volume in the context of malignancy prediction for small pulmonary nodules. Chest 2014;145(3):464.

54. Slatore CG, Baumann C, Pappas M, et al. Smoking behaviors among patients receiving computed tomography for lung cancer screening. Systematic review in support of the U.S. Preventive Services Task Force. Ann Am Thorac Soc 2014;11(4):619–27.

55. Tammemägi MC, Berg CD, Riley TL, et al. Impact of lung cancer screening results on smoking cessation. J Natl Cancer Inst 2014;106(6):dju084.

Colorectal Cancer Screening

Kjetil Garborg, MD[a,b]

KEYWORDS

- Colorectal cancer • Screening • Prevention • Adenoma • Colonoscopy

KEY POINTS

- Colorectal cancer (CRC) is the third most common malignancy worldwide.
- Screening for colorectal cancer has been shown to reduce CRC incidence and mortality and is implemented in an increasing number of countries.
- Screening modalities include noninvasive fecal tests to detect occult blood or DNA from malignant tumors and invasive tests to detect cancer and remove premalignant polyps.
- The comparative effectiveness of different screening tests to reduce CRC mortality on a population level remains to be clarified.
- Colonoscopy allowing detection of malignant tumors and removal of premalignant polyps is the only 1-step approach to CRC screening, but the magnitude of its effectiveness to reduce CRC incidence and mortality is yet to be established in randomized controlled trials.

INTRODUCTION: EXTENT OF THE DISEASE

Colorectal cancer (CRC) is the third most common cancer worldwide.[1] The estimated numbers of new CRC cases and CRC deaths in the United States in 2014 were approximately 135,000 and 50,000, respectively.[2] The life-time risk of being diagnosed with CRC is approximately 5% in the Western world. Stage at diagnosis is the most important prognostic factor for CRC, with a 5-year survival of approximately 90% for early-stage disease without regional or distant metastases but only around 10% when distant metastases are present.[3] Unlike in many other Western countries, CRC incidence rates have declined in the United States since the mid-1980s, particularly for late-stage disease.[4,5] Although the reasons for this decline are not clear, a concomitant increase in CRC screening may be an important factor (**Fig. 1**).[5]

Disclosure: The author has nothing to disclose.
[a] Department of Transplantation Medicine, Oslo University Hospital, P.b. 4950 Nydalen, 0424 Oslo, Norway; [b] Department of Medicine, Sørlandet Hospital HF, P.b. 416, 4604 Kristiansand, Norway
E-mail address: k.k.garborg@medisin.uio.no

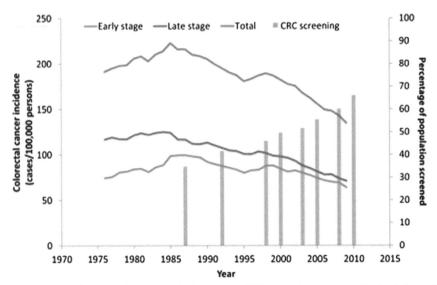

Fig. 1. CRC incidence and associated changes in CRC screening use are illustrated in US adults aged 50 years or older. (*From* Yang DX, Gross CP, Soulos PR, et al. Estimating the magnitude of colorectal cancers prevented during the era of screening: 1976 to 2009. Cancer 2014;120(18):2896; with permission.)

Risk Factors

Individuals with a strong family history of CRC, inflammatory bowel disease, and rare genetic conditions such as familial adenomatous polyposis and Lynch syndrome are at increased risk of CRC and should be referred for specialized care and surveillance.[6–8] However, most CRC cases develop in the so-called average-risk population without any of these known risk factors. In the general population, age is the most important risk factor for CRC, with 90% of cases developing in individuals more than 50 years of age.[2] The median age at CRC diagnosis in the United States is 68 years.[3]

Epidemiologic studies indicate that elements of Western lifestyle may influence the risk of CRC, but the effect of lifestyle modifications is still unclear. Factors that have been linked to a risk increase include high intake of red and processed meat, smoking, excessive alcohol consumption, and obesity,[9–12] whereas physical activity and the use of aspirin have been associated with decreased risk of CRC.[13,14] In the absence of well-defined options for primary CRC prevention, screening is currently the most widely accepted approach to reduce CRC burden.

SCREENING TECHNIQUES AND OPTIONS

Most CRCs develop slowly from well-defined precursors called adenomas through a series of genetic and epigenetic alterations: the adenoma-carcinoma sequence.[15] This transition typically takes at least 10 years. Moreover, early-stage, asymptomatic CRCs may bleed and shed cellular material into the fecal stream. The long premalignant and preclinical development allows different screening strategies to be effective in reducing CRC burden, and several screening tests are available. These tests can be broadly divided into tests for early detection of CRC to allow improved treatment outcomes, or tests for CRC prevention designed to decrease incidence and thereby also decrease mortality.

Early Detection Versus Prevention

Tests for early detection of CRC include the fecal occult blood tests (FOBTs) and stool DNA tests. These tests may detect either invisible amounts of blood or DNA from malignant tumors in stool samples before the disease becomes symptomatic. Asymptomatic CRC is generally less advanced than symptomatic disease and therefore is often curable. In contrast, prevention of CRC requires removal of premalignant polyps to interrupt the polyp-carcinoma sequence. Structural examinations that may detect both cancer and premalignant polyps include flexible sigmoidoscopy, colonoscopy, computed tomographic colonography, capsule endoscopy and double-contrast barium enema. Colonoscopy is the final common pathway for all positive screening tests to confirm or rule out the presence of CRC and remove premalignant lesions.

Stool Tests for Colorectal Cancer Screening

Guaiac-based fecal occult blood test

The first screening test that has been proved to reduce CRC mortality in randomized controlled trials (RCTs) was the guaiac-based FOBT (gFOBT). The test is performed by means of a test card with 6 windows for 2 samples from each of 3 consecutive stools. Four large-scale RCTs with long-term follow-up have shown that screening with gFOBT is associated with reduced CRC mortality compared with no screening.[16–19] The gFOBT detects peroxidase activity in the heme moiety of hemoglobin. Because heme is not specific to human hemoglobin, and because of the slow degradation of heme through the gastrointestinal tract, dietary meat and bleeding from more proximal sources may cause false-positive results.[20] However, restrictions on diet and medication are currently not advised because of limited effect on test positivity in population screening and risk of decreased screening participation.[21–23] The gFOBT has several advantages as a test for population screening: it is inexpensive, easy to use, and can be distributed and returned by mail. The major limitations of gFOBT are the low sensitivity for CRC (25%–38%) and advanced adenomas (16%–31%) and that repetitive testing every 1 to 2 years is required.[24]

Fecal immunochemical test

The fecal immunochemical test (FIT) is a newer FOBT that uses antibodies to detect the globin moiety of human hemoglobin. Globin is more rapidly degraded in the gastrointestinal tract than heme, thus the FIT is less sensitive than the gFOBT to bleeding from more proximal sources.[25] Although the effect of FIT on CRC mortality has not been evaluated in RCTs, favorable performance characteristics have been shown in comparisons with the gFOBT. The sensitivity of FIT for CRC (61%–91%) and advanced adenomas (27%–67%) is higher than for gFOBT.[24] Moreover, the easier sampling technique compared with the gFOBT, with only 1 fecal sample needed to complete the test, is associated with increased screening uptake.[26] There are 2 different FIT tests: a qualitative test with a binary outcome (positive/negative) and a quantitative test returning hemoglobin concentration in stool. The quantitative test allows for adjustments of test sensitivity and specificity for CRC and advanced adenomas, and the cutoff hemoglobin concentration for referral to colonoscopy can be adapted to available endoscopy resources.[27] However, repetitive testing is required, usually every 2 years. Although the gFOBT is still the most widely used CRC screening test in Europe, several FIT programs or pilots have been launched in Europe, Asia, Canada, and Australia.[28–30]

Stool DNA tests

Another noninvasive screening option is stool DNA testing. These tests are based on detection of 1 or more tumor-associated genetic and epigenetic markers in cells shed into the stool. In earlier studies, the sensitivity of stool DNA tests for CRC was 52% to 58% in screening populations.[31,32] In a more recent cross-sectional study, the sensitivity of a multitarget stool DNA test was 92% in a screening population.[33] Although the multitarget stool DNA test was recently approved for average-risk CRC screening by the US Food and Drug Administration, no data are yet available regarding its effect on CRC incidence and mortality, and factors such as cost-effectiveness and appropriate intervals for repeat testing remain to be clarified.

Structural Examinations of the Colon and Rectum

Flexible sigmoidoscopy

Flexible sigmoidoscopy allows direct visual inspection of the distal colon and rectum for early detection of CRC as well as interruption of the adenoma-carcinoma sequence by removal of polyps. It is currently the only screening test that has been proved to reduce both CRC incidence and mortality in large-scale RCTs.[34–37] Because flexible sigmoidoscopy is usually performed without sedation, and because bowel preparation is limited to a self-administered enema, it is a less resource demanding and burdensome procedure than colonoscopy. In a direct comparison with a 3-day gFOBT and a 1-day FIT, uptake of flexible sigmoidoscopy was considerably lower than both FOBTs, but detection rates of CRC and advanced adenomas was higher.[38] The main concern with flexible sigmoidoscopy screening is that CRCs and advanced adenomas in the proximal colon are missed. Although significant findings at flexible sigmoidoscopy should trigger a complete colonoscopy, a considerable number of patients with advanced proximal adenomas do not have a synchronous distal lesion.[39]

Colonoscopy

Colonoscopy is the final work-up examination that should follow any positive CRC screening test. It allows a complete examination of the colon and rectum, tissue sampling, and polyp removal in a single session. Thus, it is the only available 1-step approach to CRC screening and the most widely used screening test in the United States.[40] Although the magnitude of the effect of screening colonoscopy on CRC incidence and mortality is yet to be determined in RCTs, observational studies suggest that the effect of screening colonoscopy is larger than the observed effects of FOBT and flexible sigmoidoscopy screening (see **Table 2**).[41–46] Findings at colonoscopy also constitute the basis for surveillance recommendations after screening.[47,48] Nevertheless, colonoscopy is an invasive procedure, requires rigorous bowel preparation, and sedation is normally used to reduce discomfort. It is therefore an expensive test for population-based screening. Colonoscopy and polypectomy are complex technical procedures associated with possible complications such as bleeding and bowel perforation, thus proper training of endoscopists and continuous quality assurance are necessary. Quality indicators for the performance of colonoscopy were outlined in 2002 and have since been updated based on emerging evidence.[49,50]

Computed tomographic colonography

In meta-analysis of 5 screening studies, the sensitivity of computed tomographic colonography (CTC) to detect adenomas greater than or equal to 6 mm in size and adenomas and cancers greater than or equal to 10 mm was 80% and 88%, respectively.[51] In a randomized trial comparing CTC and colonoscopy, attendance was higher with CTC, but advanced neoplasia was found more frequently with colonoscopy.[52] However, if offered as an alternative to colonoscopy, total screening uptake may improve significantly.[53] Although CTC may be anticipated to be less burdensome than colonoscopy, the perceived burden may be higher.[54] Issues such as cost-effectiveness and the consequences of extracolonic findings need to be clarified before CTC can be widely implemented in population-based screening.[55]

Capsule colonoscopy

Capsule colonoscopy is a minimally invasive imaging method consisting of an ingestible capsule with a camera on both sides. Images are wirelessly transmitted to an external receiver and uploaded to a computer for image interpretation. Varying results regarding sensitivity and specificity for detection of colonic neoplasia were found in different studies.[56] In the most recent study of 884 individuals undergoing CRC screening with the latest generation of the capsule, the sensitivity of the capsule to detect polyps greater than or equal to 6 mm was 81% with a specificity of 93%.[57] In the same study, the capsule detected 3 out of 4 cancers found at colonoscopy, giving a sensitivity of 75% for CRC.[57] Although the technique is considered minimally invasive, it requires vigorous bowel cleansing before the procedure, and further ingestion of fluids is needed to propel the capsule through the intestines. Note that, in the aforementioned study, 9% of enrolled participants were excluded because of poor bowel preparation or short transit, and 11% had nonserious adverse events, mostly related to the bowel preparation.[57] Capsule colonoscopy may be appropriate when colonoscopy is either undesirable or contraindicated, but whether it is appropriate for population screening is currently uncertain.

Double-contrast barium enema

Double-contrast barium enema (DBCE) allows detection of CRC and polyps and is still endorsed as an option in 1 screening guideline.[58] However, in the era of more modern, sensitive, and less labor-intensive techniques such as computed tomography colonography, the role of DBCE in CRC screening is limited.[59]

Programmatic Versus Opportunistic Screening

Programmatic, publicly funded screening involves a central administrative apparatus to ensure equal possibility and access for all eligible individuals, systematic quality assurance, and continuous monitoring of attendance rates and outcomes. In contrast, opportunistic screening (also called spontaneous screening or case finding) denotes that the decision to undergo screening is based on patient's initiative or a recommendation from a primary care physician. In opportunistic screening, the patient may be allowed to select a screening test based on informed decision making. Although the opportunistic approach is flexible, proper evaluation of the long-term benefit, harm, and cost of screening may be difficult. In Europe, where basic health care is usually publicly funded, population-based, programmatic CRC screening is recommended.[25]

Colorectal Cancer Screening Guidelines

Several CRC screening guidelines have been published, all recommending that asymptomatic individuals at average risk for CRC should undergo screening from age 50 years.[24,25,58,60] Except for capsule colonoscopy, which is a fairly new addition to the test armamentarium, all aforementioned tests are evaluated in the most recent US guidelines. Tests with a potential for CRC prevention are preferred in 2 guidelines,[58,60] whereas in the third set of guidelines no specific test preference is stated.[24] Ultimately, the choice of test depends on availability and patient preference. A summary of test recommendations in the 3 US CRC screening guidelines are outlined in **Table 1**.

Table 1
Summary of recommendations in US CRC screening guidelines

Screening Test	Joint Guideline (American Cancer Society, US Multi-Society Task Force on CRC, American College of Radiology)[58]	US Preventive Services Task Force[24]	American College of Gastroenterology[60]
Sensitive gFOBT	+	+	+
FIT	+	+	+
Stool DNA	+	−	+
Flexible sigmoidoscopy	+	+	+
Colonoscopy	+	+	+
CT colonography	+	−	+
Double-contrast barium enema	+	−	−

Abbreviation: CT, computed tomography.
  Data from Refs.[24,58,60]

CLINICAL OUTCOMES

Major outcomes of interest in cancer screening are the effects on disease-specific incidence and mortality, the ratio of risk versus benefit, cost-effectiveness, as well as the effect on all-cause mortality. No cancer screening test has been shown to reduce all-cause mortality.[61] Compared with no screening, CRC screening has been found to be cost-effective; however, no single strategy has been found to be most effective.[62] Although ongoing screening programs and initiatives may be effective in reducing CRC incidence and mortality, the magnitude of this effect may be difficult to ascertain because of a lack of valid comparison groups. For example, the exact contribution of CRC screening to the decline in CRC incidence and mortality observed in the United States is unclear (see **Fig. 1**).[5] Therefore, previous and ongoing RCTs are the best sources of evidence regarding the effect of CRC screening. **Table 2** summarizes results from meta-analyses of RCTs (gFOBT and flexible sigmoidoscopy) and

Table 2
Results from meta-analyses of RCTs on gFOBT and flexible sigmoidoscopy screening and meta-analysis of observational studies on screening colonoscopy

Screening Test	Study Design	Relative Risk, CRC Incidence (95% CI)	Relative Risk, CRC Mortality (95% CI)
gFOBT[66]	Meta-analysis of RCTs	0.95 (0.88–1.02)	0.87 (0.82–0.92)
Flexible sigmoidoscopy[66]	Meta-analysis of RCTs	0.82 (0.74–0.90)	0.72 (0.65–0.79)
Colonoscopy[67]	Meta-analysis of observational studies	0.31 (0.12–0.77)	0.32 (0.23–0.43)

Abbreviation: CI, confidence interval.
  Data from Holme O, Bretthauer M, Fretheim A, et al. Flexible sigmoidoscopy versus faecal occult blood testing for colorectal cancer screening in asymptomatic individuals. Cochrane Database Syst Rev 2013;9:CD009259; and Brenner H, Stock C, Hoffmeister M. Effect of screening sigmoidoscopy and screening colonoscopy on colorectal cancer incidence and mortality: systematic review and meta-analysis of randomised controlled trials and observational studies. BMJ 2014;348:g2467.

observational studies (colonoscopy) reporting data on CRC incidence and mortality after screening.

Ongoing Research

Four large-scale RCTs are currently underway to evaluate the effect of screening colonoscopy on CRC incidence and mortality[63,64] (ClinicalTrials.gov: NCT01239082, NCT02078804). The Spanish COLONPREV (Colorectal Cancer Screening in Average-Risk Population: Immunochemical Fecal Occult Blood Testing versus Colonoscopy) trial started in 2008 and compares 1-time colonoscopy with biennial FIT. Baseline results have been published, but the primary end point is CRC mortality after 10 years.[63] The NordICC (Nordic-European Initiative on Colorectal Cancer) trial is an international RCT in Norway, Poland, Sweden, and The Netherlands starting in 2009 comparing 1-time colonoscopy with no screening.[64] Planned follow-up is 15 years, and baseline results can be expected in 2015. The third RCT (CONFIRM [Colonoscopy Versus Immunochemical Testing in Reducing Mortality from Colorectal Cancer]) is being conducted within the Veterans' Affairs health care system in the United States. This trial started in 2013 and compares 1-time colonoscopy with annual FIT. Planned follow-up is 10 years, and no results have been published yet (ClinicalTrials.gov number, NCT01239082). The fourth RCT (SCREESCO [Screening of Swedish Colons]) started in 2014 in Sweden and compares 1-time colonoscopy, 2 rounds of FIT, and no screening (ClinicalTrials.gov number, NCT02078804). The primary end point is CRC mortality after 15 years of follow-up. No results have yet been published.

More than 370,000 individuals are estimated to be enrolled in the 4 trials combined, and although the main results will not be available for several years, the different trial designs and interventions may provide complementary and important evidence on the effect of CRC screening by colonoscopy and FIT.

COMPLICATIONS AND CONCERNS

The life-time risk of CRC is approximately 5%. Consequently, 95% of the target population will not benefit from screening but may still risk procedural complications. Although infrequent, serious complications such as major bleeding and bowel perforation can occur during colonoscopy and polypectomy. Therefore, patients should be aware of potential risks before deciding to undergo screening. The reported rates of colonoscopic perforations varies between approximately 1 in 500 and less than 1 in 1000,[65] but the fatality of this complication has been estimated to about 5%.[50] Patients should also be informed about the risks and consequences of a false-negative or a false-positive test, which may result in false health reassurance or undue fear of serious disease.

SUMMARY

There is good evidence that CRC screening can reduce disease-specific incidence and mortality. Several tests are available, but only the gFOBT and flexible sigmoidoscopy have been evaluated in large-scale RCTs with long-term follow-up, and there is no direct evidence to show that one test is superior to another. Colonoscopy, which allows cancer detection and prevention by polyp removal, is the only 1-step approach to CRC screening and may be the most effective screening method. However, this assumption remains to be clarified, and several trials have been initiated to address this issue. Most of the population will never develop CRC with or without screening, and screening is not risk free. Patients should therefore be given balanced information about the potential benefits, limitations, and risks of screening, and continuous scrutiny of these outcomes is required to ensure that the benefits of screening outweigh the harms.

REFERENCES

1. Ferlay J, Soerjomataram I, Dikshit R, et al. Cancer incidence and mortality worldwide: sources, methods and major patterns in GLOBOCAN 2012. Int J Cancer 2015;136(5):E359–86.
2. Siegel R, Desantis C, Jemal A. Colorectal cancer statistics, 2014. CA Cancer J Clin 2014;64(2):104–17.
3. Howlader N, Noone AM, Krapcho M, et al. SEER Cancer statistics review, 1975-2011. Available at: http://seer.cancer.gov/csr/1975_2011/. Accessed January 19, 2015.
4. Ferlay J, Soerjomataram I, Ervik M, et al. GLOBOCAN 2012 v1.0, Cancer incidence and mortality worldwide: IARC CancerBase no. 11 2013; Available at: http://globocan.iarc.fr. Accessed January 26, 2015.
5. Yang DX, Gross CP, Soulos PR, et al. Estimating the magnitude of colorectal cancers prevented during the era of screening: 1976 to 2009. Cancer 2014;120(18): 2893–901.
6. Taylor DP, Burt RW, Williams MS, et al. Population-based family history-specific risks for colorectal cancer: a constellation approach. Gastroenterology 2010; 138(3):877–85.
7. Jess T, Rungoe C, Peyrin-Biroulet L. Risk of colorectal cancer in patients with ulcerative colitis: a meta-analysis of population-based cohort studies. Clin Gastroenterol Hepatol 2012;10(6):639–45.
8. Jasperson KW, Tuohy TM, Neklason DW, et al. Hereditary and familial colon cancer. Gastroenterology 2010;138(6):2044–58.
9. Chan DS, Lau R, Aune D, et al. Red and processed meat and colorectal cancer incidence: meta-analysis of prospective studies. PLoS One 2011;6(6):e20456.
10. Liang PS, Chen TY, Giovannucci E. Cigarette smoking and colorectal cancer incidence and mortality: systematic review and meta-analysis. Int J Cancer 2009; 124(10):2406–15.
11. Fedirko V, Tramacere I, Bagnardi V, et al. Alcohol drinking and colorectal cancer risk: an overall and dose-response meta-analysis of published studies. Ann Oncol 2011;22(9):1958–72.
12. Ma Y, Yang Y, Wang F, et al. Obesity and risk of colorectal cancer: a systematic review of prospective studies. PLoS One 2013;8(1):e53916.
13. Boyle T, Keegel T, Bull F, et al. Physical activity and risks of proximal and distal colon cancers: a systematic review and meta-analysis. J Natl Cancer Inst 2012;104(20):1548–61.
14. Bosetti C, Rosato V, Gallus S, et al. Aspirin and cancer risk: a quantitative review to 2011. Ann Oncol 2012;23(6):1403–15.
15. Vogelstein B, Fearon ER, Hamilton SR, et al. Genetic alterations during colorectal-tumor development. N Engl J Med 1988;319(9):525–32.
16. Shaukat A, Mongin SJ, Geisser MS, et al. Long-term mortality after screening for colorectal cancer. N Engl J Med 2013;369(12):1106–14.
17. Lindholm E, Brevinge H, Haglind E. Survival benefit in a randomized clinical trial of faecal occult blood screening for colorectal cancer. Br J Surg 2008;95(8): 1029–36.
18. Kronborg O, Jorgensen OD, Fenger C, et al. Randomized study of biennial screening with a faecal occult blood test: results after nine screening rounds. Scand J Gastroenterol 2004;39(9):846–51.
19. Scholefield JH, Moss SM, Mangham CM, et al. Nottingham trial of faecal occult blood testing for colorectal cancer: a 20-year follow-up. Gut 2012;61(7):1036–40.

20. Young GP. Population-based screening for colorectal cancer: Australian research and implementation. J Gastroenterol Hepatol 2009;24(Suppl 3):S33–42.
21. Konrad G, Katz A. Are medication restrictions before FOBT necessary?: practical advice based on a systematic review of the literature. Can Fam Physician 2012; 58(9):939–48.
22. Cole SR, Young GP. Effect of dietary restriction on participation in faecal occult blood test screening for colorectal cancer. Med J Aust 2001;175(4): 195–8.
23. Pignone M, Campbell MK, Carr C, et al. Meta-analysis of dietary restriction during fecal occult blood testing. Eff Clin Pract 2001;4(4):150–6.
24. Whitlock EP, Lin JS, Liles E, et al. Screening for colorectal cancer: a targeted, updated systematic review for the U.S. Preventive Services Task Force. Ann Intern Med 2008;149(9):638–58.
25. Segnan N, Patnick J, Karsa Lv, European Commission, Directorate-General for Health and Consumer Protection, International Agency for Research on Cancer. European guidelines for quality assurance in colorectal cancer screening and diagnosis. 1st edition. Luxembourg: Office for Official Publications of the European Communities; 2010.
26. Vart G, Banzi R, Minozzi S. Comparing participation rates between immunochemical and guaiac faecal occult blood tests: a systematic review and meta-analysis. Prev Med 2012;55(2):87–92.
27. Lee JK, Liles EG, Bent S, et al. Accuracy of fecal immunochemical tests for colorectal cancer: systematic review and meta-analysis. Ann Intern Med 2014; 160(3):171.
28. Altobelli E, Lattanzi A, Paduano R, et al. Colorectal cancer prevention in Europe: burden of disease and status of screening programs. Prev Med 2014;62:132–41.
29. Carroll MR, Seaman HE, Halloran SP. Tests and investigations for colorectal cancer screening. Clin Biochem 2014;47(10–11):921–39.
30. Major D, Bryant H, Delaney M, et al. Colorectal cancer screening in Canada: results from the first round of screening for five provincial programs. Curr Oncol 2013;20(5):252–7.
31. Imperiale TF, Ransohoff DF, Itzkowitz SH, et al, Colorectal Cancer Study Group. Fecal DNA versus fecal occult blood for colorectal-cancer screening in an average-risk population. N Engl J Med 2004;351(26):2704–14.
32. Ahlquist DA, Sargent DJ, Loprinzi CL, et al. Stool DNA and occult blood testing for screen detection of colorectal neoplasia. Ann Intern Med 2008;149(7): 441–50 W81.
33. Imperiale TF, Ransohoff DF, Itzkowitz SH, et al. Multitarget stool DNA testing for colorectal-cancer screening. N Engl J Med 2014;370(14):1287–97.
34. Atkin WS, Edwards R, Kralj-Hans I, et al. Once-only flexible sigmoidoscopy screening in prevention of colorectal cancer: a multicentre randomised controlled trial. Lancet 2010;375(9726):1624–33.
35. Segnan N, Armaroli P, Bonelli L, et al. Once-only sigmoidoscopy in colorectal cancer screening: follow-up findings of the Italian Randomized Controlled Trial–SCORE. J Natl Cancer Inst 2011;103(17):1310–22.
36. Schoen RE, Pinsky PF, Weissfeld JL, et al. Colorectal-cancer incidence and mortality with screening flexible sigmoidoscopy. N Engl J Med 2012;366(25): 2345–57.
37. Holme O, Loberg M, Kalager M, et al. Effect of flexible sigmoidoscopy screening on colorectal cancer incidence and mortality: a randomized clinical trial. JAMA 2014;312(6):606–15.

38. Hol L, van Leerdam ME, van Ballegooijen M, et al. Screening for colorectal cancer: randomised trial comparing guaiac-based and immunochemical faecal occult blood testing and flexible sigmoidoscopy. Gut 2010;59(1):62–8.

39. Dodou D, de Winter JC. The relationship between distal and proximal colonic neoplasia: a meta-analysis. J Gen Intern Med 2012;27(3):361–70.

40. Centers for Disease Control and Prevention (CDC). Vital signs: colorectal cancer screening test use–United States, 2012. MMWR Morb Mortal Wkly Rep 2013; 62(44):881–8.

41. Cotterchio M, Manno M, Klar N, et al. Colorectal screening is associated with reduced colorectal cancer risk: a case-control study within the population-based Ontario Familial Colorectal Cancer Registry. Cancer Causes Control 2005;16(7):865–75.

42. Kahi CJ, Imperiale TF, Juliar BE, et al. Effect of screening colonoscopy on colorectal cancer incidence and mortality. Clin Gastroenterol Hepatol 2009;7(7): 770–5 [quiz: 711].

43. Manser CN, Bachmann LM, Brunner J, et al. Colonoscopy screening markedly reduces the occurrence of colon carcinomas and carcinoma-related death: a closed cohort study. Gastrointest Endosc 2012;76(1):110–7.

44. Doubeni CA, Weinmann S, Adams K, et al. Screening colonoscopy and risk for incident late-stage colorectal cancer diagnosis in average-risk adults: a nested case-control study. Ann Intern Med 2013;158(5 Pt 1):312–20.

45. Nishihara R, Wu K, Lochhead P, et al. Long-term colorectal-cancer incidence and mortality after lower endoscopy. N Engl J Med 2013;369(12):1095–105.

46. Brenner H, Chang-Claude J, Jansen L, et al. Reduced risk of colorectal cancer up to 10 years after screening, surveillance, or diagnostic colonoscopy. Gastroenterology 2014;146(3):709–17.

47. Lieberman DA, Rex DK, Winawer SJ, et al. Guidelines for colonoscopy surveillance after screening and polypectomy: a consensus update by the US Multi-Society Task Force on Colorectal Cancer. Gastroenterology 2012;143(3):844–57.

48. Hassan C, Quintero E, Dumonceau JM, et al. Post-polypectomy colonoscopy surveillance: European Society of Gastrointestinal Endoscopy (ESGE) Guideline. Endoscopy 2013;45(10):842–51.

49. Rex DK, Bond JH, Winawer S, et al. Quality in the technical performance of colonoscopy and the continuous quality improvement process for colonoscopy: recommendations of the U.S. Multi-Society Task Force on Colorectal Cancer. Am J Gastroenterol 2002;97(6):1296–308.

50. Rex DK, Schoenfeld PS, Cohen J, et al. Quality indicators for colonoscopy. Am J Gastroenterol 2015;110(1):72–90.

51. de Haan MC, van Gelder RE, Graser A, et al. Diagnostic value of CT-colonography as compared to colonoscopy in an asymptomatic screening population: a meta-analysis. Eur Radiol 2011;21(8):1747–63.

52. Stoop EM, de Haan MC, de Wijkerslooth TR, et al. Participation and yield of colonoscopy versus non-cathartic CT colonography in population-based screening for colorectal cancer: a randomised controlled trial. Lancet Oncol 2012;13(1): 55–64.

53. Benson M, Pier J, Kraft S, et al. Optical colonoscopy and virtual colonoscopy numbers after initiation of a CT colonography program: long term data. J Gastrointestin Liver Dis 2012;21(4):391–5.

54. de Wijkerslooth TR, de Haan MC, Stoop EM, et al. Burden of colonoscopy compared to non-cathartic CT-colonography in a colorectal cancer screening programme: randomised controlled trial. Gut 2012;61(11):1552–9.

55. de Haan MC, Pickhardt PJ, Stoker J. CT colonography: accuracy, acceptance, safety and position in organised population screening. Gut 2015;64(2):342–50.

56. Spada C, Hassan C, Galmiche JP, et al. Colon capsule endoscopy: European Society of Gastrointestinal Endoscopy (ESGE) guideline. Endoscopy 2012;44(5): 527–36.

57. Rex DK, Adler SN, Aisenberg J, et al. Accuracy of capsule colonoscopy in detecting colorectal polyps in a screening population. Gastroenterology 2015; 148:948–57.e2.

58. Levin B, Lieberman DA, McFarland B, et al. Screening and surveillance for the early detection of colorectal cancer and adenomatous polyps, 2008: a joint guideline from the American Cancer Society, the US Multi-Society Task Force on Colorectal Cancer, and the American College of Radiology. CA Cancer J Clin 2008;58(3):130–60.

59. Levine MS, Yee J. History, evolution, and current status of radiologic imaging tests for colorectal cancer screening. Radiology 2014;273(2 Suppl):S160–80.

60. Rex DK, Johnson DA, Anderson JC, et al. American College of Gastroenterology guidelines for colorectal cancer screening 2009 [corrected]. Am J Gastroenterol 2009;104(3):739–50.

61. Saquib N, Saquib J, Ioannidis JP. Does screening for disease save lives in asymptomatic adults? Systematic review of meta-analyses and randomized trials. Int J Epidemiol 2015;44:264–77.

62. Lansdorp-Vogelaar I, Knudsen AB, Brenner H. Cost-effectiveness of colorectal cancer screening. Epidemiol Rev 2011;33(1):88–100.

63. Quintero E, Castells A, Bujanda L, et al. Colonoscopy versus fecal immunochemical testing in colorectal-cancer screening. N Engl J Med 2012;366(8):697–706.

64. Kaminski MF, Bretthauer M, Zauber AG, et al. The NordICC Study: rationale and design of a randomized trial on colonoscopy screening for colorectal cancer. Endoscopy 2012;44(7):695–702.

65. Panteris V, Haringsma J, Kuipers EJ. Colonoscopy perforation rate, mechanisms and outcome: from diagnostic to therapeutic colonoscopy. Endoscopy 2009; 41(11):941–51.

66. Holme O, Bretthauer M, Fretheim A, et al. Flexible sigmoidoscopy versus faecal occult blood testing for colorectal cancer screening in asymptomatic individuals. Cochrane Database Syst Rev 2013;(9):CD009259.

67. Brenner H, Stock C, Hoffmeister M. Effect of screening sigmoidoscopy and screening colonoscopy on colorectal cancer incidence and mortality: systematic review and meta-analysis of randomised controlled trials and observational studies. BMJ 2014;348:g2467.

Breast Cancer Screening

David Euhus, MD[a],*, Philip A. Di Carlo, MD[b], Nagi F. Khouri, MD[b]

KEYWORDS

- Breast cancer • Screening • Mammography • Breast MRI • Mammographic density

KEY POINTS

- There are ample clinical trial data demonstrating that screening mammography, using decades-old technology, reduces breast cancer mortality. Recent technological advances have significantly improved the sensitivity and specificity of screening mammography.
- Screening MRI is recommended for high-risk women, but there is currently no consensus about the best approach for women with mammographically dense breasts.
- The cancer detection rate for clinical breast examination is similar to that of many imaging modalities, but it is disappearing from clinical practice.
- The menu of available screening options is expanding, and every test will diagnose cancers missed by mammography. However, each additional test introduces the chance of harm. More screening is not necessarily better screening.

INTRODUCTION

Breast cancer is the most common cancer in women in the United States and second only to lung cancer in mortality.[1] It is estimated that there were 232,670 new breast cancer cases and 40,000 deaths in the United States in 2014. Although the incidence of breast cancer increased steadily in the United States through the 1980s and 1990s, it has now leveled off at approximately 125 cases per 100,000 per year.[2] Breast cancer survival has been steadily improving for more than 2 decades.[2,3] This improvement is attributed to a combination of early detection, greater utilization of more effective treatments, and improved supportive care. The contributions of early detection and better adjuvant therapies have been judged to be about equal.[4]

Population Screening

Population screening should only be done if the benefits of screening can be shown to outweigh the harms. Improvement in overall survival may be the most desirable

a Department of Surgery, Johns Hopkins Hospital, Johns Hopkins University, Blalock 688, 600 North Wolfe Street, Baltimore, MD 21287, USA; b Department of Radiology, Johns Hopkins Hospital, Johns Hopkins University, 600 North Caroline Street, Baltimore, MD 21287, USA
* Corresponding author.
E-mail address: deuhus1@jhmi.edu

Surg Clin N Am 95 (2015) 991–1011
http://dx.doi.org/10.1016/j.suc.2015.05.008
0039-6109/15/$ – see front matter © 2015 Elsevier Inc. All rights reserved.
surgical.theclinics.com

outcome, but reductions in disease-specific mortality and treatment morbidity also have value. Screening only works if the targeted condition is fairly common in the population, generally fatal if undetected until it is symptomatic, and generally curable if identified earlier.[5] In addition, the selected screening test must be sensitive for detecting early disease, specific for the disease (ie, have a low false-positive rate), and acceptable to most individuals.

Screening Mammography Recommendations

In 2009 the US Preventive Services Task Force recommended biennial screening mammography for women aged 50 to 74 years with individualized screening decisions for women aged 40 to 49 years.[6] These recommendations were based on a systematic review of available data, including 8 randomized prospective trials that convincingly showed a 20% to 35% reduction in breast cancer mortality for women screened between 50 and 69 years of age.[7–9] There is considerable controversy about how to interpret the available data. Consequently, several influential organizations, including the American Cancer Society, the American Congress of Obstetricians and Gynecologists (2009), and the American College of Radiology, have recommended that yearly screening mammography begin at 40 years of age.[10,11] There is no arbitrary age above which screening should cease. Women should have a life expectancy of 5 to 10 years to realize a mortality benefit from screening mammography.[12]

The Breast Cancer Screening Controversy

Much of the breast cancer screening controversy centers on interpretation of 8 randomized prospective trials,[7,13,14] but there are also concerns that the natural history of certain types of breast cancer may limit the utility of early detection. Successful population-based cancer screening depends as much on the nature of the cancer being screened for as it does on the technical performance characteristics of the selected screening test. The natural history of the cancer must be such that treatment is more effective, or significantly less morbid, for a screen-detected than a clinically apparent cancer. By the eighteenth century, breast cancer progression was envisioned as an orderly process beginning in the breast, spreading to nodal basins and then disseminating to distant sites. If this conceptual framework is accurate, then it is obvious that detecting and treating breast cancer early in the process will interrupt progression and save lives. An opposing view was articulated by Bernard Fisher and colleagues[15] in 1980 who asserted that "…breast cancer is a systemic disease, likely at its inception."[15] If this view is correct, then earlier detection of primary breast cancers would be unlikely to impact survival.

Breast cancer is a very heterogeneous disease, and the truth is somewhere in the middle. Indolent, slow-growing breast cancers are the cancers most likely to be detected by periodic screening (length bias) and also the cancers least likely to cause mortality. Screening may also detect a small primary breast cancer that is already occultly metastatic. In that case, screening will have been judged effective because it will have seemed to have increased survival by whatever time period would have been required for the cancer to become symptomatic (lead-time bias). Screening is only effective for the subset of tumors that pose a mortality risk and whereby early intervention is capable of interrupting progression. Debate centers on the size of this subset and the acceptable risk of harm from screening. Harms from screening can include cancer treatment of lesions that would never pose a mortality threat (overdiagnosis) as well as physical harm, anxiety, or financial costs imposed by false-positive screening tests.

SCREENING TECHNIQUES AND OPTIONS

The most meaningful performance measure for any breast cancer screening test is whether its application in a population improves breast cancer–specific and overall survival. This type of data is only available for mammography. Intermediate performance measures are most often related to success in identifying women with breast cancer (sensitivity and cancer detection rate) and the number of women that need to undergo additional evaluations and biopsies in order to diagnose those cancers (specificity and positive predictive value [PPV]). There are very few studies evaluating any screening modality in isolation from mammography, so results must be interpreted with caution. **Table 1** describes the performance measures most commonly reported for breast cancer screening tests.

Clinical Breast Examination and Breast Self-examination

Clinical breast examination (CBE) includes systematic palpation and visual inspection of the entire breast performed by a trained provider.[16] The American Cancer Society recommends that CBE be performed every 3 years for women in their 20s and 30s and yearly beginning at age 40 years of age.[17] Nevertheless, though the use of mammography has increased since 1990, the use of CBE has decreased.[18] Only 18% of screening facilities offer CBE along with screening mammography.[19] In addition, data for 345 breast cancer survivors responding to the National Health Interview Survey suggested that 71% of breast cancers in the United States were detected by CBE or self-examination before 1993 but only 41% after 2001.[20]

It is not clear that CBE is associated with reduced breast cancer mortality, but it is notable that among the screening trials that combined CBE with mammography 47% to 74% of the cancers were identifiable by CBE and 3% to 45% were *only* detectable by CBE and not mammography.[21–26] The National Breast and Cervical Cancer Early Detection Program performed 720,000 CBEs in 564,708 women and estimated sensitivity at 58.8% and specificity at 93.4%.[27] The cancer detection rate was 6.6 per 1000, which is similar to that of modern imaging trials. The Ontario Breast Cancer Screening program estimated the sensitivity of CBE at 47.5% and recorded a cancer detection rate of 3.8 per 1000 on the initial screen with 1.8 per 1000 on subsequent screens.[28] Of concern, however, adding CBE to screening mammography increased the false-positive rate from 7% to 13%. The investigators note that for a theoretic population of 10,000 women between 50 and 69 years of age, the addition of CBE would lead to the detection of breast cancer in only 4 women whose cancer would be missed

Table 1 Intermediate performance measures for breast cancer screening tests	
Recall rate	The fraction of women asked to return for additional imaging
Sensitivity	The fraction of all existent cancers the test successfully identified
Cancer detection rate	The number of breast cancers identified in one round of screening per 1000 women screened
Specificity	The fraction of women without cancer who had a negative screening test
PPV1	The fraction of women with a positive screening test ultimately diagnosed with cancer
PPV2	The fraction of women whose completed imaging evaluation is abnormal who are ultimately diagnosed with cancer
PPV3	The fraction of women undergoing biopsy ultimately diagnosed with cancer

by mammography. However, adding CBE would also lead to false-positive results for an additional 219 women, who would be referred for workup only to discover that they do not have cancer.

Clinical breast examination can serve an important role in breast cancer screening. Although sensitivity for cancer detection is lower than breast imaging, the specificity is reasonable. As breast cancer treatment becomes more effective, it seems reasonable to reassess the role of CBE as a primary screening modality. Much work would be required to reverse the trend toward neglect of CBE.

Breast self-examination is currently not promoted as a primary screening modality. Lack of efficacy is suggested by 2 large randomized prospective trials from Shanghai[29,30] and Russia.[31] A Cochrane review notes that breast cancer mortality was not reduced in either trial and that the probability of a benign breast biopsy was twice as high in the screened group.[32] Even though systematic breast self-examination is no longer taught or promoted, it seems reasonable to encourage breast awareness with prompt evaluation of any changes.

Mammography

A German surgeon first described radiograph images of mastectomy specimens in 1913.[33] By 1937, breast radiography was being used to diagnose breast cancer in the United States.[34] The first large randomized prospective screening mammography trial in the United States was initiated by the Health Insurance Plan of Greater New York in 1963 and reported a 25% reduction in breast cancer mortality.[35] What we know about the benefits and risks of screening mammography is largely derived from 8 large randomized prospective trials, the most recent of which was completed in the 1980s.[36] Imaging technology used in these studies was primitive compared with today's standard. Nevertheless, meta-analyses of these trials suggest a 20% to 35% reduction in mortality for women screened between 50 and 69 years of age[7–9] but less certain benefit for younger women.[6,8] The most recent independent analysis of all published data for screening mammography has estimated an overall 19% reduction in breast cancer morality.[9] This estimate varies by age and is 32% for women in their sixties but only 15% for women in their forties. The poorer performance of mammography in women younger than 50 years is related to lower breast cancer incidence, faster-growing tumors, and reduced mammographic sensitivity caused by breast density.[37] The first 2 challenges remain, but the test itself has improved dramatically over the last 2 decades.

Rapid increases in computer processing speeds, data storage capacity, and monitor resolutions have permitted a transition from film screen mammography to all digital mammography. Although not all studies have reported improved diagnostic accuracy for digital mammography, the Digital Mammographic Imaging Screening Trial, which included 49,528 asymptomatic women, found greater accuracy for women younger than 50 years, women with heterogeneously or very dense breast tissue, and premenopausal or perimenopausal women.[38]

Computer analysis of digital images, termed *computer-aided detection* (CAD), can draw attention to areas of focal density or possible microcalcifications potentially reducing the rate of missed cancers. CAD may improve cancer detection rates for general radiologists[39–41]; but a large study from the Breast Cancer Surveillance Consortium suggests that for expert breast imagers there is only a nonsignificant increase in sensitivity at the cost of significantly reduced specificity, decreased PPV, and a 20% increase in biopsy rates.[42]

Tomosynthesis, also known as 3-dimensional (3D) mammography, was patented in 1999 and approved by the Food and Drug Administration (FDA) in 2012. Multiple digital images are acquired as an x-ray tube is rotated across an arc over the breast (**Fig. 1**).

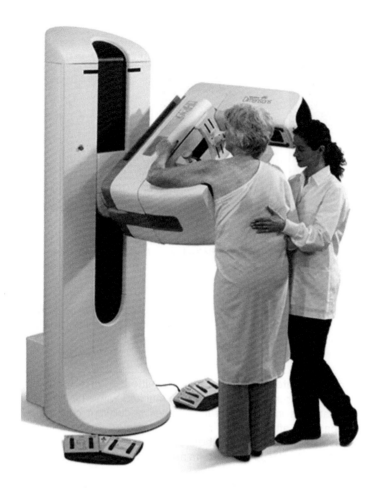

Fig. 1. Breast tomosynthesis generates multiple digital images as the x-ray tube is rotated across an arc over the breast. (*Courtesy of* Hologic, Inc, Bedford, MA.)

Computer algorithms process the digital information in a given plane of view while suppressing overlapping density from other planes. The advantage is improved sensitivity for cancer detection and also improved specificity by reducing false positives (**Fig. 2**). Tomosynthesis is currently performed in conjunction with standard 2-dimensional (2D) mammography. The available studies vary in design, but the addition of tomosynthesis seems to increase the cancer detection rate by 4% to 51% while increasing the PPV of a recall (ie, the proportion of recalls ending in a cancer diagnosis) by 0% to 147% with most studies clustering around 50% (**Table 2**). Benefit is most apparent for women less than 50 years of age.[43,44] The cancer detection rate is increased for invasive but not in situ cancers reflecting enhanced sensitivity for masses, asymmetries, and distortions rather than calcifications. This feature is desirable because ductal carcinoma in situ is at the center of the overdiagnosis controversy and early diagnosis of subtle invasive cancers is more likely to impact mortality.

Performing digital mammography and tomosynthesis sequentially doubles the radiation dose for each patient.[45,46] Newer algorithms can synthesize the tomosynthesis

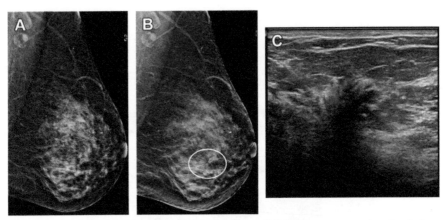

Fig. 2. Breast tomosynthesis. (*A*) Mediolateral oblique (MLO) mammogram showing heterogeneously dense breast tissue but no definite lesion. (*B*) MLO C-view from tomosynthesis clearly showing a spiculated mass (*circle*). (*C*) Sonogram confirming a hypoechoic irregular mass. This carcinoma is a small infiltrating ductal carcinoma.

data into classic cranial-caudal and medial-lateral oblique views (C-views). C-views can safely replace standard 2D digital mammography.[47,48] C-view was granted FDA approval in May of 2013.

Breast MRI

MRI images are generated from radio waves emitted by protons that have been aligned in a strong magnetic field and then stimulated with radiofrequency bursts. No ionizing radiation is involved, but intravenous gadolinium contrast is required. Enhancement patterns after contrast infusion are related to blood flow and blood vessel leakiness making contrast MRI both a structural and a functional test. Breast MRI has never been directly compared with mammography in the general population,

Table 2					
Performance of DBT plus DM compared with DM alone					
PPV1[a,Ref] PPV1 DM Alone (%)	**PPV1 DM + DBT (%)**	**PPV1 Delta[b] (%)**	**CDR/1000 DM Alone[c]**	**CDR/1000 DM + DBT**	**CDR Delta (%)**
29.0[46]	29.0	0	6.1	8.0	+27
12.0[80]	22.0	+83	5.3	8.1	+51
4.3[102]	6.4	+49	4.2	5.4	+29
6.2[43]	7.5	+21	4.6	5.5	+20
3.0[103]	4.6	+53	4.9	6.3	+29
4.4[44]	6.8	+55	5.2	5.7	+10
3.2[104]	7.9	+147	4.1	7.7	+35
—[105]	—	—	5.7	5.9	+4

Abbreviations: DBT, digital breast tomosynthesis; DM, digital mammography; CDR cancer detection rate.
   [a] PPV1: PPV of a recall. This value is the proportion of women recalled for additional imaging ultimately diagnosed with a cancer.
   [b] Delta: Change in the performance measure.
   [c] Cancer detection rate per 1000 women screened.
   Data from Refs.[43,44,46,80,102–105]

but one such trial is accruing.[49] Most studies have evaluated MRI as an adjunct to mammography in special populations, such as those at an increased risk for breast cancer (**Table 3**). The sensitivity of MRI for breast cancer detection is estimated at 71% to 100%. A woman having an MRI has about a 10% risk of being called back for additional imaging and a 5% risk of having a benign biopsy.[50] Screening MRI is recommended as an adjunct to mammography in women with a lifetime breast cancer risk of 20% to 25% or greater.[51] Indications for screening MRI are discussed further in the section on personalized breast cancer screening.

The sensitivity of MRI may be reduced in women with increased background parenchymal enhancement (BPE). BPE is largely independent of mammographic density[52,53] but is significantly greater in premenopausal than postmenopausal women[52] and also greatest during the luteal phase of the menstrual cycle.[53] The sensitivity of MRI is greatest for premenopausal women during days 7 to 14 of the menstrual cycle. The study should be timed to the menstrual cycle to maximize sensitivity. Case-control data from one study suggest that moderate to marked BPE is a risk factor for breast cancer with an odds ratio of 3.3 to 10.1.[54]

Screening breast MRI is not an option for women with pacemakers or certain other metallic implants. Claustrophobia may also limit the use of MRI. The American College of Radiology Imaging Network (ACRIN) 6666 study, which compared mammography, sonography, and MRI in increased-risk women,[55] found that 42.1% of 1215 women invited for MRI declined because of claustrophobia.[56] Pre-MRI anxiolytics can be prescribed for claustrophobic women. In addition, gadolinium can cause nephrogenic fibrosing dermopathy (also known as nephrogenic systemic fibrosis) in individuals with renal impairment. Some centers use full-dose gadolinium if the glomerular filtration rate (GFR) is greater than 60 mL/min and a half dose if it is 30 to 60 mL/min; avoid MRI all together if the GFR is less than 30 mL/min.

Screening Sonography

The American College of Radiology and the Society of Breast Imaging recommend screening sonography as an adjunct to mammography in high-risk women who

Table 3
Supplemental screening in asymptomatic women with mammographically dense breasts

Modality/Citation	Number	Sensitivity (%)		ICDR[a] (%)	Biopsied (%)	PPV3[b]
		MGM	Other			
Sonography[106]	20,864	55	100	0.24	2.6	0.11
Sonography[107,c]	14,483	82	70	0.14	0.67	0.20
Sonography[108]	9157	—	—	0.4	14.0	0.06
Sonography[58]	2659	53	52	0.53	10.2	0.11
Sonography[81]	935	—	100	0.32	5.7	0.06
MRI[58,d]	612	53	88	1.47	6.2	0.19
BSGI[61]	936	27	82	0.75	3.8	0.19

Abbreviations: BSGI, breast-specific gamma imaging; ICDR, incremental cancer detection rate; MGM, Mammography.
 [a] This value is the percentage of the screened population that had a cancer detected by the additional modality.
 [b] The proportion of biopsies that returned a cancer.
 [c] Nonfatty breasts.
 [d] Subset of women who had already had screening sonogram.
Data from Refs.[58,61,81,106–108]

cannot have an MRI.[10] Sonography is also recognized as a possible screening supplement in intermediate-risk women with mammographically dense breast tissue.

A recent review reported that screening sonography after a negative mammogram will prompt a breast biopsy in 4.2% and identify a breast cancer in 0.4%.[57] This cancer detection rate of 4 per 1000 is impressive given that the cancer detection rate generally associated with screening mammography is 6 per 1000. Most of the cancers are small, node-negative invasive cancers and are diagnosed in younger women with mammographically dense breasts. The largest blinded prospective trial of screening sonography is ACRIN 6666.[55] In this trial, radiologists performing the sonography were blinded to the results of mammography. Additional cancers were identified in 0.42% of women, but sonography disproportionately increased the number of biopsies (PPV2: 8.9% for sonography compared with 22.6% for mammography). Annual screening over a 3-year period continued to return cancers in about 0.4% each year, but the biopsy rate remained disproportionately high.[58]

Most of the available data on screening sonography were obtained from manual handheld examinations, which take 13 to 17 minutes to perform. Automated breast ultrasound (ABU) devices have been developed. The breast is immobilized in the device and 3D volumetric images are generated as a transducer systematically scans the entire breast. One multi-institutional study of ABU as an adjunct to mammography in increased-risk women with mammographically dense breasts identified additional cancers in 0.36%, which is similar to studies using handheld devices. The PPV of a biopsy recommendation was 38.4%, which is better than similar studies with handheld devices.[59] The average time to interpret the images was 8 minutes. This technology continues to improve, and several prospective studies are ongoing.

It is likely that the application of any screening modality in women with normal mammograms will incrementally increase the cancer detection rate. This increase must be balanced against increased costs as well as the risk of psychological and physical harm. Although screening sonography is relatively inexpensive, the biopsy rate per cancer detected is 3 times higher than that associated with mammography and 90% of the biopsies are benign. It is currently unclear which populations, if any, should routinely be offered screening sonography as an adjunct to mammography.

Gamma-Emitting Radioisotope Imaging

Breast-specific gamma imaging (BSGI) and molecular breast imaging (MBI) are related functional imaging tests based on preferential uptake of ^{99m}Tc-sestamibi by tumor mitochondria. Positron emission mammography (PEM) is an adaptation of PET that uses ^{18}F-flurodeoxyglucose and detectors optimized for the breast (**Fig. 3**). Recent development of very-narrow-field, high-resolution detectors has significantly improved the sensitivity of these tests for breast cancer detection. A recent meta-analysis of single-head detector BSGI that included 8 studies reported a sensitivity of 95% and specificity of 80%.[60] A study of mammography in conjunction with dual-head detector MBI in 936 women with heterogeneous or very dense breasts identified 11 breast cancers, 8 of which were only detected by MBI.[61] A comparison of PEM versus MRI for contralateral breast cancer detection in 352 evaluable women identified a contralateral breast cancer in 4.1% (15 cancers). The sensitivity of MRI was 93% but was only 20% for PEM. PPV3 was 21% and 28%, respectively.[62]

BSGI and MBI require some breast compression in order to get the cancers closer to the detector. Sensitivity for BSGI is similar across all breast density categories,[63] but PEM background is increased in women with dense breasts.[64] Image-guided biopsy systems are available for lesions that are only visible on these nuclear medicine tests.

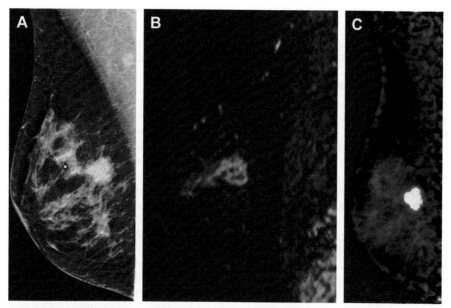

Fig. 3. PEM. (*A*) Mediolateral oblique mammogram showing a 2-cm mass. (*B*) MRI suggests 4.5 cm of abnormal enhancement. (*C*) PEM shows a 2-cm fludeoxyglucose-avid mass. Pathology confirmed a 2-cm cancer. (*Courtesy of* Stephen Seiler, MD, UT Southwestern Medical Center, Dallas, TX.)

These radioisotope tests are costly, and radiation exposure is a concern. Radiation is an established breast carcinogen. It has been estimated that the lifetime attributable risk (LAR) of a fatal breast cancer for a single BSGI examination performed in a 40 year old using 740 to 1100 MBq (20–30 mCi) of ^{99m}Tc-sestamibi is 15 to 30 times that of a digital mammogram.[65,66] PEM doses are a bit lower at 370 MBq (10 mCi), but the LAR is still estimated at 23 times that of digital mammography.[67] As the detector technology improves, radiation doses can decrease. One study has reported preservation of BSGI sensitivity and specificity at a dose of 296 MBq,[68] but it has been estimated that the dose needs to be reduced to 75 to 150 MBq to approach the benefit/risk ratio calculated for digital mammography.[66] These risks are based on calculation of mean glandular breast dose from a single injection. Risk from repeated exposure for periodic screening would be higher, and the risk to other organs is uncertain.

Other Modalities

Other screening modalities, such as digital infrared thermal imaging (thermography), sono-elastography, and electrical impedance scanning, have been evaluated in small heterogeneous case-control studies.[69] Systematic performance data for breast cancer screening are not available. These modalities are considered experimental. Dedicated breast computed tomography has been described, but no systematic screening data have been reported.[70]

PERSONALIZED BREAST CANCER SCREENING

The yield and ultimate effectiveness of breast cancer screening may be improved by tailoring screening schedules and modalities to specific populations.[71,72] For example, mammography may not be the best screening modality in women with mammographically dense breast tissue. In addition, the PPV of an abnormal screening test increases as disease prevalence increases. Targeting populations with increased near-term breast cancer risk is likely to improve the performance of any screening test.

Mammographic Density

The epithelial components of the breast are supported by a dense collagenous stroma, which is invested by variable amounts of adipose. The fibroepithelial components appear white, or dense, on a mammogram, whereas the adipose component appears black or nondense.[73] The percentage of the image area occupied by dense tissue is inversely proportional to age[74] and directly proportional to breast cancer risk.[75]

The American College of Radiology Breast Imaging Reporting and Data System (BI-RADS) includes 4 breast composition categories: (1) almost entirely fatty, (2) scattered areas of fibroglandular densities, (3) heterogeneously dense, and (4) extremely dense. Before 2013, these categories were intended to approximate the percent area occupied by dense breast tissue: (1) less than 25%, (2) 25% to 50%, (3) 51% to 75%, and (4) greater than 75%. The 2013 BI-RADS Atlas (Fifth Edition) is no longer concerned with approximating percent dense area and, instead, focuses on how the breast composition may affect the sensitivity of the test.[76] The adjectival descriptors are the same but the meaning has changed. Almost entirely fatty corresponds to high sensitivity; scattered areas of fibroglandular density suggests relatively good sensitivity; heterogeneously dense means a small breast cancer may be obscured; extremely dense tells us that the sensitivity of the test is significantly reduced.

The sensitivity of screening mammography is 85% for unselected populations[77] but 80% to 88% for women with fatty-replaced breasts as compared with only 30% to 62% for women with mammographically dense breasts.[78,79] In addition, women with extremely dense breasts are 6 times more likely to be diagnosed with a breast cancer between screens than women with primarily fatty-replaced breasts.[79] Supplemental screening using other modalities has been investigated in women with mammographically dense breast tissue. **Table 3** shows the performance characteristics for mammography and other tests, performed in addition to mammography, for asymptomatic women with reduced mammographic sensitivity. There are no systematic studies of digital breast tomosynthesis in women with mammographic dense breasts. Most of the studies that included a subgroup analysis by breast density found that improvements in cancer detection and recall rates were evenly distributed across density categories,[43,46,80] though one study reported a nonsignificant trend for reduced recall rates.[44] Breast density does not seem to be a useful criterion for selecting women for tomosynthesis. MRI and BSGI have excellent sensitivity in women with dense mammograms, generate biopsy recommendations in 4% to 6%, and diagnose mammographically occult breast cancer in 0.75% to 1.5% (about 1 in 5 biopsies). Screening sonography is arguably the least expensive supplemental screening test in women with dense breasts; but partly because of its relatively low PPV, it has been estimated to cost $60,267 per breast cancer detected.[81] In addition, though the sensitivity of MRI and BSGI is independent of mammographic density,[63,82] it is not clear whether this is true for sonography. One study suggested that the sensitivity of screening sonography is reduced in fatty breasts,[83] whereas another found that tumors in fatty regions of the breast were more readily detected by sonography.[84] There are currently no generally accepted supplemental screening recommendations for women with low mammographic sensitivity and no randomized prospective trial data to inform such guidelines. Supplemental screening decisions are individualized based on the preferences of patients and their breast imagers as well as the willing-ness of patients or insurers to pay for additional testing.

Enhanced Surveillance in Increased Risk Populations

The potential net benefit for population screening increases as the prevalence of the disease of interest increases. Consequently, special screening is often recommended for individuals with increased breast cancer risk. These individuals can be recognized based on gene mutations, cancer family history, personal history of mantle radiation for lymphoma, or a diagnosis of high-risk preneoplasia, such as atypical hyperplasia or lobular carcinoma in situ. Apart from a deleterious mutation in a breast cancer pre-disposition gene or a personal history of mantle radiation, published guidelines and, consequently, third-party payer reimbursement policies have required quantitative measures of breast cancer risk. For example, the American Cancer Society has endorsed screening MRI for women with a life-time breast cancer risk that exceeds 20%[51]; this has been adopted in the National Comprehensive Cancer Network's (NCCN) breast cancer screening guidelines.[85] Near-term risk (eg, 5-year risk) is more closely related to disease prevalence than lifetime risk, but most third-party payers have adopted the 20% lifetime risk criterion. Clinicians who identify and manage increased-risk women are encouraged to consider near-term risk in their screening recommendations. There are several mathematical models available for calculating breast cancer risk (**Table 4**).

The current NCCN guidelines for breast cancer screening in women with hereditary breast ovarian cancer syndrome include (1) encourage breast awareness at 18 years of age, (2) clinical breast examination every 6 to 12 months beginning at 25 years of age, (3) annual MRI beginning at 25 years of age (consider mammography if MRI is not possible), and (4) annual mammography and MRI beginning at 30 years of age.[85] Annual mammography before 30 years of age must be carefully considered in BRCA gene mutation carriers as there some evidence that medical x-ray exposure early in life increases breast cancer risk in these women.[86–88]

The sensitivity of MRI ranges from 77% to 100% in high-risk women (as compared with 12.5%–40.0% for mammography) and the specificity from 81.0% to 98.9% (as compared with 93%–100% for mammography, **Table 5**). The false-positive rate is higher for MRI than mammography but not excessively so.

Screening MRI increases the diagnosis of smaller, lymph-node-negative breast cancers[89] but has not yet been shown to improve survival.[90,91] One recent study found that 10-year cancer-specific survival was only 69% for MRI-detected breast cancers in BRCA1 mutation carriers[91] suggesting that early detection with MRI may not trans-late into survival benefits. In addition, MRI is expensive. Modeling studies have suggested that the cost ranges from $43,000 to greater than $700,000 per quality-adjusted life-year gained depending on the specific population selected for screening, the age when screening starts, and the duration of screening.[92,93]

COMPLICATIONS AND CONCERNS

The harms of screening mammography are mostly related to false positives and the potential for overdiagnosis of breast cancer. A false-positive screening mammogram is one that prompts a recall for additional imaging and sometimes a biopsy, without terminating in a breast cancer diagnosis. This scenario can result in significant anxiety, economic harm, or even physical harm. It has been estimated that the 10-year cumu-lative risk for at least one false-positive mammogram is 61.3% for women starting screening at 40 to 50 years of age and 49.7% for women who start at 66 to 74 years

Table 4
Cohort validation of mathematical models for breast cancer risk stratification

Model	Calibration[a] (E:O Ratio)	Discrimination (C-Statistic)	Strengths and Weaknesses
BCRT[109–112]	0.81–1.03	0.58–0.67	The Gail model is a general risk assessment model best adapted to Caucasian women who participate in screening (http://www.cancer.gov/bcrisktool/).
IBIS[112]	1.08	0.65	It includes more risk factors than any other model (eg, BMI and HRT use). It may overestimate risk in women with atypical hyperplasia[113] (http://www.ems-trials.org/riskevaluator/).
Claus[114]	1.05	—	It is a family history model. It does not include ovarian or male breast cancer.
BRCAPRO[112]	0.59	0.6	It is a genetic model designed for families with hereditary breast-ovarian cancer. These poor validation statistics are from a more general population (http://bcb.dfci.harvard.edu/bayesmendel/software.php).
BOADICEA[115]	0.92	0.7	It is a genetic model designed for families with hereditary breast-ovarian cancer. These good validation statistics are from a familial cancer population (http://ccge.medschl.cam.ac.uk/boadicea/boadicea-web-application/).

Includes only cohort studies with at least 100 incident breast cancers.
Abbreviations: BMI, body mass index; HRT, hormone replacement therapy.
[a] Expected to observed ratio for incident breast cancers.
Data from Refs.[109–115]

of age.[94,95] One investigator has suggested that, among 1000 US women aged 50 years who are screened annually for a decade, 0.3 to 3.2 will avoid a breast cancer death, whereas 490 to 670 will have at least 1 false alarm.[96]

Overdiagnosis is the detection of a breast cancer with little or no potential to cause significant symptoms or death. Quantifying overdiagnosis is difficult and controversial. One compelling observation supporting the concept of overdiagnosis is that after

Table 5
Performance of screening MRI in asymptomatic high-risk women

Number Screened[Ref]	Number of Cancers	Sensitivity (%) MGM	Sensitivity (%) MRI	Specificity (%) MGM	Specificity (%) MRI
1909[89]	51	33.3	79.5	95.0	89.8
649[116]	35	40.0	77.0	93.0	81.0
529[117]	43	33.0	91.0	96.8	97.2
367[118]	4	25.0	100	98.1	92.6
236[119]	22	36.0	77.0	99.8	95.4
105[120]	8	12.5	100.0	100.0	98.9

Abbreviations: MGM, Mammography; MRI, Magnetic Resonance Imaging.
Data from Refs.[89,116–120]

more than 3 decades of screening mammography, there has been a large increase in the detection of early stage breast cancer but only a small decrease in the diagnosis of node-positive or metastatic disease.[97] In addition, there is some evidence that some screen-detected breast cancers can regress or become undetectable over time.[98,99] Estimates of the magnitude of overdiagnosis are derived by comparing cancer incidence in screened women with incidence in women who were never screened but were followed for a long period of time. A recent meta-analysis estimated that 19% of screen-detected breast cancers are overdiagnosed.[100,101] One investigator has suggested that, among 1000 US women aged 50 years who are screened annually for a decade, 0.3 to 3.2 will avoid a breast cancer death, whereas 3 to 14 will be overdiagnosed and treated needlessly.[96] Nevertheless, there is currently no way to know which screen-detected cancers pose a threat and which do not.

Ionizing radiation is an established carcinogen for the breast, thyroid, bone marrow, and other organs. There is great variation in individual susceptibility, but higher doses earlier in life carry the greatest risk. It has been estimated that annual mammography between 40 and 80 years of age could cause 20 to 25 fatal breast cancers per 100,000 screened.[65] This risk is likely increased significantly for tests requiring higher radiation doses, such as BSGI, MBI, and PEM, and also for earlier ages at initiation of screening. There are some data to suggest that annual screening mammography in BRCA gene mutation carriers between 25 and 30 years of age provides enough early age radiation exposure to increase breast cancer incidence.[86–88] This concern is much less after 30 years of age.

SUMMARY

Randomized prospective screening mammography trials using primitive, decades-old technology demonstrated reduced breast cancer mortality especially for women older than 50 years of age. Recent advances in mammography, notably the introduction of digital mammography and tomosynthesis, have improved the sensitivity and specificity of the test, even for younger women. Annual screening mammography beginning at 40 years of age is recommended by most professional societies. There are no established guidelines for adjunctive screening in women with mammographically dense breast tissue, but screening MRI is endorsed for high-risk women. The menu of available screening tests is expanding, and each will diagnose cancers missed by mammography. It is important to recognize that each additional test will introduce a certain risk of harm that could include financial costs, anxiety from false alarms, physical harm from medical procedures, physical and emotional harm from overdiagnosis, and risk from radiation exposure. Clinical breast examination, which is gradually disappearing, may have a revitalized role in the era of effective treatment of established breast cancers.

REFERENCES

1. Siegel R, Ma J, Zou Z, et al. Cancer statistics, 2014. CA Cancer J Clin 2014; 64(1):9–29.
2. Howlader N, Noone AM, Krapcho M, et al. SEER cancer statistics review, 1975-2011. 2014. Available at: http://seer.cancer.gov/csr/1975_2011/. Accessed June 21, 2015.
3. Edwards BK, Noone AM, Mariotto AB, et al. Annual report to the nation on the status of cancer, 1975-2010, featuring prevalence of comorbidity and impact on survival among persons with lung, colorectal, breast, or prostate cancer.

Cancer 2014;120(9):1290–314. Available at: http://onlinelibrary.wiley.com/doi/10.1002/cncr.28509/abstract.

4. Berry DA, Cronin KA, Plevritis SK, et al. Effect of screening and adjuvant therapy on mortality from breast cancer. N Engl J Med 2005;353(17):1784–92.

5. Croswell JM, Ransohoff DF, Kramer BS. Principles of cancer screening: lessons from history and study design issues. Semin Oncol 2010;37(3):202–15. Available at: http://www.ncbi.nlm.nih.gov/pmc/articles/PMC2921618/pdf/nihms204926.pdf.

6. US Preventive Services Task Force. Screening for breast cancer: U.S. Preventive Services Task Force recommendation statement. Ann Intern Med 2009; 151(10):716–26 W-236.

7. Fletcher SW, Elmore JG. Clinical practice. Mammographic screening for breast cancer. N Engl J Med 2003;348(17):1672–80. Available at: http://www.ncbi.nlm.nih.gov/pmc/articles/PMC3157308/pdf/nihms-306428.pdf.

8. Humphrey LL, Helfand M, Chan BK, et al. Breast cancer screening: a summary of the evidence for the U.S. Preventive Services Task Force. Ann Intern Med 2002;137(5 Part 1):347–60.

9. Pace LE, Keating NL. A systematic assessment of benefits and risks to guide breast cancer screening decisions. JAMA 2014;311(13):1327–35. Available at: http://jama.jamanetwork.com/data/Journals/JAMA/929938/jrv140002.pdf.

10. Lee CH, Dershaw DD, Kopans D, et al. Breast cancer screening with imaging: recommendations from the Society of Breast Imaging and the ACR on the use of mammography, breast MRI, breast ultrasound, and other technologies for the detection of clinically occult breast cancer. J Am Coll Radiol 2010;7(1):18–27. Available at: http://www.jacr.org/article/S1546-1440(09)00480-3/pdf.

11. Smith RA, Cokkinides V, Brooks D, et al. Cancer screening in the United States, 2010: a review of current American Cancer Society guidelines and issues in cancer screening. CA Cancer J Clin 2010;60(2):99–119.

12. Lee SJ, Boscardin WJ, Stijacic-Cenzer I, et al. Time lag to benefit after screening for breast and colorectal cancer: meta-analysis of survival data from the United States, Sweden, United Kingdom, and Denmark. BMJ 2013;346:e8441. Available at: http://www.bmj.com/content/bmj/346/bmj.e8441.full.pdf.

13. Gotzsche PC, Olsen O. Is screening for breast cancer with mammography justifiable? Lancet 2000;355(9198):129–34. Available at: http://www.thelancet.com/journals/lancet/article/PIIS0140-6736(99)06065-1/abstract.

14. Olsen O, Gotzsche PC. Cochrane review on screening for breast cancer with mammography. Lancet 2001;358(9290):1340–2. Available at: http://www.thelancet.com/journals/lancet/article/PIIS0140-6736(01)06449-2/abstract.

15. Fisher B, Redmond C, Fisher ER. The contribution of recent NSABP clinical trials of primary breast cancer therapy to an understanding of tumor biology–an overview of findings. Cancer 1980;46(4 Suppl):1009–25.

16. Barton MB, Harris R, Fletcher SW. The rational clinical examination. Does this patient have breast cancer? The screening clinical breast examination: should it be done? How? JAMA 1999;282(13):1270–80. Available at: http://jama.jamanetwork.com/article.aspx?articleid=191969.

17. Saslow D, Hannan J, Osuch J, et al. Clinical breast examination: practical recommendations for optimizing performance and reporting. CA Cancer J Clin 2004;54(6):327–44.

18. Meissner HI, Breen N, Yabroff KR. Whatever happened to clinical breast examinations? Am J Prev Med 2003;25(3):259–63. Available at: http://www.ajpmonline.org/article/S0749-3797(03)00189-2/abstract.

19. Hendrick RE, Cutter GR, Berns EA, et al. Community-based mammography practice: services, charges, and interpretation methods. AJR Am J Roentgenol 2005;184(2):433–8.
20. Breen N, Yabroff KR, Meissner HI. What proportion of breast cancers are detected by mammography in the United States? Cancer Detect Prev 2007; 31(3):220–4.
21. Shapiro S, Venet W, Strax P, et al. Periodic screening for breast cancer: the health insurance plan project and its sequelae, 1963-1986. Baltimore (MD): The Johns Hopkins Press; 1988.
22. Roberts MM, Alexander FE, Anderson TJ, et al. Edinburgh trial of screening for breast cancer: mortality at seven years. Lancet 1990;335(8684):241–6.
23. Miller AB, Baines CJ, To T, et al. Canadian National Breast Screening Study: 1. Breast cancer detection and death rates among women aged 40 to 49 years. CMAJ 1992;147(10):1459–76.
24. Miller AB, Baines CJ, To T, et al. Canadian National Breast Screening Study: 2. Breast cancer detection and death rates among women aged 50 to 59 years. CMAJ 1992;147(10):1477–88.
25. Baker LH. Breast cancer detection demonstration project: five-year summary report. CA Cancer J Clin 1982;32(4):194–225.
26. Chamberlain J, Clifford RE, Nathan BE, et al. Error-rates in screening for breast cancer by clinical examination and mammography. Clin Oncol 1979;5(2): 135–46.
27. Bobo JK, Lee NC, Thames SF. Findings from 752,081 clinical breast examinations reported to a national screening program from 1995 through 1998. J Natl Cancer Inst 2000;92(12):971–6. Available at: http://jnci.oxfordjournals. org/content/92/12/971.full.pdf.
28. Chiarelli AM, Majpruz V, Brown P, et al. The contribution of clinical breast examination to the accuracy of breast screening. J Natl Cancer Inst 2009;101(18): 1236–43.
29. Thomas DB, Gao DL, Self SG, et al. Randomized trial of breast self-examination in Shanghai: methodology and preliminary results. J Natl Cancer Inst 1997; 89(5):355–65. Available at: http://jnci.oxfordjournals.org/content/89/5/355.full. pdf.
30. Thomas DB, Gao DL, Ray RM, et al. Randomized trial of breast self-examination in Shanghai: final results. J Natl Cancer Inst 2002;94(19):1445–57. Available at: http://jnci.oxfordjournals.org/content/94/19/1445.full.pdf.
31. Semiglazov VF, Sagaidak VN, Moiseyenko VM, et al. Study of the role of breast self-examination in the reduction of mortality from breast cancer. The Russian Federation/World Health Organization Study. Eur J Cancer 1993;29A(14): 2039–46.
32. Kosters JP, Gotzsche PC. Regular self-examination or clinical examination for early detection of breast cancer. Cochrane Database Syst Rev 2003;(2). CD003373. Available at: http://onlinelibrary.wiley.com/doi/10.1002/14651858. CD003373/abstract.
33. Salomon A. Beiträge zur Pathologie und Klinik der Mammakarzinome. Arch Klin Chir 1913;101:573–668.
34. Gershon-Cohen J, Colcher AE. Evaluation of roentgen diagnosis of early carcinoma of breast. JAMA 1937;108:867–71.
35. Shapiro S. Periodic screening for breast cancer: the HIP randomized controlled trial. Health insurance plan. J Natl Cancer Inst Monogr 1997;(22):27–30.

36. Duffy SW, Tabar L, Smith RA. The mammographic screening trials: commentary on the recent work by Olsen and Gotzsche. CA Cancer J Clin 2002;52(2):68–71.

37. Buist DS, Porter PL, Lehman C, et al. Factors contributing to mammography failure in women aged 40-49 years. J Natl Cancer Inst 2004;96(19):1432–40.

38. Pisano ED, Gatsonis C, Hendrick E, et al. Diagnostic performance of digital versus film mammography for breast-cancer screening. N Engl J Med 2005;353(17): 1773–83. Available at: http://www.nejm.org/doi/pdf/10.1056/NEJMoa052911.

39. Brem RF, Baum J, Lechner M, et al. Improvement in sensitivity of screening mammography with computer-aided detection: a multi-institutional trial. AJR Am J Roentgenol 2003;181(3):687–93. Available at: http://www.ncbi.nlm.nih.gov/pubmed/12933460.

40. Warren Burhenne LJ, Wood SA, D'Orsi CJ, et al. Potential contribution of computer-aided detection to the sensitivity of screening mammography. Radiology 2000;215(2):554–62.

41. Birdwell RL, Ikeda DM, O'Shaughnessy KF, et al. Mammographic characteristics of 115 missed cancers later detected with screening mammography and the potential utility of computer-aided detection. Radiology 2001;219(1):192–202. Available at: http://www.ncbi.nlm.nih.gov/pubmed/11274556.

42. Fenton JJ, Taplin SH, Carney PA, et al. Influence of computer-aided detection on performance of screening mammography. N Engl J Med 2007;356(14): 1399–409. Available at: http://www.nejm.org/doi/pdf/10.1056/NEJMoa066099.

43. McCarthy AM, Kontos D, Synnestvedt M, et al. Screening outcomes following implementation of digital breast tomosynthesis in a general-population screening program. J Natl Cancer Inst 2014;106(11) [pii:dju316].

44. Haas BM, Kalra V, Geisel J, et al. Comparison of tomosynthesis plus digital mammography and digital mammography alone for breast cancer screening. Radiology 2013;269(3):694–700. Available at: http://www.ncbi.nlm.nih.gov/pubmed/23901124.

45. Conant EF. Clinical implementation of digital breast tomosynthesis. Radiol Clin North Am 2014;52(3):499–518. Available at: http://www.sciencedirect.com/science/article/pii/S0033838913002315.

46. Skaane P, Bandos AI, Gullien R, et al. Comparison of digital mammography alone and digital mammography plus tomosynthesis in a population-based screening program. Radiology 2013;267(1):47–56.

47. Skaane P, Bandos AI, Eben EB, et al. Two-view digital breast tomosynthesis screening with synthetically reconstructed projection images: comparison with digital breast tomosynthesis with full-field digital mammographic images. Radiology 2014;271(3):655–63.

48. Zuley ML, Guo B, Catullo VJ, et al. Comparison of two-dimensional synthesized mammograms versus original digital mammograms alone and in combination with tomosynthesis images. Radiology 2014;271(3):664–71.

49. Saadatmand S, Rutgers EJ, Tollenaar RA, et al. Breast density as indicator for the use of mammography or MRI to screen women with familial risk for breast cancer (FaMRIsc): a multicentre randomized controlled trial. BMC Cancer 2012;12:440.

50. Lehman CD. Role of MRI in screening women at high risk for breast cancer. J Magn Reson Imaging 2006;24(5):964–70. Available at: http://onlinelibrary.wiley.com/doi/10.1002/jmri.20752/abstract.

51. Saslow D, Boetes C, Burke W, et al. American Cancer Society guidelines for breast screening with MRI as an adjunct to mammography. CA Cancer

J Clin 2007;57(2):75–89 [Erratum appears in CA Cancer J Clin 2007;57(3): 185]. Available at: http://ovidsp.ovid.com/ovidweb.cgi?T=JS&CSC=Y&NEWS =N&PAGE=fulltext&D=med4&AN=17392385 http://linksource.ebsco.com/ linking.aspx?sid=OVID:medline&id=pmid:17392385&id=doi:&issn=0007-9235 &isbn=&volume=57&issue=2&spage=75&date=2007&title=CA%3A+a+ Cancer+Journal+for+Clinicians&atitle=American+Cancer+Society+guidelines +for+breast+screening+with+MRI+as+an+adjunct+to+mammography. &aulast=Saslow&pid=%3CAN%3E17392385%3C%2FAN%3E.

52. Scaranelo AM, Carrillo MC, Fleming R, et al. Pilot study of quantitative analysis of background enhancement on breast MR images: association with menstrual cycle and mammographic breast density. Radiology 2013;267(3):692–700.

53. Uematsu T, Kasami M, Watanabe J. Should breast MRI be performed with adjustment for the phase in patients' menstrual cycle? Correlation between mammographic density, age, and background enhancement on breast MRI without adjusting for the phase in patients' menstrual cycle. Eur J Radiol 2012;81(7):1539–42.

54. King V, Brooks JD, Bernstein JL, et al. Background parenchymal enhancement at breast MR imaging and breast cancer risk. Radiology 2011;260(1):50–60.

55. Berg WA, Blume JD, Cormack JB, et al. Combined screening with ultrasound and mammography vs mammography alone in women at elevated risk of breast cancer. JAMA 2008;299(18):2151–63.http://jama.jamanetwork.com/data/Journals/ JAMA/4415/joc80037_2151_2163.pdf.

56. Berg WA, Blume JD, Adams AM, et al. Reasons women at elevated risk of breast cancer refuse breast MR imaging screening: ACRIN 6666. Radiology 2010;254(1):79–87. Available at: http://www.ncbi.nlm.nih.gov/pmc/articles/ PMC2811274/pdf/2541090953.pdf.

57. Merry GM, Mendelson EB. Update on screening breast ultrasonography. Radiol Clin North Am 2014;52(3):527–37. Available at: http://www.sciencedirect.com/ science/article/pii/S0033838913002340.

58. Berg WA, Zhang Z, Lehrer D, et al. Detection of breast cancer with addition of annual screening ultrasound or a single screening MRI to mammography in women with elevated breast cancer risk. JAMA 2012;307(13):1394–404.

59. Kelly KM, Dean J, Lee SJ, et al. Breast cancer detection: radiologists' performance using mammography with and without automated whole-breast ultrasound. Eur Radiol 2010;20(11):2557–64. Available at: http://www.ncbi.nlm.nih. gov/pmc/articles/PMC2948156/pdf/330_2010_Article_1844.pdf.

60. Sun Y, Wei W, Yang HW, et al. Clinical usefulness of breast-specific gamma imaging as an adjunct modality to mammography for diagnosis of breast cancer: a systemic review and meta-analysis. Eur J Nucl Med Mol Imaging 2013;40(3): 450–63. Available at: http://link.springer.com/article/10.1007%2Fs00259-012-2279-5.

61. Rhodes DJ, Hruska CB, Phillips SW, et al. Dedicated dual-head gamma imaging for breast cancer screening in women with mammographically dense breasts. Radiology 2011;258(1):106–18.

62. Berg WA, Madsen KS, Schilling K, et al. Comparative effectiveness of positron emission mammography and MRI in the contralateral breast of women with newly diagnosed breast cancer. AJR Am J Roentgenol 2012;198(1):219–32.

63. Rechtman LR, Lenihan MJ, Lieberman JH, et al. Breast-specific gamma imaging for the detection of breast cancer in dense versus nondense breasts. AJR Am J Roentgenol 2014;202(2):293–8.

64. Koo HR, Moon WK, Chun IK, et al. Background (1)(8)F-FDG uptake in positron emission mammography (PEM): correlation with mammographic density and background parenchymal enhancement in breast MRI. Eur J Radiol 2013; 82(10):1738–42.

65. Hendrick RE. Radiation doses and cancer risks from breast imaging studies. Radiology 2010;257(1):246–53.

66. O'Connor MK, Li H, Rhodes DJ, et al. Comparison of radiation exposure and associated radiation-induced cancer risks from mammography and molecular imaging of the breast. Med Phys 2010;37(12):6187–98. Available at: http://www.ncbi.nlm.nih.gov/pmc/articles/PMC2997811/pdf/MPHYA6-000037-006187_1.pdf.

67. Hendrick RE, Pisano ED, Averbukh A, et al. Comparison of acquisition parameters and breast dose in digital mammography and screen-film mammography in the American College of Radiology Imaging Network digital mammographic imaging screening trial. AJR Am J Roentgenol 2010;194(2):362–9. Available at: http://www.ncbi.nlm.nih.gov/pmc/articles/PMC2854416/pdf/nihms176331.pdf.

68. Hruska CB, Weinmann AL, Tello Skjerseth CM, et al. Proof of concept for low-dose molecular breast imaging with a dual-head CZT gamma camera. Part II. Evaluation in patients. Med Phys 2012;39(6):3476–83.

69. Vreugdenburg TD, Willis CD, Mundy L, et al. A systematic review of elastography, electrical impedance scanning, and digital infrared thermography for breast cancer screening and diagnosis. Breast Cancer Res Treat 2013;137(3):665–76.

70. O'Connell AM, Karellas A, Vedantham S. The potential role of dedicated 3D breast CT as a diagnostic tool: review and early clinical examples. Breast J 2014;20(6):592–605. Available at: http://onlinelibrary.wiley.com/doi/10.1111/tbj.12327/abstract.

71. Onega T, Beaber EF, Sprague BL, et al. Breast cancer screening in an era of personalized regimens: a conceptual model and National Cancer Institute initiative for risk-based and preference-based approaches at a population level. Cancer 2014;120(19):2955–64. Available at: http://onlinelibrary.wiley.com/doi/10.1002/cncr.28771/abstract.

72. Venturini E, Losio C, Panizza P, et al. Tailored breast cancer screening program with microdose mammography, US, and MR imaging: short-term results of a pilot study in 40-49-year-old women. Radiology 2013;268(2):347–55.

73. Pike MC, Pearce CL. Mammographic density, MRI background parenchymal enhancement and breast cancer risk. Ann Oncol 2013;24(Suppl 8):viii37–41. Available at: http://www.ncbi.nlm.nih.gov/pmc/articles/PMC3894109/pdf/mdt310.pdf.

74. Stomper PC, D'Souza DJ, DiNitto PA, et al. Analysis of parenchymal density on mammograms in 1353 women 25-79 years old. AJR Am J Roentgenol 1996; 167(5):1261–5.

75. Pettersson A, Graff RE, Ursin G, et al. Mammographic density phenotypes and risk of breast cancer: a meta-analysis. J Natl Cancer Inst 2014;106(5). Available at: http://jnci.oxfordjournals.org/content/106/5/dju078.

76. Sickles E, D'Orsi CJ, Bassett LW, et al. ACR BI-RADS mammography. ACR BI-RADS atlas, breast imaging reporting and data system. Reston (VA): American College of Radiology; 2013.

77. Rosenberg RD, Hunt WC, Williamson MR, et al. Effects of age, breast density, ethnicity, and estrogen replacement therapy on screening mammographic sensitivity and cancer stage at diagnosis: review of 183,134 screening mammograms in Albuquerque, New Mexico. Radiology 1998;209(2):511–8.

78. Carney PA, Miglioretti DL, Yankaskas BC, et al. Individual and combined effects of age, breast density, and hormone replacement therapy use on the accuracy of screening mammography. Ann Intern Med 2003;138(3):168–75. Available at: http://annals.org/article.aspx?articleid=716007.
79. Mandelson MT, Oestreicher N, Porter PL, et al. Breast density as a predictor of mammographic detection: comparison of interval- and screen-detected cancers. J Natl Cancer Inst 2000;92(13):1081–7.
80. Ciatto S, Houssami N, Bernardi D, et al. Integration of 3D digital mammography with tomosynthesis for population breast-cancer screening (STORM): a prospective comparison study. Lancet Oncol 2013;14(7):583–9.
81. Hooley RJ, Greenberg KL, Stackhouse RM, et al. Screening US in patients with mammographically dense breasts: initial experience with Connecticut public act 09-41. Radiology 2012;265(1):59–69.
82. Sardanelli F, Giuseppetti GM, Panizza P, et al. Sensitivity of MRI versus mammography for detecting foci of multifocal, multicentric breast cancer in Fatty and dense breasts using the whole-breast pathologic examination as a gold standard. AJR Am J Roentgenol 2004;183(4):1149–57.
83. Kopans DB, Meyer JE, Lindfors KK. Whole-breast US imaging: four-year follow-up. Radiology 1985;157(2):505–7.
84. Saarenmaa I, Salminen T, Geiger U, et al. The effect of age and density of the breast on the sensitivity of breast cancer diagnostic by mammography and ultrasonography. Breast Cancer Res Treat 2001;67(2):117–23.
85. National Comprehensive Cancer Network. Breast cancer version 3. 2014. Available at: http://www.nccn.org/professionals/physician_gls/pdf/breast.pdf. Accessed July 10, 2014.
86. Gronwald J, Pijpe A, Byrski T, et al. Early radiation exposures and BRCA1-associated breast cancer in young women from Poland. Breast Cancer Res Treat 2008;112(3):581–4. Available at: http://ovidsp.ovid.com/ovidweb.cgi?T=JS&CSC=Y&NEWS=N&PAGE=fulltext&D=medl&AN=18205043. http://linksource.ebsco.com/linking.aspx?sid=OVID:medline&id=pmid:18205043&id=doi:&issn=0167-6806&isbn=&volume=112&issue=3&spage=581&date=2008&title=Breast+Cancer+Research+%26+Treatment&atitle=Early+radiation+exposures+and+BRCA1-associated+breast+cancer+in+young+women+from+Poland.&aulast=Gronwald&pid=%3CAN%3E18205043%3C%2FAN%3E.
87. Pijpe A, Andrieu N, Easton DF, et al. Exposure to diagnostic radiation and risk of breast cancer among carriers of BRCA1/2 mutations: retrospective cohort study (GENE-RAD-RISK). BMJ 2012;345:e5660.
88. Berrington de Gonzalez A, Berg CD, Visvanathan K, et al. Estimated risk of radiation-induced breast cancer from mammographic screening for young BRCA mutation carriers. J Natl Cancer Inst 2009;101(3):205–9.
89. Kriege M, Brekelmans CT, Boetes C, et al. Efficacy of MRI and mammography for breast-cancer screening in women with a familial or genetic predisposition. N Engl J Med 2004;351(5):427–37.
90. Gareth ED, Nisha K, Yit L, et al. MRI breast screening in high-risk women: cancer detection and survival analysis. Breast Cancer Res Treat 2014;145(3):663–72. Available at: http://link.springer.com/article/10.1007%2Fs10549-014-2931-9.
91. Moller P, Stormorken A, Jonsrud C, et al. Survival of patients with BRCA1-associated breast cancer diagnosed in an MRI-based surveillance program. Breast Cancer Res Treat 2013;139(1):155–61. Available at: http://link.springer.com/article/10.1007%2Fs10549-013-2540-z.

92. Plevritis SK, Kurian AW, Sigal BM, et al. Cost-effectiveness of screening BRCA1/2 mutation carriers with breast magnetic resonance imaging. JAMA 2006; 295(20):2374–84. Available at: http://jama.jamanetwork.com/data/Journals/JAMA/5025/JOC60058.pdf.

93. Moore SG, Shenoy PJ, Fanucchi L, et al. Cost-effectiveness of MRI compared to mammography for breast cancer screening in a high risk population. BMC Health Serv Res 2009;9:9. Available at: http://www.ncbi.nlm.nih.gov/pmc/articles/PMC2630922/pdf/1472-6963-9-9.pdf.

94. Hubbard RA, Kerlikowske K, Flowers CI, et al. Cumulative probability of false-positive recall or biopsy recommendation after 10 years of screening mammography: a cohort study. Ann Intern Med 2011;155(8):481–92.

95. Braithwaite D, Zhu W, Hubbard RA, et al. Screening outcomes in older US women undergoing multiple mammograms in community practice: does interval, age, or comorbidity score affect tumor characteristics or false positive rates? J Natl Cancer Inst 2013;105(5):334–41.

96. Welch HG, Passow HJ. Quantifying the benefits and harms of screening mammography. JAMA Intern Med 2014;174(3):448–54. Available at: http://archinte.jamanetwork.com/article.aspx?articleid=1792915.

97. Bleyer A, Welch HG. Effect of three decades of screening mammography on breast-cancer incidence. N Engl J Med 2012;367(21):1998–2005.

98. Zahl PH, Maehlen J, Welch HG. The natural history of invasive breast cancers detected by screening mammography. Arch Intern Med 2008;168(21): 2311–6.

99. Zahl PH, Gotzsche PC, Maehlen J. Natural history of breast cancers detected in the Swedish mammography screening programme: a cohort study. Lancet Oncol 2011;12(12):1118–24.

100. Independent UK Panel on Breast Cancer Screening. The benefits and harms of breast cancer screening: an independent review. Lancet 2012;380(9855): 1778–86.

101. Marmot MG, Altman DG, Cameron DA, et al. The benefits and harms of breast cancer screening: an independent review. Br J Cancer 2013;108(11):2205–40.

102. Friedewald SM, Rafferty EA, Rose SL, et al. Breast cancer screening using tomosynthesis in combination with digital mammography. JAMA 2014; 311(24):2499–507. Available at: http://jama.jamanetwork.com/data/Journals/JAMA/930408/joi140069.pdf.

103. Greenberg JS, Javitt MC, Katzen J, et al. Clinical performance metrics of 3D digital breast tomosynthesis compared with 2D digital mammography for breast cancer screening in community practice. AJR Am J Roentgenol 2014;203: 687–93.

104. Rose SL, Tidwell AL, Bujnoch LJ, et al. Implementation of breast tomosynthesis in a routine screening practice: an observational study. AJR Am J Roentgenol 2013;200(6):1401–8.

105. Durand MA, Haas BM, Yao X, et al. Early clinical experience with digital breast tomosynthesis for screening mammography. Radiology 2015;274(1):85–92.

106. Chae EY, Kim HH, Cha JH, et al. Evaluation of screening whole-breast sonography as a supplemental tool in conjunction with mammography in women with dense breasts. J Ultrasound Med 2013;32(9):1573–8. Available at: http://www.jultrasoundmed.org/content/32/9/1573.full.pdf.

107. Korpraphong P, Limsuwarn P, Tangcharoensathien W, et al. Improving breast cancer detection using ultrasonography in asymptomatic women with

non-fatty breast density. Acta Radiol 2014;55(8):903–8. Available at: http://acr. sagepub.com/content/55/8/903.long.

108. Corsetti V, Houssami N, Ferrari A, et al. Breast screening with ultrasound in women with mammography-negative dense breasts: evidence on incremental cancer detection and false positives, and associated cost. Eur J Cancer 2008;44(4):539–44.

109. Costantino JP, Gail MH, Pee D, et al. Validation studies for models projecting the risk of invasive and total breast cancer incidence. J Natl Cancer Inst 1999;91: 1541–8.

110. Rockhill B, Spiegelman D, Byrne C, et al. Validation of the Gail, et al. model of breast cancer risk prediction and implications for chemoprevention. J Natl Cancer Inst 2001;93:358–66.

111. Tice JA, Cummings SR, Ziv E, et al. Mammographic breast density and the Gail model for breast cancer risk prediction in a screening population. Breast Cancer Res Treat 2005;94(2):115–22.

112. Powell M, Jamshidian F, Cheyne K, et al. Assessing breast cancer risk models in Marin County, a population with high rates of delayed childbirth. Clin Breast Cancer 2014;14(3):212–20.e1. Available at: http://www.sciencedirect.com/science/article/pii/S1526820913002851.

113. Boughey JC, Hartmann LC, Anderson SS, et al. Evaluation of the Tyrer-Cuzick (International Breast Cancer Intervention Study) model for breast cancer risk prediction in women with atypical hyperplasia. J Clin Oncol 2010;28(22): 3591–6. Available at: http://jco.ascopubs.org/content/28/22/3591.full.pdf.

114. Evans DG, Ingham S, Dawe S, et al. Breast cancer risk assessment in 8,824 women attending a family history evaluation and screening programme. Fam Cancer 2014;13(2):189–96.

115. MacInnis RJ, Bickerstaffe A, Apicella C, et al. Prospective validation of the breast cancer risk prediction model BOADICEA and a batch-mode version BOADICEA Centre. Br J Cancer 2013;109(5):1296–301.

116. Leach MO, Boggis CR, Dixon AK, et al. Screening with magnetic resonance imaging and mammography of a UK population at high familial risk of breast cancer: a prospective multicentre cohort study (MARIBS). Lancet 2005;365(9473): 1769–78.

117. Kuhl CK, Schrading S, Leutner CC, et al. Mammography, breast ultrasound, and magnetic resonance imaging for surveillance of women at high familial risk for breast cancer. J Clin Oncol 2005;23(33):8469–76. Available at: http://jco. ascopubs.org/content/23/33/8469.full.pdf.

118. Lehman CD, Blume JD, Weatherall P, et al. Screening women at high risk for breast cancer with mammography and magnetic resonance imaging. Cancer 2005; 103(9):1898–905. Available at: http://onlinelibrary.wiley.com/store/10.1002/cncr. 20971/asset/20971_ftp.pdf?v=1&t=i31j63l3&s=9abb545f0a1983acddeddeba00 202ae7f1012ac4.

119. Warner E, Plewes DB, Hill KA, et al. Surveillance of BRCA1 and BRCA2 mutation carriers with magnetic resonance imaging, ultrasound, mammography, and clinical breast examination. JAMA 2004;292(11):1317–25. Available at: http://jama. jamanetwork.com/data/Journals/JAMA/4944/JOC32405.pdf.

120. Podo F, Sardanelli F, Canese R, et al. The Italian multi-centre project on evaluation of MRI and other imaging modalities in early detection of breast cancer in subjects at high genetic risk. J Exp Clin Cancer Res 2002;21(3 Suppl):115–24.

Screening for Viral Hepatitis and Hepatocellular Cancer

Andrew M. Cameron, MD, PhD

KEYWORDS

- Screening • Surveillance • Hepatitis B virus • Hepatitis C virus
- Hepatocellular carcinoma

KEY POINTS

- Accurate tests for at-risk populations are available for hepatitis B virus, hepatitis C virus (HCV), and hepatocellular carcinoma (HCC).
- Effective treatments for all three diseases exist if diagnosed early.
- New antivirals are making a significant impact on HCV.
- Liver transplant is curative for early HCC and is prioritized by the United Network for Organ Sharing in the United States.

Screening and surveillance for deadly disease only makes sense if:

1. There are identifiable populations at risk for the condition.
2. There are sensitive and specific low-cost tests available for the condition.
3. There are effective treatments for the condition on diagnosis that result in decreased mortality.

Hepatitis B virus (HBV) infection, hepatitis C virus (HCV) infection, and hepatocellular carcinoma (HCC) are each important clinical conditions that meet all of these criteria and therefore have screening recommendations that are standard of care.

SCREENING FOR HEPATITIS B VIRUS INFECTION

HBV infection is a global health problem with an estimated 350 million persons chronically infected.[1] In the United States there are estimated to be more than 1 million carriers (defined as positive for HBV surface antigen for more than 6 months).[2–4] HBV carriers in the United States or abroad are at risk for developing cirrhosis, hepatic decompensation, and HCC (25% lifetime risk of serious sequelae).[5–7] Because

Department of Surgery, The Johns Hopkins Hospital, Ross 765, 720 Rutland Avenue, Baltimore, MD 21205, USA
E-mail address: acamero5@jhmi.edu

Surg Clin N Am 95 (2015) 1013–1021
http://dx.doi.org/10.1016/j.suc.2015.05.005
surgical.theclinics.com

effective medicines are available for HBV treatment, the following guidelines exist from the American Association for the Study of Liver Diseases (AASLD) to direct screening.

HBV is transmitted by perinatal transmission, percutaneous and sexual exposure, as well as by close personal contact.[3] In countries like the United States where vaccination of most infants and adolescents is the rule, the risk of transmission in schools or day care is low.

The tests used to screen for HBV infection include hepatitis B surface antigen (HBsAg) and anti–hepatitis B surface antibodies (anti-HBs). Alternatively hepatitis B core antibody can be used for screening as long as positive tests are followed by HBsAg and anti-HBs to determine infection versus prior exposure and immunity.

The following should be screened for HBV status (**Box 1**): persons born in endemic areas (eg, Asia, Africa, South Pacific Islands, Middle East); those born in the United States who were not vaccinated and are children of parents from an endemic area; patients with chronically increased liver function tests of unclear cause; immunosuppressed patients; men who have sex with men, have multiple partners, or a history of sexually transmitted diseases; inmates of correctional facilities; those who have ever used injection drugs; dialysis patients; those infected with HCV or human immunodeficiency virus (HIV); pregnant women; and household contacts of someone with HBV.

Box 1
Groups at high risk for HBV who should be screened

Patients from areas of endemic HBV:

- Asia
- Africa
- South Pacific Islands
- Middle East
- Mediterranean: Spain and Malta
- Indigenous arctic populations: Canada, Greenland, Alaska
- South America
- Eastern Europe
- Caribbean
- Central America

Others recommended for screening:

- US born, unvaccinated, with parents from endemic areas
- Household contacts of those with HBV
- Intravenous drug users
- Sexual contacts of those with HBV, those with multiple sexual partners, history of sexually transmitted diseases
- Inmates of correctional facilities
- Individuals with increased aminotransferase levels, HCV, human immunodeficiency virus (HIV), or cirrhosis
- Pregnant women
- Patients on hemodialysis

Organ donors, live or deceased, are tested for HBV as well. Anyone tested for HBV who is seronegative should be vaccinated.

SCREENING FOR HEPATITIS C VIRUS INFECTION

HCV infects 1% of the US population: 3 million people, less than half of whom know they are infected.[8] Because highly effective directly acting antivirals are now available for hepatitis C (ie, sofosbuvir, semipravir, ledipasvir) and liver disease is usually slowly progressive, there is a long period for detection and treatment.[9] High-risk groups who are most likely to benefit from screening have been identified. HCV transmission occurs inefficiently and usually only by direct exposure to blood (eg, via sharing of intravenous drug needles, which accounts for 60% of HCV in the United States). Blood transfusion before 1992 is the second most common route of exposure and other less common routes include maternal fetal transmission; transfer via medical device, such as endoscope; sexual intercourse, although usually only in the case of HIV-coinfected gay men; long-term hemodialysis; or needle-stick injuries in the health care setting.[10]

Testing for HCV infection is accomplished by screening for antibodies against viral proteins (anti-HCV) followed by nucleic acid testing using a polymerase chain reaction (PCR)–based test for viral RNA (reverse transcription PCR [RT-PCR]). HCV antibodies are usually not detected during the first 2 months following infection but are almost always detected by 6 months. These antibodies usually do not neutralize the virus, and do not provide immunity against subsequent viral infections. HCV antibodies may be lost several years after spontaneous clearance of virus, which occurs in approximately 20% of cases. Current screening serologic tests include electroimmunoassay and chemiluminescence immunoassay. These tests are delayed in their positivity, as described earlier; can show false-positives; do not distinguish between acute or chronic infection; and do not allow measurement of response to treatment.

Nucleic acid testing for HCV is straightforward: both genotype and quantitative viral load can be determined. RT-PCR HCV tests may remain negative for up to weeks after an exposure but are positive thereafter. Viral load (and its disappearance) is now used to determine efficacy of antiviral therapy.

Class I evidence exists for testing the following groups for HCV infection (**Box 2**): people with high-risk behavior (injection or intranasal drug use, historic or current), those with high-risk exposure (long-term hemodialysis [ever]); getting a tattoo in an unregulated setting; health care, emergency medical, and public safety workers after needle sticks, sharps, or mucosal exposures to HCV-infected blood; children born to women infected with HCV; prior recipients of transfusions or organ transplants, including persons who were notified that they received blood from a donor who later tested positive for HCV infection, received a transfusion of blood or blood components, or underwent an organ transplant before July 1992; those who received clotting factor concentrates produced before 1987; or persons who were ever incarcerated. Others for whom there is strong evidence for testing include those infected with HIV, those with unexplained liver disease or increase of liver function tests, and solid organ donors, deceased or living.

In addition, 1-time HCV testing is now recommended for any persons born between 1945 and 1965, regardless of risk status.

Annual HCV testing is recommended for persons who inject drugs and for HIV-seropositive men who have unprotected sex with men. Periodic testing should be also offered to other persons with ongoing risk factors for exposure to HCV.

Box 2
Persons who should get tested for HCV

- Those with high-risk behaviors
  - Injection drug use
  - Intranasal illicit drug use
- Those with high-risk exposures
  - Hemodialysis
  - Unprofessional tattoo
  - Health care worker with needle-stick exposure
  - Children born to HCV-positive women
  - Recipients of blood transfusion or solid organ transplant before 1992
  - Incarceration, prior or present
- Other
  - HIV infection
  - Chronic liver disease or increase of serum aminotransferase levels
  - Solid organ donors, deceased or living

DIAGNOSING OTHER VIRAL HEPATITIDES
Hepatitis A

Hepatitis A infection almost universally results in an acute, self-limited illness and can produce either icteric or anicteric syndromes. The incubation period is 28 days. The anicteric prodrome lasts from 2 days to 3 weeks and typically consists of fatigue, malaise, nausea, vomiting, anorexia, fever, and right upper quadrant pain. The diagnosis may be missed in cases that do not progress to jaundice. In cases in which jaundice becomes manifest, it persists for 1 to 6 weeks. Transaminase levels are typically more than 1000 IU/mL and serum bilirubin (>10 mg/dL) and alkaline phosphatase values are increased as well. Serum immunoglobulin (Ig) M antibodies are detected in 95% of patients and are the gold standard of diagnosis. IgG antibody levels become increased as jaundice subsides and may persist for years.

Hepatitis D

The hepatitis D virus (HDV), or delta agent, is an incomplete RNA virus that requires the concomitant presence of HBV for viral assembly and propagation. The only enzymatic activity of HDV is a ribozyme that autocleaves circular RNA and makes it linear. The HDV genome is a 1680-nucleotide, single-stranded circular RNA. Eight genotypes have been proposed. A single HDV antigen is encoded, it is a structural component of the virion, and a lipoprotein envelope is provided by HBV.

It is estimated that HDV is found in approximately 5% of HBV carriers. Because of its dependence on HBV, HDV always occurs in association with HBV infection. Transmission is similar to that of HBV, via parenteral or sexual exposure to blood or body fluids. HDV hepatitis occurs only in HBsAg-positive patients.

Acute infection is diagnosed by the presence of anti-HDV IgM. Anti-HBcore IgM distinguishes coinfection from superinfection. The diagnosis in patients with chronic liver disease is made by the presence of HBsAg and antibodies against HDV in the serum and is confirmed by the presence of HDV antigen in the liver or HDV RNA in the serum.

Hepatitis E

Hepatitis E virus (HEV) is a nonenveloped single-stranded RNA virus. It is 30 nm in diameter and is most similar to other viruses of the Caliciviridae family. There are thought to be 4 genotypes.

Hepatitis E is enterically transmitted (waterborne hepatitis or enterically transmitted non-A, non-B hepatitis) and is epidemiologically similar to hepatitis A virus. Infection has been prominently observed in Asia, Africa, the Middle East, and Central America. In addition, vertical transmission from mother to child has been documented and can be a source of perinatal morbidity and mortality. HEV generally causes a self-limited acute infection, although chronic infection has been described in organ transplant recipients. The incubation period usually lasts 3 to 8 weeks, and most individuals recover without chronic findings after a transient cholestatic episode. However, young adults and women in late stages of pregnancy may develop fulminant hepatitis E. Mortality from HEV is 0.5% to 4% in the general population but up to 20% in pregnant women. Diagnosis is aided by detection of serum or fecal genomes during the acute phase. In addition, anti-HEV IgM or IgG can be shown in follow-up.

Cytomegalovirus

Cytomegalovirus (CMV) is a member of the Beta Herpes Viridae family. It is usually associated with mild hepatitis but occasionally causes acute liver failure. Transmission can be intrauterine, perinatal, or postnatal; through intimate contact of infected fluids such as blood, saliva, or urine, or through transplanted organs. Infection is lifelong because of the latency of the virus and can be detected in up to 70% of individuals in US cities. Organ injury can occur as a result of primary infection or because of reactivation of latent infection. In the neonatal period, congenital infection can be severe and fatal. In immunocompetent adults, liver dysfunction tends to be found in association with CMV mononucleosis. In immunosuppressed adults, infection leads to liver dysfunction with jaundice and at times liver failure. Acalculous cholecystitis is another presentation. CMV antigenemia and PCR detection have made diagnosis rapid. Liver biopsy is important to establish the diagnosis of hepatitis. Pathologic examination shows inflammation and injury ranging from fatty changes to necrosis to fibrosis. Giant multinucleated cells and large nuclear inclusions can be encountered in hepatocytes and bile duct and epithelial cells.

Epstein-Barr Virus

Epstein-Barr virus (EBV) is a DNA virus and member of the Herpesviridae family. Infection persists for life because of the latency of the virus and it is usually transmitted by close personal or intimate contact via oral secretions. Some degree of liver involvement is encountered in almost all cases of EBV mononucleosis. It is usually mild with no major clinical manifestations and resolves spontaneously. The presence of jaundice may reflect either more severe hepatitis or an associated hemolytic anemia. Occasional cases of acute liver failure have been reported in both the immunocompetent and immunodeficient populations. Leukocytosis is usually present, with lymphocytosis and monocytosis. The monospot test is sensitive but not specific, but there is a reliable PCR test.

Herpes Simplex Virus

The prevalence of antibodies to herpes simplex virus (HSV)-1 is around 75% in most populations and around 20% have antibodies to HSV-2. Fulminant hepatitis is a rare complication of HSV infection; those at risk include neonates, the immunocompromised, the malnourished, and pregnant adults. Fulminant hepatitis is usually associated with multiorgan failure and is associated with a high mortality. Clinical features include high fever, anorexia with nausea, abdominal pain, leucopenia, and coagulopathy. Liver biopsy is important in establishing the diagnosis. Microscopic examination shows diffuse eosinophilic intranuclear inclusion bodies, multinucleated cells, widespread necrosis, and inflammation. Cowdry A–type intranuclear inclusions are typical. Confirmation is by PCR.

Varicella Zoster Virus

Herpesvirus varicella (also called varicella zoster virus) is usually associated with mild hepatitis but occasionally causes acute liver failure. Up to one-fourth of children with varicella (chickenpox) show temporary mild biochemical liver abnormalities. Reye syndrome may be encountered during the convalescence period, especially in patients who receive aspirin. In such cases mortality can be as high as 30%. Fulminant fatal hepatic failure is uncommon, but generally affects immunocompromised patients. Confirmation of the diagnosis can be achieved by isolation of the virus from affected tissues.

SCREENING FOR HEPATOCELLULAR CARCINOMA

The incidence of HCC is variable across the world but is increasing in many countries.[11] In a few areas, like Japan and Singapore, it may even have decreased slightly.[12] Involvement of a multidisciplinary team in managing liver cancer is important because the disease most often arises in the setting of underlying liver disease and its management depends on assessing degree of liver decompensation, which is different from that of most other cancers.

Although there are now agreed-on guidelines, and screening has become widely accepted, there is only a single randomized controlled trial of surveillance versus no surveillance that has shown benefit of a strategy of 6-month surveillance with Ultrasound and alpha-fetoprotein.[13] In the cohort of patients that were followed as described, mortality was reduced by 37%. The goal of surveillance is to decrease mortality from the disease, or provide meaningful improvement in survival duration for those diagnosed. Surveillance can be recommended in HCC for certain high-risk groups, the goal being to detect early stage disease that has shown survival benefit with treatments like resection and especially transplant.

AASLD guidelines specify which groups are appropriate for screening based on increased risk: surveillance is deemed cost-effective if expected HCC risk exceeds 1.5%/y in patients with HCV infection and 0.2%/y in patients with hepatitis B. Some recent studies show that alpha-fetoprotein level alone lacks adequate sensitivity and specificity for effective surveillance, thus surveillance is based on US. The recommended screening interval is 6 months. Diagnosis is based on imaging characteristics and biopsy. Arterial uptake by a lesion with subsequent washout on dynamic imaging is the radiographically validated standard. Other studies have shown that screening with AFP alone is the most cost-effective, although most conclude that US and AFP are the most effective overall.[14]

Ultimately, surveillance is clearly beneficial and thus recommended for (**Box 3**): Asian hepatitis B carriers aged more than 40 years, any hepatitis B carrier with a family history of HCC, African or North American black people with hepatitis B, cirrhotic HBV carriers, hepatitis C cirrhotics, stage 4 patients with primary biliary cirrhosis, those with genetic hemochromatosis and cirrhosis, those with alpha1-antitrypsin deficiency and cirrhosis, and those patients with cirrhosis of any or unknown cause. For those

Box 3
Who should undergo HCC surveillance
• Asian hepatitis carriers more than 40 years of age
• HBV carriers with family history of HCC
• African/North American black people with HBV
• Cirrhotics
• Stage 4 primary biliary cirrhosis
Probable benefit from surveillance:
• HBV carriers less than 40 years of age
• Hepatitis C with stage 3 fibrosis
• Noncirrhotic nonalcoholic fatty liver disease

hepatitis B carriers younger than 40 years old, those with HCV and stage 3 fibrosis or less, and patients with noncirrhotic nonalcoholic fatty liver disease, the benefit of surveillance remains uncertain.

Current recommendations also vary with the size of a detected lesion or nodule: lesions less than 1 cm may be followed with ultrasonography examinations at 3-month intervals. If stable, this level of surveillance is all that is required. If growth in lesion size is appreciable, then computed tomography (CT) scan with contrast to further characterize the lesion is indicated. If a lesion is discovered that is greater than 1 cm, it is investigated with multiphase CT or contrast-enhanced magnetic resonance, and if lesions show the stereotypic pattern of arterial enhancement and venous washout, then the diagnosis of HCC is made. If imaging features are not diagnostic, biopsy may be considered, although sometimes small lesions (less than 2 cm) can be closely followed with attention to changes in their size or imaging characteristics.

WHEN TO OBTAIN A LIVER BIOPSY TO DIAGNOSE HEPATOCELLULAR CARCINOMA

Percutaneous liver biopsy for lesions suspicious for HCC is controversial and is in general not recommended, because the diagnosis can almost always be made confidently based on radiographic criteria: a new nodular-appearing cirrhotic liver that displays arterial enhancement and venous washout. In addition, concerns have been raised about the possibility of bleeding and spread of tumor along the needle track. The risk of these complications is estimated to be around 2% to 5%.[15–19] Other investigators have not observed an increased risk of tumor spread.[20–22] Cases should be considered individually and biopsy may prove useful in cases in which imaging is not diagnostic or even in cases of large liver tumors that would be considered for transplant if the tumor grade was well differentiated.[23] In addition, concerns over sampling bias still remain.[24]

REFERENCES

1. Lavanchy D. Hepatitis B virus epidemiology, disease burden, treatment, and current emerging prevention and control measures. J Viral Hepat 2004;11(2): 97–107.
2. McQuillan GM, Coleman PJ, Kruszon-Moran D, et al. Prevalence of hepatitis B virus infection in the United States: the National Health and Nutrition Examination Surveys. 1976 through 1994. Am J Public Health 1999;89(1):14–8.

3. Mast EE, Margolis HS, Fiore AE, et al. A comprehensive immunization strategy to eliminate transmission of hepatitis B virus in the United States: recommendations of the Advisory Committee on Immunization Practices (ACIP) part I: immunizations of infants, children and adolescents. MMWR Recomm Rep 2005;54(RR-16):1–31.

4. Mast EE, Weinbaum CM, Fiore AE, et al. A comprehensive immunization strategy to eliminate transmission of hepatitis B virus in the United States: recommendations of the Advisory Committee on Immunization Practices (ACIP) part II: immunizations of adults. MMWR Recomm Rep 2006;55(RR-16):1–33.

5. Beasley RP. Hepatitis B virus. The major etiology of hepatocellular carcinoma. Cancer 1988;61(10):1942–56.

6. Bosch FX, Ribes J, Cleries R, et al. Epidemiology of hepatocellular carcinoma. Clin Liver Dis 2005;9(2):191–211.

7. Weinbaum CM, Williams I, Mast EE, et al. Recommendations for identification and public health management of persons with chronic Hepatitis B virus infection. MMWR Recomm Rep 2008;57(RR-8):1–20.

8. Denniston MM, Jiles RB, Drobeniuc J, et al. Chronic hepatitis C virus infection in the United States, National Health and Nutrition Examination Survey 2003 to 2010. Ann Intern Med 2014;160(5):293–300.

9. Smith BD, Morgan RL, Beckett GA, et al. Recommendations for the identification of chronic hepatitis C virus infection among persons born during 1945–1965. MMWR Recomm Rep 2012;61(RR-4):1–32.

10. Schmidt AJ, Falcato L, Zahno B, et al. Prevalence of hepatitis C in a Swiss sample of men who have sex with men: whom to screen for HCV infection? BMC Public Health 2014;14(1):3.

11. Bosch FX, Ribes J, Diaz M, et al. Primary liver cancer: worldwide incidence and trends. Gastroenterology 2004;127:S5–16.

12. Umemura T, Ichijo T, Yoshizawa K, et al. Epidemiology of hepatocellular carcinoma in Japan. J Gastroenterol 2009;44(Suppl 19):102–7.

13. Zhang BH, Yang BH, Tang ZY. Randomized controlled trial of screening for hepatocellular carcinoma. J Cancer Res Clin Oncol 2004;130:417–22.

14. Thompson Coon J, Rogers G, Hewson P, et al. Surveillance of cirrhosis for hepatocellular carcinoma: a cost utility analysis. Br J Cancer 2008;98(1):1166–75.

15. John TG, Garden OJ. Needle track seeding of primary and secondary liver carcinoma after percutaneous liver biopsy. HPB Surg 1993;6(3):199.

16. Durand F, Regimbeau JM, Belghiti J, et al. Assessment of the benefits and risks of percutaneous biopsy before surgical resection of hepatocellular carcinoma. J Hepatol 2001;35(2):254.

17. Huang GT, Sheu JC, Yang PM, et al. Ultrasound-guided cutting biopsy for the diagnosis of hepatocellular carcinoma–a study based on 420 patients. J Hepatol 1996;25(3):334.

18. Kim SH, Lim HK, Lee WJ, et al. Needle-tract implantation in hepatocellular carcinoma: frequency and CT findings after biopsy with a 19.5-gauge automated biopsy gun. Abdom Imaging 2000;25(3):246.

19. Ohlsson B, Nilsson J, Stenram U, et al. Percutaneous fine-needle aspiration cytology in the diagnosis and management of liver tumours. Br J Surg 2002;89(6):757.

20. Bialecki ES, Ezenekwe AM, Brunt EM, et al. Comparison of liver biopsy and noninvasive methods for diagnosis of hepatocellular carcinoma. Clin Gastroenterol Hepatol 2006;4(3):361.

21. Ng KK, Poon RT, Lo CM, et al. Impact of preoperative fine-needle aspiration cyto-logic examination on clinical outcome in patients with hepatocellular carcinoma in a tertiary referral center. Arch Surg 2004;139(2):193.

22. Liu YW, Chen CL, Chen YS, et al. Needle tract implantation of hepatocellular car-cinoma after fine needle biopsy. Dig Dis Sci 2007;52(1):228.

23. DuBay D, Sandroussi C, Sandhu L, et al. Liver transplantation for advanced he-patocellular carcinoma using poor tumor differentiation on biopsy as an exclusion criterion. Ann Surg 2011;253(1):166–72.

24. Pawlik TM, Gleisner AL, Anders RA, et al. Preoperative assessment of hepatocel-lular carcinoma tumor grade using needle biopsy: implications for transplant eligibility. Ann Surg 2007;245(3):435–42.

Prostate Cancer Screening and the Associated Controversy

William Tabayoyong, MD, PhD, Robert Abouassaly, MD, MSc*

KEYWORDS

- Prostate cancer • Prostate specific antigen • Screening

KEY POINTS

- Prostate-specific antigen (PSA) screening has reduced prostate cancer mortality but has also led to overdiagnosis and overtreatment.
- In May 2012 the US Preventive Services Task Force (USPSTF) recommended against prostate cancer screening.
- In response to the USPSTF, professional organizations issued updated guidelines advocating for shared decision making between patients and physicians regarding the risks and benefits of screening.
- Active surveillance is a feasible strategy to reduce the harms of overtreatment.

INTRODUCTION

Extent of Disease

Prostate cancer is the most common cancer diagnosed in males in the United States. In 2014, the American Cancer Society estimated that 233,000 patients would be diagnosed with prostate cancer and that prostate cancer alone would account for 27% of all new incident cases of cancer in men. Prostate cancer is also the second leading cause of cancer death for men with an estimated 29,480 deaths in 2014, accounting for 10% of all male cancer deaths.[1]

Natural History of Prostate Cancer

The aggressiveness of prostate cancer is highly variable and largely depends on initial grade at diagnosis. Patients with a Gleason score of 8 to 10 cancers can progress from localized disease to metastasis and death within a relatively short time period,

Urology Institute, University Hospitals Case Medical Center, 11100 Euclid Avenue, Cleveland, OH 44106, USA
* Corresponding author.
E-mail address: Robert.Abouassaly@UHhospitals.org

Surg Clin N Am 95 (2015) 1023–1039
http://dx.doi.org/10.1016/j.suc.2015.05.001
0039-6109/15/$ – see front matter © 2015 Elsevier Inc. All rights reserved.
surgical.theclinics.com

whereas patients with a Gleason score of 6 or lower disease may never experience symptoms or disease progression and ultimately die of causes other than prostate cancer.[2] In fact, autopsy studies have identified clinically insignificant prostate cancers in up to 75% of men 85 years or older who died of causes other than prostate cancer.[3]

Johansson and colleagues[4–7] have published a series of reports from 1989 to 2013 on a cohort of 223 patients with untreated prostate cancer in Sweden and have documented the trends in disease progression, disease-free survival, and prostate cancer–specific mortality.[8] Importantly, prostate-specific antigen (PSA) was not available at the time the cohort was assembled, so the results of these studies are representative of a population that has not been screened for prostate cancer. Initial findings at 5 and 10 years showed a low mortality rate with disease-specific survivals of 94% and 87%, respectively, suggesting that aggressive treatment was unnecessary for patients with a less than 10-year life expectancy.[4,5] Further follow-up, however, has revealed an increasing prostate cancer mortality rate for men surviving 15 to 20 years after diagnosis.[6,7] The final report encompassing over 30 years of follow-up showed an overall 41% local progression rate, 18% progression to distant metastases, and overall mortality rate of 17% owing to prostate cancer.[8] The mean time to development of metastases was 9.2 years and the mean time to prostate cancer death was 9.5 years.[8] Patients with higher grade disease had higher mortality rates; 55% for a Gleason score of 8 to 10, 23% for a Gleason score of 3 + 4 = 7, and 20% for a Gleason score of 4 + 3 = 7.[8]

Albertsen and colleagues[9,10] published a similar series of reports on a cohort of 767 untreated prostate cancer patients identified in the Connecticut Tumor Registry who were diagnosed with prostate cancer before the availability of PSA. After 15 years of follow-up, men with low-grade Gleason (a score of 2–4 or 5) prostate cancer had low mortality rates ranging between 4% and 7% and 6% and 11%, respectively.[9] Men with Gleason 6 disease had intermediate mortality ranging from 18% to 30%. Regardless of age at presentation, men with Gleason 7 or Gleason 8 to 10 prostate cancer had high mortality rates ranging between 42% to 70% and 60% to 87%, respectively. These trends remained consistent at 20 years of follow-up.[10]

Together, the findings of Johansson and Albertsen and their colleagues demonstrate a high mortality rate for patients with Gleason 7 or higher prostate cancer. Their findings suggest that patients with a life expectancy of greater than 10 years with Gleason 7 or higher prostate cancer would benefit the most from a screening protocol and definitive therapy.

Risk Factors

Age, African-American race, and family history are all significant risk factors for developing prostate cancer. Prostate cancer is a disease that afflicts older men, with the median age of diagnosis at 67 years.[11] African-American males have the highest incidence of prostate cancer with an incident rate 1.6 times higher than that of Caucasian men in the United States, and African-American males also have a 2.4 times greater risk of death from prostate cancer compared with Caucasian males in the United States.[2]

Family history is also an important risk factor for the development of prostate cancer, especially with regard to number of first-degree relatives affected. Men with 1 first-degree relative with prostate cancer have a 2-fold increased lifetime risk of developing prostate cancer. This lifetime risk increases to fourfold if there are 2 first-degree relatives with prostate cancer. Age at diagnosis of first-degree relatives is also important, because the lifetime risk is increased 3-fold if the relative was 60 years of age or younger when diagnosed.[12]

Key points on risk factors

- Prostate cancer is the most common malignancy diagnosed in men and is the second leading cause of cancer death for men in the United States.

- Men with a Gleason score of 7 or higher prostate cancer would benefit the most from a screening protocol and definitive therapy.

- Risk factors for prostate cancer include age, African-American race, and family history.

SCREENING TECHNIQUES AND OPTIONS
Prostate-Specific Antigen

PSA is a serine protease released into the seminal fluid that lyses the seminal fluid protein seminogelin during the process of semen liquefaction.[2,13] Production of PSA is restricted to the prostatic epithelium and transcription of PSA is driven by androgens.[13] PSA levels in the blood are typically low, but can be increased owing to disruption of normal prostatic architecture, which occurs with malignant processes such as cancer or benign processes that include benign prostatic hyperplasia, inflammation, infection, or trauma.[2,13]

PSA was first purified in 1979 and the first assay to detect PSA in human serum was developed in 1980.[14,15] The first commercially available PSA assay was approved by the US Food and Drug Administration (FDA) in 1986.[13] In 1987, Stamey and colleagues[16] demonstrated that increased levels of PSA were associated with advanced clinical stage prostate cancers and that the measured serum PSA level was proportional to the estimated tumor volume, confirming that PSA could be used as a serum marker for prostate cancer. In 1991, Catalona and colleagues[17] reported the first study using serum PSA as a screening test for prostate cancer. Using a PSA cutoff of 4 ng/mL as the trigger for initiating prostate biopsy, Catalona and associates demonstrated that the combination of PSA with digital rectal examination (DRE) was superior to DRE alone for the detection of prostate cancer. Without the addition of PSA, DRE alone would have missed the diagnosis of prostate cancer in 32% of cases. Brawer and colleagues[18] performed a similar study using a PSA cutoff of 4 ng/mL and confirmed that 37.5% of prostate cancer diagnoses would have been missed using DRE alone as the only screening tool. Shortly thereafter, use of PSA for the screening of prostate cancer became widespread in the United States, albeit without the benefit of a large, prospective trial to guide optimal screening strategies.

Impact of Prostate-Specific Antigen Screening on the Epidemiology of Prostate Cancer

The introduction of PSA screening has had a profound impact on the incidence and mortality of prostate cancer.[1,11,19] Prostate cancer incidence increased at a steady rate of approximately 2% per year from 1975 to 1987 (**Fig. 1**).[20] With the widespread introduction of PSA screening in the late 1980s and early 1990s, a dramatic increase in prostate cancer incidence occurred with a peak in 1992, attributed to earlier detection of cases and to detection of cases that would never have been diagnosed or treated. After 1992 the incidence of prostate cancer declined until 1995, attributed to the cull effect resulting from the number of earlier detected cases as a consequence of PSA screening. Incidence then increased at a rate similar to the pre-PSA era until 2001 when rates began trending downward, although there has been considerable fluctuation over recent years, a likely reflection of the variation in use of PSA testing.

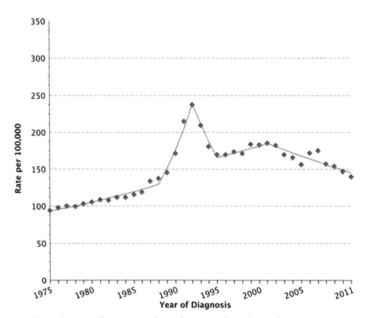

Fig. 1. Age-adjusted Surveillance, Epidemiology, and End Results 9 prostate cancer incidence rates for all ages and races from 1975 to 2011. (*From* Surveillance, Epidemiology, and End Results Program, 1975–2011. National Cancer Institute. 2015. Available at: http://seer.cancer.gov/faststats/selections.php?series=cancer. Accessed January 17, 2015.)

Prostate cancer mortality rates increased slowly between 1975 and the early 1990s with a peak in 1992, and has continued to decline steadily, such that today prostate cancer mortality rates are lower than that observed before the introduction of PSA screening (**Fig. 2**).[1,19–21] In addition, since the introduction of PSA, 5-year survival rates for all races have improved significantly, up to 100% from the years 2003 to 2009 compared with a pre-PSA era rate of just 68% during the years 1975 through 1977.[1] The decline in prostate cancer mortality and improvement in 5-year survival is felt to be due to a combination of factors: PSA screening, a change in the biology of the disease over time, more aggressive treatment of prostate cancer, and attribution of death to causes other than prostate cancer.[22–25] Etzioni and colleagues[26] used 2 mathematical models to quantify the association between PSA screening and prostate cancer mortality trends and demonstrated that PSA screening contributed more than 45% to 70% toward the reduction in mortality outcomes.

In addition to significant changes in prostate cancer incidence and mortality, PSA screening has led to a more favorable pathologic stage migration with a significantly increased proportion of men identified with organ confined disease at the time of diagnosis.[27] From 1984 to 2005, the incidence of men with non–organ-confined prostate cancer decreased from 79.3% to 24.7% and this decrease was largely accounted for by PSA screening, although this decreasing trend in pathologic stage migration has slowed toward the latter years of the PSA era.[28]

PSA screening has also led to a decrease in the mean age at diagnosis from 72.2 years in 1988 and 1989 down to 67.2 years in 2004 and 2005.[29] Compared with 1986, the relative incidence rate of prostate cancer diagnoses in 2005 was 0.56 for men aged 80 years and older, 1.09 in 70- to 79-year-old males, 1.91 in men ages 60 to 69, 3.64 in men aged 50 to 59 years, and 7.23 in men less than 50 years old.[30]

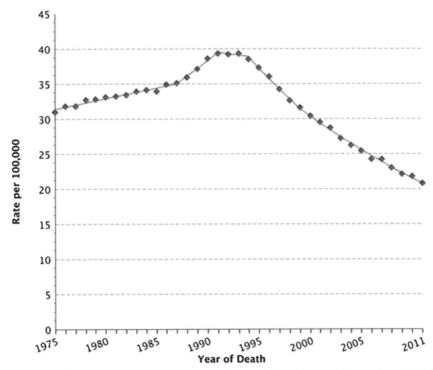

Fig. 2. Age-adjusted US prostate cancer mortality rates for all ages and races from 1975 to 2011. (*From* Surveillance, Epidemiology, and End Results Program, 1975–2011. National Cancer Institute. 2015. Available at: http://seer.cancer.gov/faststats/selections.php?series=cancer. Accessed January 17, 2015.)

Limitations of Prostate-Specific Antigen

Although PSA has been validated as a prostate cancer marker and its use in screening has been well-documented, its greatest limitation is that it is not specific for prostate cancer. Indeed, benign processes such as benign prostatic hyperplasia, acute urinary retention, prostatitis and inflammation, and prostatic trauma can all increase serum PSA levels.[2] The optimal upper limit of the normal range for PSA is unclear, and currently there is no consensus cutoff value for PSA that is specific for prostate cancer. Historically, a PSA value of 4 ng/mL was used as the cutoff to initiate prostate biopsy; however, it has been documented that high-grade cancers are also associated with PSA values of less than 4 ng/mL. For example, Thompson and colleagues[31] reported that, among men with a median age of 72 years, biopsy-proven prostate cancer was detected in 6.6% of men with a PSA of less than 0.5 ng/mL, 10% of men with a PSA between 0.6 and 1 ng/mL, 17% of men with a PSA between 1.1 and 2.0 ng/mL, 24% of men with a PSA between 2.1 and 3.0 ng/mL, and 27% of men with a PSA between 3.1 and 4 ng/mL. A PSA cutoff of 4 ng/mL has a calculated sensitivity of 78.7% and a specificity of 59.2%.[32] Increasing the PSA cutoff to 5 ng/mL achieves an increase in specificity to 95%; however, it decreases the sensitivity to 33% which is inadequate for an effective screening test.[33] PSA concentration is also a poor discriminator of low- and high-risk disease, and clinically insignificant prostate cancer is common.[13] As a result, PSA screening has led to a concern for overdiagnosis and overtreatment of clinically indolent prostate cancers that ultimately pose no harm to the patient and subject men to the morbidity of prostate cancer treatment.

Key points on prostate specific antigen

- Expression of PSA is restricted to the prostatic epithelium and is driven by androgens.
- Malignant processes such as cancer or benign processes that include benign prostatic hyperplasia, inflammation, infection, or trauma can cause increased PSA levels.
- PSA screening has led to a reduction in prostate cancer mortality and a more favorable pathologic stage migration, with more men diagnosed with organ-confined disease.
- PSA screening has led to the overdiagnosis and overtreatment of many cases of clinically insignificant prostate cancer.

CLINICAL OUTCOMES
Prostate Cancer Screening Trials: Prostate, Lung, Colorectal, and Ovarian and European Randomized Study of Screening for Prostate Cancer

Two large, randomized trials assessing the effect of PSA screening on prostate cancer were recently published. The first trial was the Prostate, Lung, Colorectal, and Ovarian (PLCO) cancer screening trial conducted at 10 centers in the United States.[34] The study reported on 76,693 men ages 55 to 74 years old who were randomized to either annual screening or usual care. Men in the screening group were offered annual PSA and DRE, whereas the usual care group served as the control group and received the care offered by their primary care physician. Men with a PSA of greater than 4 ng/mL or a positive DRE were advised to undergo prostate biopsy. In the screening group, compliance rates for PSA testing and DRE were 85% and 86%, respectively. Within the first year, 40% of patients in the control group received PSA screening and by the sixth year, a total of 52% of the patients in the control group received PSA screening. Additionally, 44% of all patients enrolled into the study regardless of group designation had received a baseline PSA screening test before enrollment. After 7 years of follow-up, no difference in prostate cancer mortality between groups was identified, with an incidence of 2.0 deaths per 10,000 person-years (50 deaths) in the screening group and 1.7 deaths per 10,000 person-years (44 deaths) in the control group (rate ratio, 1.13; 95% CI, 0.75–1.70). The PLCO trial results with follow-up extended to 13 years were published recently.[35] These extended follow-up results again demonstrated no significant difference in mortality rates between the screening group and the control group.

The European Randomized Study of Screening for Prostate Cancer (ERSPC) was the second trial, and it included 162,243 men ages 55 to 69 years old from 7 European countries who were randomized to a screening group that was offered PSA screening at an average of once every 4 years or to a control group that was not offered screening.[36] Owing to variation in screening protocols in each country, the PSA cutoff that indicated biopsy was variable. Some protocols initiated ancillary tests such as DRE or transrectal ultrasonography if PSA levels were close to but not exceeding PSA cutoff levels and if those ancillary tests were positive, biopsy was indicated. The compliance rate for PSA testing in the screening group was 82%. Owing to the use of PSA tests outside the protocol assignment in the control group, there was a 20% contamination rate in the control group. The average rate of compliance with biopsy when indicated was 85.8%. After 9 years of follow-up, results demonstrated that PSA-based screening reduced the rate of prostate cancer mortality by 20% (rate ratio, 0.80; 95% CI, 0.65–0.98, adjusted $P = .04$). Additionally, the authors concluded that a total of 1410 men would need to be screened and 48 men would need to be treated to prevent 1 prostate cancer death, suggesting that PSA screening is associated with a high risk of overdiagnosis. Updated ERSPC results with follow-up extended to 11 and 13 years were recently published.[37,38] After 11 years of follow-up, the relative reduction in the risk of death from prostate cancer in the group receiving PSA screening increased to 21%, and the number needed to screen decreased to 1055 and the number needed to treat decreased to 37 to prevent 1 death from prostate cancer. After 13 years of follow-up, the risk reduction of prostate cancer mortality owing to screening increased to 29%, the number needed to screen decreased to 781, and the number needed to treat decreased to 27.

US Preventive Services Task Force 2012 Recommendation

Until 2009, there were no prospective data available to guide the use of PSA screening for prostate cancer, and the results of the PLCO and ERSPC trials were highly anticipated. This was reflected in the guideline statements of many agencies including the US Preventive Services Task Force (USPSTF). The 2008 USPSTF position on prostate cancer screening was that there was insufficient evidence to assess the balance of benefits and harms of screening for prostate cancer in men younger than age 75, although screening was not recommended for men age 75 years or older.[39] After publication of the PLCO and ERSPC data, in May 2012 the USPSTF issued an updated recommendation statement regarding screening for prostate cancer.[40] In this update, the USPSTF gave PSA screening a Grade D recommendation, indicating that the USPSTF recommended against the use of PSA for prostate cancer screening and that they believed with moderate or high certainty that PSA screening had no net benefit or that the harms outweighed the benefits. These recommendations were based largely on the insignificant difference in mortality rate between the screening and usual care group in the PLCO trial and the high numbers needed to screen and treat to prevent 1 prostate cancer death as determined by the ERSPC trial. The USPSTF concluded that PSA-based screening would lead inevitably to a substantial overdiagnosis and overtreatment of men who would have otherwise remained asymptomatic and thus would subject these men unnecessarily to the adverse effects of prostate cancer diagnosis and treatment.

Key points on clinical outcomes

- The PLCO trial did not show a significant reduction in prostate cancer mortality between the screening group and the usual care group.
- The ERSPC trial demonstrated a significantly reduced rate of prostate cancer mortality by 20% after 9 years of follow-up with a number needed to screen of 1410.
- The USPSTF recommended against the use of PSA for prostate cancer screening based on the negative results of the PLCO and the high number needed to screen reported by the ERSPC.

COMPLICATIONS AND CONCERNS
Critique of the US Preventive Services Task Force Recommendation

The USPSTF recommendation against prostate cancer screening was met with criticism from several professional organizations including the American Urologic Association (AUA) and the Society of Urologic Oncology owing to concerns that the recommendation was a disservice to men that could cause more harm than intended.[41,42] Furthermore, analysis of the USPSTF recommendation statement[40] and the USPSTF's evidence review[43] upon which their recommendations were formulated demonstrates that the USPSTF misinterpreted the key data and did not consider appropriately the significant methodologic flaws of the PLCO and ERSPC trials.[44,45] A major argument by the USPSTF was that the PLCO trial failed to demonstrate a significant reduction in prostate cancer mortality in the screened group compared with the control group; however, a critical flaw of the PLCO trial was that it was not a true comparison between a screened population and an unscreened population. Before the study, 44% of all enrollees, regardless of whether they were randomized ultimately into the screening group or the control group, had at least 1 PSA test before enrollment.[34] Furthermore, men in the control group were offered PSA screening by their primary care physicians while enrolled in the control arm of the study at a rate of 40% to 52% per year,[34] and at the conclusion of the trial, 79% of the men in the control arm had received at least 1 PSA test at some point during the trial.[46] In addition, only 41% of the patients in the screening arm with positive PSA values underwent prompt biopsy within 1 year.[47] Overall, the issues with enrollment of a high number of pre-screened participants, the high degree of contamination in the control arm, and the lack of biopsy in a high percentage of PSA positive participants in the screening group impair the ability to conclude definitively from the PLCO data whether PSA screening provides a benefit.[48]

The USPSTF acknowledged that the ERSPC trial at 9 years of follow-up demonstrated a significant reduction in prostate cancer mortality for men in the screening group; however, because the risk of overdiagnosis was as high as 50% and the number needed to screen to prevent 1 prostate cancer death was greater than 1400, the USPSTF ultimately concluded that the risks of overdiagnosis and overtreatment as a result of PSA screening outweighed the benefits of early detection and potential cure.[40] When considering these data, it is important to remember that prostate cancer has a long natural history with greater than 9 years mean time to development of metastases and mean time to prostate cancer death in the absence of prostate cancer screening.[8] Moreover, the introduction of PSA screening has led to an earlier diagnosis of prostate cancers, several years before they would have become apparent clinically, and this lead-time bias due to PSA screening has been estimated to be 11 to 12 years.[49] In light of these facts, the significant decrease in prostate cancer mortality seen at 9 years in the ERSPC trial is even more remarkable. Given the lead-time bias of 11 to 12 years, we should expect that any positive impact of PSA screening on prostate cancer mortality will become more evident with further follow-up. This is indeed what has occurred, with the 11- and 13-year ERSPC results showing continued improvement in the risk reduction of prostate cancer mortality and continued decrease in the number needed to screen to prevent 1 prostate cancer death.[37,38] At 13 years of follow-up, the number needed to screen decreased to 781, a 45% reduction from the original 1410 reported at 9 years.[36,38] This new number compares favorably with breast and colon cancers, 2 malignancies for which screening is encouraged by the USPSTF.[50,51] For example, the number of women ages 50 to 59 years needed to screen with mammography to prevent 1 death from breast cancer was 1339, and the number needed to screen to prevent 1 death from colon cancer with the Hemoccult fecal occult blood test was 1173.[50,52]

Another important prostate cancer screening trial that was largely ignored by the USPSTF was the Göteborg trial. The Göteborg trial was an independent Swedish trial conceived and initiated before the ERSPC trial. It included 20,000 men ages 50 to 64 years old who were randomized to a screening group that was offered PSA screening every 2 years until the age of 69 or to a control group that was not offered screening.[53] Men ages 55 to 64 were eventually included in the ERSPC analysis, but the men ages 50 to 54 were excluded. Despite the addition of a subset of the Göteborg trial participants to the ERSPC, the overall results of the entire Göteborg trial were always planned to be reported separately. The initial PSA cutoff value that initiated DRE and transrectal ultrasound-guided prostate biopsy was 3.4 ng/mL. In 1999, this value was decreased to 2.9 ng/mL to achieve consistency with other ERSPC sites, and decreased again to 2.5 ng/mL in 2005 to account for a change in the assay calibrator. The compliance rate for PSA testing in the screening group was 76% and the average rate of compliance with biopsy was 93%. The estimated rate of prescreening before initiation of the trial was only 3% and contamination of the control group was negligible, in comparison with the 20% contamination in the ERSPC trial and the 50% contamination in the PLCO trial. After 14 years of follow-up, PSA-based screening reduced significantly the rate of prostate cancer mortality by 44% (rate ratio, 0.56; 95% CI, 0.39–0.82, $P = .002$). Additionally, the authors concluded that a total of 293 men would need to be screened and 12 men would need to be treated to prevent 1 prostate cancer death.

Impact of the US Preventive Services Task Force Recommendation

Before the adoption of PSA screening, the majority of prostate cancers were diagnosed at an advanced stage and were fatal.[54] Using current population data, Scosyrev and colleagues[55] estimated that without the benefit of PSA screening, the total number of men presenting with metastatic prostate cancer would be approximately 3 times greater than the actual number observed. This raises concerns that abandoning PSA screening as suggested by the USPSTF will result in a high number of prostate cancer deaths that could be prevented. Indeed, Gulati and colleagues[56] used statistical models to predict prostate cancer incidence and mortality rates for the period from 2013 through 2025 if PSA screening was discontinued. The models predicted that although discontinued screening eliminated all cases of overdiagnosis, it also failed to prevent 100% of avoidable cancer deaths.

Several recent studies have evaluated the impact of the USPSTF recommendation statement on the use of PSA screening. After the release of the USPSTF recommendations, Aslani and colleagues[57] demonstrated a dramatic decrease in the number of screening tests performed in academic and community hospitals in Northeastern Ohio, and Cohn and colleagues[58] reported that fewer PSA tests were being ordered by primary care providers. Bhindi and colleagues[59] took the analysis 1 step further and examined biopsy and cancer detection rates. They found a significant decrease in the number of first-time biopsies as a result of PSA screening from 42.5 per month in the year preceding the USPSTF recommendations to 24 per month in the year after the recommendation statement was issued. In addition, there was a significant decrease in the number of Gleason score 7 to 10 prostate cancers detected per month, suggesting that several cases of clinically significant prostate cancer were going undiagnosed and that opportunities for early intervention and cure were being missed. In contrast, Perez and colleagues[60] found no significant decrease in the number of patients referred for evaluation of elevated PSA to a tertiary center in New York in the year before or the year after the USPSTF recommendation was released. The differences in these studies may reflect differences in practice patterns and application of new guidelines in different geographic regions.

It is also important to emphasize that patients' perceptions of prostate cancer screening are influenced by the USPSTF recommendations. A recent patient survey demonstrated that a majority of patients were in favor of prostate cancer screening; however after reading a document based on AUA patient education materials in favor of screening and then reading another document based on patient education materials from the USPSTF opposing screening, 13% of patients changed their minds and adopted a less favorable opinion of screening.[61]

Addressing the Concerns: Strategies to Prevent Overdiagnosis and Overtreatment

Overdiagnosis is the detection of a clinically insignificant prostate cancer owing to PSA screening that would not have caused any morbidity or mortality in the patient's lifetime had the patient not been screened.[48] Despite the limitations of PSA that it is not specific for prostate cancer and that it can not discriminate between low-grade versus high-grade disease, data from the Malmö Preventive Medicine Study show that an early baseline PSA value could risk stratify patients into high- or low-risk groups.[62–65] The Malmö Preventive Medicine Study was a Swedish population based study on cardiovascular risk factors from 1974 to 1986. It included 21,277 men ages 27 to 52 years who gave a blood sample at baseline. Participants' records were then linked to the cancer registry at the National Board of Health and Welfare in Sweden to identify men diagnosed with incident prostate cancer. PSA levels in archived, previously unthawed anticoagulated blood samples obtained at baseline from participants were then analyzed retrospectively. Importantly, the Malmö Preventive Medicine cohort was enrolled before the PSA era and there was no subsequent recommendation for prostate cancer screening in this region; therefore, this cohort provides a natural experiment for investigating the association between PSA and long-term prostate cancer outcomes.[62,65] Using these data, Ulmert and colleagues[62] and Lilja and colleagues[63] demonstrated that a baseline PSA value obtained between the ages of 44 and 50 years could estimate the probability of developing clinically significant prostate cancer by the age of 75. Their analyses showed that men between the ages of 44 and 50 years with a total PSA ranging between 0.5 and 1 ng/mL had the same low risk of developing advanced prostate cancer as the general population with a mean risk of 3.5%; however, for men with a PSA of 2 ng/mL or greater the risk of developing advanced prostate cancer increased to 12%, more than 3 times the population mean. Similarly, Vickers and colleagues[64] demonstrated that a single PSA value at the age of 60 years could predict the development of prostate cancer metastases or death by the age of 85, with 90% of prostate cancer deaths occurring in men that had a PSA of more than 2 ng/mL at the age of 60. Furthermore, men with a PSA of less than 1 ng/mL at the age of 60 had a 0.5% probability of developing prostate cancer and a 0.2% risk of dying from prostate cancer at the age of 85. Taken together, these data demonstrate that a baseline PSA between the ages of 44 and 50 and a follow-up screen at 60 years could help to stratify patients into low- and high-risk groups for developing clinically significant prostate cancer. Using this strategy, men at high risk could be offered more rigorous screening and treatment and men at low risk could be spared the risks and harms of prostate biopsy, overdiagnosis, and unnecessary treatment.

The primary harm of overdiagnosis is unnecessary treatment, or overtreatment. The potential harms of prostate cancer overtreatment include impotence, incontinence, and death for radical prostatectomy, and impotence, urgency, painful defecation, radiation enteritis, and an increased risk of secondary malignancy for radiotherapy.[30] An alternate treatment strategy aimed to reduce overtreatment of patients diagnosed with low-risk prostate cancer is active surveillance, which involves deferring definitive therapy in favor of continued observation with routine follow-up PSA tests and prostate biopsies and proceeding toward definitive treatment only if there is evidence of disease progression.[66] Several recent trials have reported on the feasibility of active surveillance as an effective treatment alternative for men with low-risk prostate cancer. Roemeling and colleagues[67] reported that for 278 men under active surveillance with a median follow-up of 3.4 years, overall survival was 89% after 8 years and cause-specific survival was 100%. Similarly, Soloway and colleagues[68] also reported a 100% cause specific survival for 99 men undergoing active surveillance at a median follow-up of 45 months, with a probability that 85% of men would remain treatment free at 5 years. The outcomes of the largest active surveillance cohort with the longest follow-up were published recently by Klotz and colleagues.[66] This was a study of 993 men with a median follow-up of 6.4 years, including more than 200 patients with greater than 10 years of follow-up and 50 patients with greater than 15 years of follow-up. The 10- and 15-year cause-specific survivals in this cohort were 98% and 94%, respectively. At 5, 10, and 15 years, 75.7%, 63.5%, and 55% of patients remained untreated and on active surveillance, respectively. For those men who ultimately had disease progression and required definitive therapy, the 5- and 10-year post-treatment recurrence-free survivals were 77% and 60%, respectively. These values compare favorably with the 5-year recurrence-free survival of 81% and the 10 year recurrence-free survival of 66% reported for men treated promptly with radical prostatectomy who would have been candidates for active surveillance.[69] Overall, these data suggest that active surveillance can reduce overtreatment by almost 50% at 15 years and that men on active surveillance are not at immediate risk of death from prostate cancer if definitive therapy is deferred until signs of disease progression are observed.

Professional Organizations' Recommendations

After publication of the PLCO and ERSPC trials and in response to the USPSTF 2012 PSA recommendation statement, the AUA and other professional organizations including the American College of Physicians (ACP), the American Society of Clinical Oncology (ASCO), and the National Comprehensive Cancer Network (NCCN) updated their guidelines regarding prostate cancer screening. In a departure from their 2009 Best Practice Statement where yearly PSA screening was advocated for all men starting at the age of 40,[70] the 2013 AUA Early Detection of Prostate Cancer Guidelines recommend against screening for men under age 40 years, for men at average risk of developing prostate cancer age 40 to 54 years, and for men older than 70 years or any man with less than a 10- to 15-year life expectancy.[71] Men at average risk were defined as men who did not have a family history of prostate cancer or men who are not of African-American race. For men ages 55 to 69 years, the AUA advocates for shared decision making between the patient and physician with appropriate discussion of the risks and benefits involved with PSA screening. The theme of shared decision making introduced by the AUA is echoed in both the 2013 ACP Guidelines and the 2012 ASCO Guidelines, with the only differences being that the ACP recommends shared decision making for patients ages 50 to 69 years and the ASCO limits its recommendation to men with a greater than 10-year life expectancy.[72,73] The ACP does not recommend screening for men under 50 years of age, and similar to the AUA, the ACP and ASCO guidelines do not recommend screening for men older than 69 years of age or with less than a 10- to 15-year life expectancy. In contrast, the 2014 NCCN guidelines continue to advocate that a baseline PSA be available to men aged 45 to 49 years, that a baseline PSA should be offered to men aged 50 to 70 years, and that PSA testing should be individualized only when patients reach 70 years of age depending on life expectancy,[74] a strategy supported by data from the Malmö Preventive Medicine Study discussed.

Future Directions

Current efforts are underway to identify new biomarkers that can supplement or replace PSA as a screening test for prostate cancer. One promising test is the Prostate Health Index (PHI). The PHI is a new formula that combines all 3 known isoforms of

PSA (total PSA, free PSA, and p2PSA) into a single score.[75] PHI is calculated using the following formula: ([-2]proPSA/free PSA) × $\sqrt{PSA}$. In a large, multicenter trial to evaluate the utility of PHI for prostate cancer detection in 892 men undergoing prostate biopsy with total PSA levels from 2 to 10 ng/mL and normal DRE, PHI demonstrated a greater specificity for distinguishing prostate cancer on biopsy compared with PSA or percentage free PSA.[75] PHI has been approved recently by the FDA and is available now commercially in the United States.

Another promising test is the 4 Kallikrein (4K) Score Test. The 4K Score Test is a statistical algorithm that uses blood levels of 4 kallikrein markers—total PSA, free PSA, intact PSA, and kallikrein-related peptidase 2—to predict the presence of clinically significant prostate cancer.[76] In a recent cohort study of 392 men who previously had received radical prostatectomy, archived blood was thawed and assayed for the 4 kallikrein markers. The calculated 4K score demonstrated good accuracy distinguishing pathologically insignificant from aggressive disease on radical prostatectomy specimens with an area under the curve of 0.84.[76]

These novel biomarkers show great promise in their potential to improve prostate cancer screening and reduce overdiagnosis; however, their utility must first be validated in large, prospective trials to avoid the controversial fate of PSA.

Key points on complications and concerns

- Some believe that the USPSTF misinterpreted key data and overlooked critical flaws of the PLCO and ERSPC when formulating their recommendation statement.
- The PLCO trial was not a true comparison between a screened group and a nonscreened control group as contamination in the control group was as high as 50%.
- ERSPC data with follow-up out to 13 years show continued improvement in the risk reduction of prostate cancer mortality and continued decline in the number needed to screen to prevent one prostate cancer death.
- The Göteborg trial was not hampered by the flaws of the PLCO or ERSCP and after 14 years of follow-up, PSA-based screening significantly reduced the rate of prostate cancer mortality by 44%. The number needed to screen to prevent 1 cancer death was 293, which compares favorably to breast cancer and colorectal cancer, 2 malignancies for which the USPSTF encourages screening.
- The use of PSA for prostate cancer screening has not been altogether abandoned; however, its use has dramatically reduced since the release of the USPSTF recommendation statement in 2012.
- Complete abandonment of PSA screening will eliminate all cases of overdiagnosis, but will also fail to prevent 100% of avoidable cancer deaths.
- A baseline PSA between ages 44 and 50 and a follow-up screen at 60 years could help to stratify patients into low- or high-risk groups for developing clinically significant prostate cancer.
- Active surveillance is a feasible strategy to reduce the harms of overtreatment.
- The AUA, ACP, and ASCO advocate for shared decision making between patient and physician with appropriate discussion of the risks and benefits involved with PSA screening.
- The PHI and 4K are promising novel prostate cancer biomarkers.

SUMMARY

PSA screening has decreased prostate cancer mortality; however, there is concern that PSA screening has led to overdiagnosis and overtreatment of clinically insignificant prostate cancers. The USPSTF recently released a controversial statement recommending against the use of PSA for prostate cancer screening. Prostate cancer is the most common malignancy diagnosed in men and is the second leading cause of cancer death for men in the United States, accounting for 30,000 deaths per year. Abandoning PSA screening would be a disservice to these men and would result in failure to prevent avoidable cancer deaths. In response to the USPSTF, the AUA and other professional organizations have acknowledged the high rate of overdiagnosis and overtreatment and now advocate for shared decision making between patient and physician regarding the risks and benefits of screening. Currently, active surveillance is a feasible strategy to reduce overtreatment without compromising the therapeutic window and chance for cure. Future efforts should emphasize strategies to distinguish between clinically insignificant and aggressive prostate cancers so that definitive therapy can be disseminated appropriately.

REFERENCES

1. Siegel R, Ma J, Zou Z, et al. Cancer statistics, 2014. CA Cancer J Clin 2014;64(1): 9–29.
2. Gjertson CK, Albertsen PC. Use and assessment of PSA in prostate cancer. Med Clin North Am 2011;95(1):191–200.
3. Sakr WA, Haas GP, Cassin BF, et al. The frequency of carcinoma and intraepithelial neoplasia of the prostate in young male patients. J Urol 1993;150(2 Pt 1): 379–85.
4. Johansson JE, Adami HO, Andersson SO, et al. Natural history of localised prostatic cancer. A population-based study in 223 untreated patients. Lancet 1989; 1(8642):799–803.
5. Johansson JE, Adami HO, Andersson SO, et al. High 10-year survival rate in patients with early, untreated prostatic cancer. JAMA 1992;267(16):2191–6.
6. Johansson JE, Holmberg L, Johansson S, et al. Fifteen-year survival in prostate cancer. A prospective, population-based study in Sweden. JAMA 1997;277(6): 467–71.
7. Johansson JE, Andrén O, Andersson SO, et al. Natural history of early, localized prostate cancer. JAMA 2004;291(22):2713–9.
8. Popiolek M, Rider JR, Andrén O, et al. Natural history of early, localized prostate cancer: a final report from three decades of follow-up. Eur Urol 2013;63(3): 428–35.
9. Albertsen PC, Hanley JA, Gleason DF, et al. Competing risk analysis of men aged 55 to 74 years at diagnosis managed conservatively for clinically localized prostate cancer. JAMA 1998;280(11):975–80.
10. Albertsen PC, Hanley JA, Fine J. 20-year outcomes following conservative management of clinically localized prostate cancer. JAMA 2005;293(17):2095–101.
11. Brawley OW. Prostate cancer epidemiology in the United States. World J Urol 2012;30(2):195–200.
12. Bratt O. Hereditary prostate cancer: clinical aspects. J Urol 2002;168(3):906–13.
13. Lilja H, Ulmert D, Vickers AJ. Prostate-specific antigen and prostate cancer: prediction, detection and monitoring. Nat Rev Cancer 2008;8(4):268–78.
14. Wang MC, Valenzuela LA, Murphy GP, et al. Purification of a human prostate specific antigen. Invest Urol 1979;17(2):159–63.
15. Kuriyama M, Wang MC, Papsidero LD, et al. Quantitation of prostate-specific antigen in serum by a sensitive enzyme immunoassay. Cancer Res 1980;40(12): 4658–62.

16. Stamey TA, Yang N, Hay AR, et al. Prostate-specific antigen as a serum marker for adenocarcinoma of the prostate. N Engl J Med 1987;317(15):909–16.

17. Catalona WJ, Smith DS, Ratliff TL, et al. Measurement of prostate-specific antigen in serum as a screening test for prostate cancer. N Engl J Med 1991;324(17): 1156–61.

18. Brawer MK, Chetner MP, Beatie J, et al. Screening for prostatic carcinoma with prostate specific antigen. J Urol 1992;147(3 Pt 2):841–5.

19. Merrill RM, Stephenson RA. Trends in mortality rates in patients with prostate cancer during the era of prostate specific antigen screening. J Urol 2000;163(2): 503–10.

20. National Cancer Institute, Surveillance, Epidemiology, and End Results Program. 2015. Available at: http://seer.cancer.gov/faststats/selections.php?series=cancer. Accessed January 17, 2015.

21. Tarone RE, Chu KC, Brawley OW. Implications of stage-specific survival rates in assessing recent declines in prostate cancer mortality rates. Epidemiology 2000; 11(2):167–70.

22. Etzioni R, Legler JM, Feuer EJ, et al. Cancer surveillance series: interpreting trends in prostate cancer–part III: Quantifying the link between population prostate-specific antigen testing and recent declines in prostate cancer mortality. J Natl Cancer Inst 1999;91(12):1033–9.

23. Walsh PC. Cancer surveillance series: interpreting trends in prostate cancer–part I: evidence of the effects of screening in recent prostate cancer incidence, mortality, and survival rates. J Urol 2000;163(1):364–5.

24. Feuer EJ, Merrill RM, Hankey BF. Cancer surveillance series: interpreting trends in prostate cancer–part II: cause of death misclassification and the recent rise and fall in prostate cancer mortality. J Natl Cancer Inst 1999;91(12):1025–32.

25. Etzioni R, Gulati R, Tsodikov A, et al. The prostate cancer conundrum revisited: treatment changes and prostate cancer mortality declines. Cancer 2012; 118(23):5955–63.

26. Etzioni R, Tsodikov A, Mariotto A, et al. Quantifying the role of PSA screening in the US prostate cancer mortality decline. Cancer Causes Control 2008;19(2): 175–81.

27. Catalona WJ, Smith DS, Ratliff TL, et al. Detection of organ-confined prostate cancer is increased through prostate-specific antigen-based screening. JAMA 1993; 270(8):948–54.

28. Dong F, Reuther AM, Magi-Galluzzi C, et al. Pathologic stage migration has slowed in the late PSA era. Urology 2007;70(5):839–42.

29. Li J, Djenaba JA, Soman A, et al. Recent trends in prostate cancer incidence by age, cancer stage, and grade, the United States, 2001-2007. Prostate Cancer 2012;2012:691380.

30. Welch HG, Albertsen PC. Prostate cancer diagnosis and treatment after the introduction of prostate-specific antigen screening: 1986-2005. J Natl Cancer Inst 2009;101(19):1325–9.

31. Thompson IM, Pauler DK, Goodman PJ, et al. Prevalence of prostate cancer among men with a prostate-specific antigen level < or =4.0 ng per milliliter. N Engl J Med 2004;350(22):2239–46.

32. Carter HB, Pearson JD, Metter EJ, et al. Longitudinal evaluation of prostate-specific antigen levels in men with and without prostate disease. JAMA 1992; 267(16):2215–20.

33. Holmstrom B, Johansson M, Bergh A, et al. Prostate specific antigen for early detection of prostate cancer: longitudinal study. BMJ 2009;339:b3537.

34. Andriole GL, Crawford ED, Grubb RL 3rd, et al. Mortality results from a randomized prostate-cancer screening trial. N Engl J Med 2009;360(13):1310–9.
35. Andriole GL, Crawford ED, Grubb RL 3rd, et al. Prostate cancer screening in the randomized Prostate, Lung, Colorectal, and Ovarian Cancer Screening Trial: mortality results after 13 years of follow-up. J Natl Cancer Inst 2012;104(2):125–32.
36. Schroder FH, Hugosson J, Roobol MJ, et al. Screening and prostate-cancer mortality in a randomized European study. N Engl J Med 2009;360(13):1320–8.
37. Schroder FH, Hugosson J, Roobol MJ, et al. Prostate-cancer mortality at 11 years of follow-up. N Engl J Med 2012;366(11):981–90.
38. Schroder FH, Hugosson J, Roobol MJ, et al. Screening and prostate cancer mortality: results of the European Randomised Study of Screening for Prostate Cancer (ERSPC) at 13 years of follow-up. Lancet 2014;384(9959):2027–35.
39. U.S. Preventive Services Task Force. Screening for prostate cancer: U.S. Preventive Services Task Force recommendation statement. Ann Intern Med 2008; 149(3):185–91.
40. Moyer VA, U.S. Preventive Services Task Force. Screening for prostate cancer: U.S. Preventive Services Task Force recommendation statement. Ann Intern Med 2012;157(2):120–34.
41. AUA Health Policy Brief, AUA Response to USPSTF PSA Recommendations. 2011. Available at: http://www.auanet.org/advnews/hpbrief/view.cfm?i=649&a=1806. Accessed January 17, 2015.
42. Messing E, Albertson P, Andriole GL Jr, et al. SUO's response to the USPSTF. 2011. Available at: http://suonet.org/news/SUO%20precon%20news%202011.pdf. Accessed January 17, 2015.
43. Chou R, Croswell JM, Dana T, et al. Screening for prostate cancer: a review of the evidence for the U.S. Preventive Services Task Force. Ann Intern Med 2011; 155(11):762–71.
44. Cooperberg MR. Implications of the new AUA guidelines on prostate cancer detection in the U.S. Curr Urol Rep 2014;15(7):420.
45. Catalona WJ, D'Amico AV, Fitzgibbons WF, et al. What the U.S. Preventive Services Task Force missed in its prostate cancer screening recommendation. Ann Intern Med 2012;157(2):137–8.
46. Pinsky PF, Blacka A, Kramer BS, et al. Assessing contamination and compliance in the prostate component of the Prostate, Lung, Colorectal, and Ovarian (PLCO) Cancer Screening Trial. Clin Trials 2010;7(4):303–11.
47. Pinsky PF, Andriole GL, Kramer BS, et al. Prostate biopsy following a positive screen in the prostate, lung, colorectal and ovarian cancer screening trial. J Urol 2005;173(3):746–50 [discussion: 750–1].
48. Etzioni RD, Thompson IM. What do the screening trials really tell us and where do we go from here? Urol Clin North Am 2014;41(2):223–8.
49. Draisma G, De Koning HJ. MISCAN: estimating lead-time and over-detection by simulation. BJU Int 2003;92(Suppl 2):106–11.
50. US Preventive Services Task Force. Screening for breast cancer: U.S. Preventive Services Task Force recommendation statement. Ann Intern Med 2009;151(10): 716–26, W-236.
51. U.S. Preventive Services Task Force. Screening for colorectal cancer: U.S. Preventive Services Task Force recommendation statement. Ann Intern Med 2008; 149(9):627–37.
52. Towler B, Irwig L, Glasziou P, et al. A systematic review of the effects of screening for colorectal cancer using the faecal occult blood test, Hemoccult. BMJ 1998; 317(7158):559–65.

53. Hugosson J, Carlsson S, Aus G, et al. Mortality results from the Goteborg randomised population-based prostate-cancer screening trial. Lancet Oncol 2010; 11(8):725–32.

54. Ganz PA, Barry JM, Burke W, et al. National Institutes of Health State-of-the-Science Conference: role of active surveillance in the management of men with localized prostate cancer. Ann Intern Med 2012;156(8):591–5.

55. Scosyrev E, Wu G, Mohile S, et al. Prostate-specific antigen screening for prostate cancer and the risk of overt metastatic disease at presentation: analysis of trends over time. Cancer 2012;118(23):5768–76.

56. Gulati R, Tsodikov A, Etzioni R, et al. Expected population impacts of discontinued prostate-specific antigen screening. Cancer 2014;120(22):3519–26.

57. Aslani A, Minnillo BJ, Johnson B, et al. The impact of recent screening recommendations on prostate cancer screening in a large health care system. J Urol 2014;191(6):1737–42.

58. Cohn JA, Wang CE, Lakeman JC, et al. Primary care physician PSA screening practices before and after the final U.S. Preventive Services Task Force recommendation. Urol Oncol 2014;32(1):41.e23–30.

59. Bhindi B, Mamdani M, Kulkarni GS, et al. Impact of the U.S. Preventive Services Task Force Recommendations Against PSA Screening on Prostate Biopsy and Cancer Detection Rates. J Urol 2015;193(5):1519–24.

60. Perez TY, Danzig MR, Ghandour RA, et al. Impact of the 2012 United States Preventive Services Task Force statement on prostate-specific antigen screening: analysis of urologic and primary care practices. Urology 2015;85(1):85–91.

61. Maurice MJ, Abouassaly R. Patient opinions on prostate cancer screening are swayed by the United States Preventative Services Task Force recommendations. Urology 2014;84(2):295–9.

62. Ulmert D, Cronin AM, Björk T, et al. Prostate-specific antigen at or before age 50 as a predictor of advanced prostate cancer diagnosed up to 25 years later: a case-control study. BMC Med 2008;6:6.

63. Lilja H, Cronin AM, Dahlin A, et al. Prediction of significant prostate cancer diagnosed 20 to 30 years later with a single measure of prostate-specific antigen at or before age 50. Cancer 2011;117(6):1210–9.

64. Vickers AJ, Cronin AM, Björk T, et al. Prostate specific antigen concentration at age 60 and death or metastasis from prostate cancer: case-control study. BMJ 2010;341:c4521.

65. Vickers AJ, Ulmert D, Sjoberg DD, et al. Strategy for detection of prostate cancer based on relation between prostate specific antigen at age 40-55 and long term risk of metastasis: case-control study. BMJ 2013;346:f2023.

66. Klotz L, Vesprini D, Sethukavalan P, et al. Long-term follow-up of a large active surveillance cohort of patients with prostate cancer. J Clin Oncol 2015;33(3):272–7.

67. Roemeling S, Roobol MJ, de Vries SH, et al. Active surveillance for prostate cancers detected in three subsequent rounds of a screening trial: characteristics, PSA doubling times, and outcome. Eur Urol 2007;51(5):1244–50 [discussion: 1251].

68. Soloway MS, Soloway CT, Williams S, et al. Active surveillance; a reasonable management alternative for patients with prostate cancer: the Miami experience. BJU Int 2008;101(2):165–9.

69. Kane CJ, Im R, Amling CL, et al. Outcomes after radical prostatectomy among men who are candidates for active surveillance: results from the SEARCH database. Urology 2010;76(3):695–700.

70. Greene KL, Albertsen PC, Babaian RJ, et al. Prostate specific antigen best practice statement: 2009 update. J Urol 2009;182(5):2232–41.

71. Carter HB, Albertsen PC, Barry MJ, et al. Early detection of prostate cancer: AUA Guideline. J Urol 2013;190(2):419–26.
72. Qaseem A, Barry MJ, Denberg TD, et al. Screening for prostate cancer: a guidance statement from the Clinical Guidelines Committee of the American College of Physicians. Ann Intern Med 2013;158(10):761–9.
73. Basch E, Oliver TK, Vickers A, et al. Screening for prostate cancer with prostate-specific antigen testing: American Society of Clinical Oncology Provisional Clinical Opinion. J Clin Oncol 2012;30(24):3020–5.
74. Carroll PR, Parsons JK, Andriole G, et al. Prostate cancer early detection, version 1.2014. Featured updates to the NCCN Guidelines. J Natl Compr Cancer Netw 2014;12(9):1211–9 [quiz: 1219].
75. Loeb S, Catalona WJ. The Prostate Health Index: a new test for the detection of prostate cancer. Ther Adv Urol 2014;6(2):74–7.
76. Carlsson S, Maschino A, Schröder F, et al. Predictive value of four kallikrein markers for pathologically insignificant compared with aggressive prostate cancer in radical prostatectomy specimens: results from the European Randomized Study of Screening for Prostate Cancer section Rotterdam. Eur Urol 2013;64(5): 693–9.

Screening for Pancreatic Cancer

Keita Wada, MD, PhD[a], Kyoichi Takaori, MD, PhD, FMAS(H)[b],*, L. William Traverso, MD[c]

KEYWORDS

- Familial pancreatic cancer • Pancreatic cancer • Pancreatic intraepithelial neoplasia
- Intraductal papillary mucinous neoplasm • Screening

KEY POINTS

- Neither extended resection nor extended indication for surgical resection alone improves survival of patients with pancreatic cancer.
- Early detection followed by resection of pancreatic cancer at an early stage, preferably before invasion, is the optimal chance for a cure.
- High-grade pancreatic intraepithelial neoplasia (PanIN) and intraductal papillary mucinous neoplasm (IPMN) are the targets for early detection of pancreatic cancer.
- Screening of pancreatic cancer is practical and cost-effective only in high-risk individuals, including familial pancreatic cancer kindred, multiple genetic syndrome (eg, Peutz-Jeghers syndrome), familial atypical multiple mole melanoma, hereditary pancreatitis, Lynch syndrome, and so forth.
- Screening in high-risk individuals with endoscopic ultrasound and MRI may lead to detection of lobular atrophy or localized fibrosis associated with PanIN and cystic lesions and duct dilatation associated with IPMN.
- Surgical treatments for high-grade PanIN are not well established at this time, whereas clinical management of IPMN is commonly based on the existing consensus guidelines.

INTRODUCTION

Pancreatic cancer (PC) is becoming, more and more, a serious health problem worldwide. In 2014, it was estimated that there were 337,872 newly diagnosed patients with PC in the world and 330,391 patients died of the disease in the same year.[1] In the United States, as many as 39,590 patients died of PC, making it the fourth most common cause of death.[2] Unfortunately, the incidence of PC is increasing year by year in the most developed countries, including the United States and Japan. Furthermore,

[a] Department of Surgery, Teikyo University School of Medicine, 2-11-1 Kaga, Itabashi-ku, Tokyo 173-8605, Japan; [b] Division of Hepato-Biliary-Pancreatic Surgery and Transplantation, Department of Surgery, Kyoto University Graduate School of Medicine, 54 Kawahara-cho, Shogoin, Sakyo-ku, Kyoto 606-5807, Japan; [c] St. Luke's Center for Pancreatic and Liver Disease, 100 E, Idaho St, Boise, ID 83712, USA
* Corresponding author.
E-mail address: takaori@kuhp.kyoto-u.ac.jp

Surg Clin N Am 95 (2015) 1041–1052
http://dx.doi.org/10.1016/j.suc.2015.05.010
0039-6109/15/$ – see front matter © 2015 Elsevier Inc. All rights reserved.
surgical.theclinics.com

PC is also emerging as a serious health problem in developing countries. Even more devastating is that the mortality, as high as 98% according to the worldwide statistics, remains essentially unchanged despite the tremendous efforts to cure PC.[1]

Surgery is commonly cited as the only chance for cure although a larger proportion of patients with PC are deemed unresectable due to systemic metastasis and/or local involvements at the time of presentation. Concerned surgeons have advocated extended resection, including retroperitoneal tissue clearing and en bloc resection of the nerve plexus around the superior mesenteric artery.[3–5] However, these attempts have completely failed as affirmed by all randomized control trials carried out in the United States, Japan, and Korea.[6–9] The subjects did not survive any longer but suffered from intractable diarrhea after extended resection. Another attempt, by surgeons, to improve survival of patients with PC was extending the indication for surgical resections. En bloc resection of portal vein is now practicable owing to the introduction of safe techniques for vascular reconstruction and certainly extends the indication. The outcome of portal vein resection seems to be satisfactory according to data from the PC registry of the Japan Pancreas Society (JPS).[10] However, there is no concrete evidence that portal vein resection improves survival outcomes. Further attempts to remove a major artery, as in a distal pancreatectomy with celiac artery resection, may extend the surgical indication but has failed to demonstrate prolonged survival.[11] These findings imply that those patients with locally extended tumor are also metastatic and that local therapy by surgery alone does not help them. According to autopsy studies, approximately 90% of patients with PC, including resectable and unresectable, at the time of manifestation are metastatic.[12,13] Even in patients who are eligible for resection, 80% die with metastatic recurrence. Therefore, although it is true that surgical resection may allow a chance for cure, it should be acknowledged that few patients do not have metastatic disease at the onset.

In reality, most patients with PC are diagnosed late with metastatic and/or locally advanced disease. Therefore, the best way to improve the cure rate is to screen the individuals at a risk of developing PC and detect earlier disease or precursors, which are curable by surgical resection. In this article, the state-of-the-art of screening for PC is reviewed and the best management for patients at a high-risk of developing PC is discussed.

HOW EARLY DOES PANCREATIC CANCER HAVE TO BE DETECTED FOR CURE?

PC smaller than 2 cm is associated with significantly better survival compared with that larger than 2 cm. However, even the tumors less than 2 cm are often associated with distant metastasis and dismal prognosis.[14] The 5-year survival in patients with PC smaller than 1 cm in historic studies did not reach 50%,[15,16] suggesting that invasion process of PC may occur when it is even smaller than 1 cm. This implies the need to detect PC in its process before invasion to achieve absolute cure.

TARGET LESIONS

It is now believed that most PC arises from pancreatic intraepithelial neoplasia (PanIN). PanIN lesions are presently classified into PanIN-1A, PanIN-1B, PanIN-2, and PanIN-3. Briefly, PanIN-1A and PanIN-1B are proliferative lesions without remarkable nuclear abnormality of flat and papillary architectures, respectively. PanIN-3 is associated with severe architectural and cytonuclear abnormalities but invasion through the basement membrane is absent. PanIN-2 is an intermediate category between PanIN-1 and PanIN-3 and associated with a moderate degree of architectural and cytonuclear abnormality. Alternatively, PanINs may be classified into 2 categories of low-grade PanIN and high-grade PanIN. PanIN lesions harbor stepwise accumulations of genetic abnormalities that are identified in PC (**Fig. 1**).[17] Point mutations of K-RAS at codon 12, inactivation of p16 (INK4A), abnormal expression of p53 (TP53), and inactivation of smad4 (SMAD4) are the hallmarks of PC.[18] Whereas K-RAS mutation and p16 inactivation are common features in low-grade PanINs, abnormal expression of p53 and inactivation of smad4 are exclusively detected in high-grade PanINs and it is assumed that these are late events that are involved in the mechanisms of invasion. About 30% of individuals older than 70 years harbor low-grade PanINs and such common lesions cannot be the target of invasive treatments.[19] In contrast, PanIN-3 lesions, or high-grade PanINs, are extremely rare conditions and are considered the stage when the lesion is ready to invade. Therefore, high-grade PanINs are the target lesions for early detection and curative treatments.

It had been suggested by one author (KT) that PanINs could arise from any part of the pancreatic duct system.[20–22] This means that some PanINs may arise from large ducts, including the main pancreatic duct, and that others may be extremely small lesions originating from the peripheral intralobular ducts.[22] Small PanINs arising from the peripheral ducts have been challenging targets for screening due to the difficulty in identifying them by imaging. In contrast, PanINs involving the larger ducts are often associated with localized fibrosis and/or caliber changes of the duct, which can be identified by imaging studies such as endoscopic ultrasonography (EUS) and MRI.[23]

Intraductal papillary mucinous neoplasm (IPMN) is another precursor of PC. Morphologically, IPMN is classified into main-duct type and branch-duct type according to the location or tumor. Some IPMNs extend into both the main and branch pancreatic ducts and are often called mixed type or combined type.[24] About half of the main-duct IPMNs are associated with high-grade dysplasia and 30% are invasive.[25] Most (but not all) of branch-duct IPMNs are benign without high-grade dysplasia. Only when the branch-duct IPMNs are associated with mural nodules on imaging, greater than 3 cm in size, or symptomatic, are they are more likely to harbor high-grade dysplasia. Invasive carcinoma can develop from the branch-duct IPMN and it is also acknowledged that invasive cancer may develop from different sites in the pancreata involved by branch-duct IPMNs.[26] Such a complicated situation has created much debate about how these IPMNs should be treated. There is international consensus about managements of IPMN and, currently, the treatment of IPMN is practiced according to the international consensus guidelines in many institutions.[27] Remember that these criteria are dynamic and are constantly being challenged.

WHO IS AT RISK OF DEVELOPING PANCREATIC CANCER? WHO SHOULD BE SCREENED?

The literature suggests that both nongenetic and genetic factors may contribute to developing PC (**Tables 1** and **2**).[28–46] Risk level of each nongenetic factor is low (relative risk [RR] 1.2–4.0). In addition, given a low incidence of PC, which is 8.5 to 12 per 100,000 per year,[2] screening for individuals with nongenetic factors is not practical nor cost-effective,[47] although some of these nongenetic factors as smoking, alcohol, and Helicobacter pylori infection are controllable.

Genetic risk factors such as Peutz-Jeghers syndrome (PJS), hereditary pancreatitis, familial atypical multiple mole melanoma, and Lynch syndrome (hereditary nonpolyposis colorectal cancer [HNPCC]) are not controllable and have a high risk level (RR: 34–132) to develop PC.[38,40,43,48] In addition, it has been reported that up to 10% of PC is associated with family history,[49] which implies that PC screening for high-risk individuals (HRIs) based on family history or known genetic syndrome would be more practical; but who should be screened?

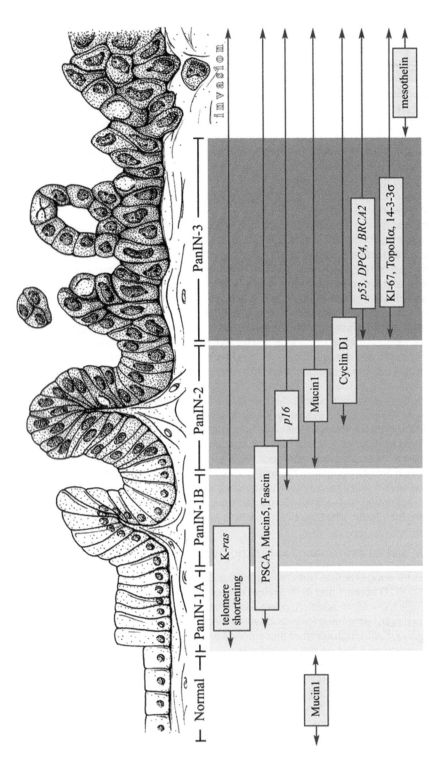

Fig. 1. PanINs with multicomponent tissue-microarray analysis of immunohistochemical abnormalities in PanIN lesions. (*From* Maitra A, Adsay NV, Argani P, et al. Multicomponent analysis of the pancreatic adenocarcinoma progression model using a pancreatic intraepithelial neoplasia tissue microarray. Mod Pathol 2003;16:909; with permission).

Table 1
Nongenetic risk factors of developing pancreatic cancer

Risk Factors	Risk Level
Tobacco[28]	1.7
Alcohol $\geq$9 drinks per day[29]	1.6
Obesity, 5 kg/m^2 increase in body mass index[30]	1.12
Diabetes[31]	1.9
Type II diabetes[32]	1.8
Non-O blood type[33]	1.4
H pylori infection[34]	1.4
Chronic pancreatitis[35]	14–16
IPMN[36,37]	16–26

Data from Refs.[28–37]

A recent consensus-based guideline suggested that patients with increased risk of developing disease (ie, greater than 5% lifetime risk or fivefold increase RR) should be screened.[50] Strong agreement, which is defined as greater than or equal to 75% of vote, was achieved in patients with strong family history and gene mutation carriers, including PJS, BRCA2, PALB2, p16, and HNPCC. A consensus was also achieved in patients whose documented cystic or solid lesions in the pancreas or indeterminate main duct stricture without a mass should be followed periodically by imaging (**Box 1**).[50] Thus, family history is still the main tool to quantify risk of developing PC. A prospective study demonstrated that the risk of developing PC was 9 times higher in familial

Table 2
Genetic risk factors of developing pancreatic cancer

Syndrome	Gene	Relative Risk	Risk by Age 70	Other Associated Cancers
Peutz-Jeghers syndrome[38,39]	SKT11, LKB1	132	11%–36%	Esophagus, stomach, small intestine, colon, lung, breast, uterus, ovary
Hereditary pancreatitis[41,42]	PRSS1, SPink1, CTFR	50–70	40%–55%	—
Familial atypical multiple-mole melanoma[43,44]	p16INK4a/MTS1	34–39	17%	Melanoma, breast
Lynch syndrome (hereditary nonpolyposis colorectal cancer)[48]	MSH2, MLH1, MSH6, PMS2, EPCAM	4.7–8.6	3.7%	Colon, endometrium, stomach, ovary, ureter, kidney, biliary tract, brain
Hereditary breast ovarian cancer[70–72]	BRCA1, BRCA2	4.5	2%–7%	Breast, ovary, prostate
Cystic fibrosis[73]	CFTR	6.9	<5%	Digestive cancers
Ataxia-telangiectasia[74]	ATM	3	Unknown	Leukemia, lymphoma
Von Hippel-Lindau syndrome[75]	VHL	Unknown	5%–17%	Kidney
Familial PC[51,74,76,77]	Unknown	9.0	4%	—

Data from Refs.[38,39,41–44,48,51,70–77]

Box 1
Consensus-based high-risk individuals for pancreatic cancer screening

- Individuals with 3 or more affected blood relatives, with at least one affected FDR
- Individuals with at least 2 affected FDRs with PC
- Individuals with 2 or more affected blood relatives with PC, with at least one affected FDR
- All patients with Peutz-Jeghers syndrome
- *p16* mutation carriers with one affected FDR
- *BRCA2* mutation carriers with one affected FDR
- *BRCA2* mutation carriers with 2 affected family members (no FDR) with PC
- *PALB2* mutation carriers with one affected FDR
- Mismatch repair gene mutation carriers (Lynch syndrome) with one affected FDR
- Patients with a cystic lesion without worrisome features for malignancy
- Patients with solid tumors who are not able to perform immediate surgery
- Patients with an indeterminate main pancreatic duct stricture without a mass.

Abbreviation: FDR: first-degree relative.

PC (FPC) kindred, which is defined as those having 2 or more affected first-degree relatives (FDRs) with PC compared with the general population. This risk in FPC kindreds was elevated according to the number of affected relatives. That is, individuals with 2 affected FDRs with PC have 6.4-fold increased risk (95% CI 1.8–16.4) and individuals with 3 or more FDRs with PC have a 32.0-fold increased risk (95% CI 10.4–74.7).[51]

The age to start screening is also a matter of debate. It has been reported that the average age at diagnosis in FPC kindreds is younger than in kindreds with sporadic PC or the general population.[52,53] However, there was no consensus recommendation about the age to initiate screening for HRIs without pancreatic lesions.[50] The general calculation is that the age to begin screening is 10 years younger than the earliest member of affected FDRs.

How Should Individuals at Risk Be Screened?

Screening for healthy individuals carries the assumption of high risk for developing PC and, it is hoped, should be performed based on clinical trials. Several clinical trials have used different imaging modalities to detect small lesions, including computed tomography (CT); MRI or magnetic resonance cholangiopancreatography (MRI/MRCP), with or without secretin enhancement; endoscopic retrograde cholangiopancreatography (ERCP); and EUS. A diagnostic yield among studies was highly variable, ranging between 1.3% and 50% due to heterogeneity of the study populations, diagnostic modality, and target lesions (**Table 3**).[54–66]

A multicenter prospective cohort study, Cancer of the Pancreas Screening 3 (CAPS3) Study was conducted to compare diagnostic modalities between standardized pancreatic-protocol enhanced CT, secretin-enhanced MRI/MRCP, and EUS for one-time screening for HRI. The study showed that EUS (42.5%) and MRI/MRCP (33.3%) are better than CT (11%) for detecting small pancreatic lesions that are predominantly cystic rather than solid mass.[66] In addition, considering that screening is long-term (>10 years) for healthy subjects, repeated radiation exposure with CT should be indicated only for individuals with documented or suspected lesions by MRI/MRCP and/or EUS.[50]

Table 3
Summary of screening programs in the literature

Author, Year	Number of Subjects	High-Risk Group	Imaging Tests	Resection (%)	Diagnostic yield[†] (%)
Brentnall et al,[54] 1999	14	FPC	EUS + ERCP + CT	7 (50)	7 (50)
Kimmey et al,[55] 2002	46	FPC	EUS +/− ERCP	12 (26)	12 (26)
Canto et al,[56] 2004	38	FPC, PJS	EUS + CT +/− ERCP, EUS-FNA	7 (21)	2 (5.3)
Canto et al,[57] 2006	78	FPC, PJS	EUS + CT +/− ERCP, EUS-FNA	7 (9)	8[a] (10)
Langer et al,[58] 2009	76	FPC, BRCA, FAMMM	EUS + MRI/MRCP	6 (8)	1 (1.3)
Poley et al,[59] 2009	44	FPC, FAMMM, PJS, BRCA, LFS, HP	EUS	10 (23)	10 (23)
Verna et al,[60] 2010	51	FPC, BRCA, HNPCC, FAMMM	EUS + MRI +/− ERCP, EUS-FNA	5 (10)	6[a] (12)
Luding et al,[61] 2011	109	FPC, BRCA	MRI/MRCP +/− EUS-FNA	6 (5.5)	6 (5.5)
Vasen et al,[62] 2011	79	FAMMM	MRI/MRCP	5 (6.3)	5 (6.3)
Zubarik et al,[63] 2011	27	FPC with elevated CA19-9	EUS	3 (11)	2 (7.4)
Schneider et al,[64] 2011	72	FPC, BRCA, PALB2	EUS + MRI/MRCP	9 (13)	6 (8.3)
Al-Sukhni et al,[65] 2012	262	FPC, p16, PJS, STK11, BRCA, HP	MRI/MRCP +/− CT, EUS	4 (1.5)	6 (2.3)
Canto et al,[66] 2012	216	FPC, BRCA, PJS	CT, MRI, EUS	5 (2.2)	5 (2.3)

Abbreviations: CT, computed tomography; ERCP, endoscopic retrograde cholangiopancreatography; EUS, endoscopic ultrasonography; FAMMM, familial atypical multiple mole melanoma; FNA, fine-needle aspiration; FPC, familial PC; HNPCC, hereditary nonpolyposis colorectal cancer; HP, hereditary pancreatitis; LFS, Li-Fraumeni syndrome; MRI/MRCP, MRI or magnetic resonance cholangiopancreatography; PJS, Peutz-Jeghers syndrome.

[†] Defined as pathologically proven (pre)malignant lesion (pancreatic adenocarcinoma, IPMN, MCN, PanIN-2/3, and neuroendocrine tumor).
[a] Included biopsy results.
Data from Refs.[54–66]

HOW SHOULD SUSPECTED LESIONS BE MANAGED?

Previous studies included 1022 subjects with heterogeneous definition of HRIs for developing PC. Surgical resection was performed in 64 (6.3%, range 2%–26%) based on various surgical indications during a limited follow-up period.[55–57,59–66] Invasive ductal adenocarcinomas were identified in 20 (1.9%), which is higher than the general population, whereas 8 of 20 (40%) were detected during the follow-up period. Other pathologic results obtained by surgical resection included various degrees of IPMNs and PanINs, and some serous cystic neoplasms or neuroendocrine tumors. Multiple studies have described that HRIs have a higher incidence of pancreatic abnormalities, predominantly cystic neoplasms and dysplasia.[60,66,67] It is uncertain whether surgical resection for those suspected lesions would improve survival. Although pancreatectomy has become a safe procedure with a mortality rate of around 2% in most high-volume centers,[68,69] the risk–benefit ratio of pancreatectomy for precursor lesions in HRIs should be carefully evaluated and considered because it has not helped most patients. If screening is negative, prophylactic pancreatectomy is not recommended.

If screening is positive, the type of surgery is matter of debate in the screening program. Initial experience from the University of Washington group reported the use of total pancreatectomy based on significant findings by EUS and ERCP.[54,55] This approach has the advantage of removing all at-risk pancreatic parenchyma of dysplastic lesions shown as multicentric by the studies.[54,55] However, it should be remembered that total pancreatectomy has long-term significant sequelae, such as brittle diabetes and malnutrition. Another approach is partial pancreatectomy, either distal pancreatectomy or pancreaticoduodenectomy, for the lesions detected by imaging followed by surveillance for the remnant parenchyma left behind, which has been favored in recent clinical trials.[56–66]

Patients who are identified as having suspicious small lesions, which are most likely branch-duct IPMNs, are being followed by various criteria at each center. Most sporadic branch-duct IPMNs without worrisome features, including a cyst greater than or equal to 3 cm, mural nodules, main duct involvement, have a low risk for malignancy and can be followed safely according to the consensus guidelines.[27] However, it is uncertain if these criteria are also appropriate for HRIs. Given the observation that, even in patients who are involved in intensive screening programs, some were diagnosed as PC at an advanced stage (eg, node-positive and/or metastatic) during the follow-up period.[57,60,62,65] This implies the difficulty in detecting early, curable PC even in the screening program. Thus, it must be considered that the goal of screening program should be set to treat precursors rather than asymptomatic PC.

Currently, evidence and experience is limited for achieving the goal of screening for HRIs, which is prevention of PC. However, clinical trial-based screening programs will give a better understanding of precursor lesions and the natural history of PC. Will these studies affect the disease by decrease in mortality from PC? The conundrum of screening is that the patient who is successfully screened never develops the disease and, therefore, never knows whether they would have lost! Cohort trials are required to discover a way to decrease population mortality from PC.

REFERENCES

1. Ferlay J, Soerjomataram I, Dikshit R, et al. Cancer incidence and mortality worldwide: sources, methods and major patterns in GLOBOCAN 2012. Int J Cancer 2015;136:E359–86.
2. American Cancer Society Facts and Figures 2014. 2014; Available at: http://www.cancer.org/research/cancerfactsstatistics/cancerfactsfigures2014/. Accessed April 25, 2015.

3. Fortner JG, Kim DK, Cubilla A, et al. Regional pancreatectomy: en bloc pancreatic, portal vein and lymph node resection. Ann Surg 1977;186:42–50.
4. Ishikawa O, Ohhigashi H, Sasaki Y, et al. Practical usefulness of lymphatic and connective tissue clearance for the carcinoma of the pancreas head. Ann Surg 1988;208:215–20.
5. Manabe T, Ohshio G, Baba N, et al. Radical pancreatectomy for ductal cell carcinoma of the head of the pancreas. Cancer 1989;64:1132–7.
6. Yeo CJ, Cameron JL, Lillemoe KD, et al. Pancreaticoduodenectomy with or without distal gastrectomy and extended retroperitoneal lymphadenectomy for periampullary adenocarcinoma, part 2: randomized controlled trial evaluating survival, morbidity, and mortality. Ann Surg 2002;236:355–66 [discussion: 366–8].
7. Farnell MB, Pearson RK, Sarr MG, et al. A prospective randomized trial comparing standard pancreatoduodenectomy with pancreatoduodenectomy with extended lymphadenectomy in resectable pancreatic head adenocarcinoma. Surgery 2005;138:618–28 [discussion: 628–30].
8. Nimura Y, Nagino M, Takao S, et al. Standard versus extended lymphadenectomy in radical pancreatoduodenectomy for ductal adenocarcinoma of the head of the pancreas: long-term results of a Japanese multicenter randomized controlled trial. J Hepatobiliary Pancreat Sci 2012;19:230–41.
9. Jang JY, Kang MJ, Heo JS, et al. A prospective randomized controlled study comparing outcomes of standard resection and extended resection, including dissection of the nerve plexus and various lymph nodes, in patients with pancreatic head cancer. Ann Surg 2014;259:656–64.
10. Egawa S, Toma H, Ohigashi H, et al. Japan Pancreatic Cancer Registry; 30th year anniversary: Japan Pancreas Society. Pancreas 2012;41:985–92.
11. Hirano S, Kondo S, Hara T, et al. Distal pancreatectomy with en bloc celiac axis resection for locally advanced pancreatic body cancer: long-term results. Ann Surg 2007;246:46–51.
12. Kamisawa T, Isawa T, Koike M, et al. Hematogenous metastases of pancreatic ductal carcinoma. Pancreas 1995;11:345–9.
13. Iacobuzio-Donahue CA, Fu B, Yachida S, et al. DPC4 gene status of the primary carcinoma correlates with patterns of failure in patients with pancreatic cancer. J Clin Oncol 2009;27:1806–13.
14. Egawa S, Takeda K, Fukuyama S, et al. Clinicopathological aspects of small pancreatic cancer. Pancreas 2004;28:235–40.
15. Ishikawa O, Ohigashi H, Imaoka S, et al. Minute carcinoma of the pancreas measuring 1 cm or less in diameter–collective review of Japanese case reports. Hepatogastroenterology 1999;46:8–15.
16. Tsuchiya R, Tsunoda T. Tumor size as a predictive factor. Int J Pancreatol 1990;7: 117–23.
17. Maitra A, Adsay NV, Argani P, et al. Multicomponent analysis of the pancreatic adenocarcinoma progression model using a pancreatic intraepithelial neoplasia tissue microarray. Mod Pathol 2003;16:902–12.
18. Yachida S, Jones S, Bozic I, et al. Distant metastasis occurs late during the genetic evolution of pancreatic cancer. Nature 2010;467:1114–7.
19. Kozuka S, Sassa R, Taki T, et al. Relation of pancreatic duct hyperplasia to carcinoma. Cancer 1979;43:1418–28.
20. Hruban RH, Takaori K, Klimstra DS, et al. An illustrated consensus on the classification of pancreatic intraepithelial neoplasia and intraductal papillary mucinous neoplasms. Am J Surg Pathol 2004;28:977–87.

21. Takaori K, Hruban RH, Maitra A, et al. Pancreatic intraepithelial neoplasia. Pancreas 2004;28:257–62.
22. Takaori K, Hruban RH, Maitra A, et al. Current topics on precursors to pancreatic cancer. Adv Med Sci 2006;51:23–30.
23. Brune K, Abe T, Canto M, et al. Multifocal neoplastic precursor lesions associated with lobular atrophy of the pancreas in patients having a strong family history of pancreatic cancer. Am J Surg Pathol 2006;30:1067–76.
24. Tanaka M, Chari S, Adsay V, et al. International consensus guidelines for management of intraductal papillary mucinous neoplasms and mucinous cystic neoplasms of the pancreas. Pancreatology 2006;6:17–32.
25. Crippa S, Fernandez-Del Castillo C, Salvia R, et al. Mucin-producing neoplasms of the pancreas: an analysis of distinguishing clinical and epidemiologic characteristics. Clin Gastroenterol Hepatol 2010;8:213–9.
26. Yamaguchi K, Ohuchida J, Ohtsuka T, et al. Intraductal papillary-mucinous tumor of the pancreas concomitant with ductal carcinoma of the pancreas. Pancreatology 2002;2:484–90.
27. Tanaka M, Fernandez-del Castillo C, Adsay V, et al. International consensus guidelines 2012 for the management of IPMN and MCN of the pancreas. Pancreatology 2012;12:183–97.
28. Iodice S, Gandini S, Maisonneuve P, et al. Tobacco and the risk of pancreatic cancer: a review and meta-analysis. Langenbecks Arch Surg 2008;393:535–45.
29. Lucenteforte E, La Vecchia C, Silverman D, et al. Alcohol consumption and pancreatic cancer: a pooled analysis in the International Pancreatic Cancer Case-Control Consortium (PanC4). Ann Oncol 2012;23:374–82.
30. Larsson SC, Orsini N, Wolk A. Body mass index and pancreatic cancer risk: a meta-analysis of prospective studies. Int J Cancer 2007;120:1993–8.
31. Ben Q, Xu M, Ning X, et al. Diabetes mellitus and risk of pancreatic cancer: a meta-analysis of cohort studies. Eur J Cancer 2011;47:1928–37.
32. Huxley R, Ansary-Moghaddam A, Berrington de Gonzalez A, et al. Type-II diabetes and pancreatic cancer: a meta-analysis of 36 studies. Br J Cancer 2005; 92:2076–83.
33. Wolpin BM, Kraft P, Gross M, et al. Pancreatic cancer risk and ABO blood group alleles: results from the pancreatic cancer cohort consortium. Cancer Res 2010; 70:1015–23.
34. Trikudanathan G, Philip A, Dasanu CA, et al. Association between *Helicobacter pylori* infection and pancreatic cancer. A cumulative meta-analysis. JOP 2011; 12:26–31.
35. Lowenfels AB, Maisonneuve P, Cavallini G, et al. Pancreatitis and the risk of pancreatic cancer. International Pancreatitis Study Group. N Engl J Med 1993; 328:1433–7.
36. Uehara H, Nakaizumi A, Ishikawa O, et al. Development of ductal carcinoma of the pancreas during follow-up of branch duct intraductal papillary mucinous neoplasm of the pancreas. Gut 2008;57:1561–5.
37. Tanno S, Nakano Y, Koizumi K, et al. Pancreatic ductal adenocarcinomas in long-term follow-up patients with branch duct intraductal papillary mucinous neoplasms. Pancreas 2010;39:36–40.
38. Giardiello FM, Brensinger JD, Tersmette AC, et al. Very high risk of cancer in familial Peutz-Jeghers syndrome. Gastroenterology 2000;119:1447–53.
39. van Lier MG, Wagner A, Mathus-Vliegen EM, et al. High cancer risk in Peutz-Jeghers syndrome: a systematic review and surveillance recommendations. Am J Gastroenterol 2010;105:1258–64 [author reply: 1265].

40. Lowenfels AB, Maisonneuve P, DiMagno EP, et al. Hereditary pancreatitis and the risk of pancreatic cancer. International Hereditary Pancreatitis Study Group. J Natl Cancer Inst 1997;89:442–6.
41. Howes N, Lerch MM, Greenhalf W, et al. Clinical and genetic characteristics of hereditary pancreatitis in Europe. Clin Gastroenterol Hepatol 2004;2:252–61.
42. Rebours V, Boutron-Ruault MC, Schnee M, et al. Risk of pancreatic adenocarcinoma in patients with hereditary pancreatitis: a national exhaustive series. Am J Gastroenterol 2008;103:111–9.
43. Borg A, Sandberg T, Nilsson K, et al. High frequency of multiple melanomas and breast and pancreas carcinomas in CDKN2A mutation-positive melanoma families. J Natl Cancer Inst 2000;92:1260–6.
44. Vasen HF, Gruis NA, Frants RR, et al. Risk of developing pancreatic cancer in families with familial atypical multiple mole melanoma associated with a specific 19 deletion of p16 (p16-Leiden). Int J Cancer 2000;87:809–11.
45. Goldstein AM, Chan M, Harland M, et al. Features associated with germline CDKN2A mutations: a GenoMEL study of melanoma-prone families from three continents. J Med Genet 2007;44:99–106.
46. Lynch HT, Fusaro RM, Lynch JF, et al. Pancreatic cancer and the FAMMM syndrome. Fam Cancer 2008;7:103–12.
47. Ikeda M, Sato T, Morozumi A, et al. Morphologic changes in the pancreas detected by screening ultrasonography in a mass survey, with special reference to main duct dilatation, cyst formation, and calcification. Pancreas 1994;9:508–12.
48. Lynch HT, Voorhees GJ, Lanspa SJ, et al. Pancreatic carcinoma and hereditary nonpolyposis colorectal cancer: a family study. Br J Cancer 1985;52:271–3.
49. Klein AP, de Andrade M, Hruban RH, et al. Linkage analysis of chromosome 4 in families with familial pancreatic cancer. Cancer Biol Ther 2007;6:320–3.
50. Canto MI, Harinck F, Hruban RH, et al. International Cancer of the Pancreas Screening (CAPS) Consortium summit on the management of patients with increased risk for familial pancreatic cancer. Gut 2013;62:339–47.
51. Klein AP, Brune KA, Petersen GM, et al. Prospective risk of pancreatic cancer in familial pancreatic cancer kindreds. Cancer Res 2004;64:2634–8.
52. Petersen GM, de Andrade M, Goggins M, et al. Pancreatic cancer genetic epidemiology consortium. Cancer Epidemiol Biomarkers Prev 2006;15:704–10.
53. Brune KA, Lau B, Palmisano E, et al. Importance of age of onset in pancreatic cancer kindreds. J Natl Cancer Inst 2010;102:119–26.
54. Brentnall TA, Bronner MP, Byrd DR, et al. Early diagnosis and treatment of pancreatic dysplasia in patients with a family history of pancreatic cancer. Ann Intern Med 1999;131:247–55.
55. Kimmey MB, Bronner MP, Byrd DR, et al. Screening and surveillance for hereditary pancreatic cancer. Gastrointest Endosc 2002;56:S82–6.
56. Canto MI, Goggins M, Yeo CJ, et al. Screening for pancreatic neoplasia in high-risk individuals: an EUS-based approach. Clin Gastroenterol Hepatol 2004;2:606–21.
57. Canto MI, Goggins M, Hruban RH, et al. Screening for early pancreatic neoplasia in high-risk individuals: a prospective controlled study. Clin Gastroenterol Hepatol 2006;4:766–81 [quiz: 665].
58. Langer P, Kann PH, Fendrich V, et al. Five years of prospective screening of high-risk individuals from families with familial pancreatic cancer. Gut 2009;58:1410–8.
59. Poley JW, Kluijt I, Gouma DJ, et al. The yield of first-time endoscopic ultrasonography in screening individuals at a high risk of developing pancreatic cancer. Am J Gastroenterol 2009;104:2175–81.

60. Verna EC, Hwang C, Stevens PD, et al. Pancreatic cancer screening in a prospective cohort of high-risk patients: a comprehensive strategy of imaging and genetics. Clin Cancer Res 2010;16:5028–37.

61. Ludwig E, Olson SH, Bayuga S, et al. Feasibility and yield of screening in relatives from familial pancreatic cancer families. Am J Gastroenterol 2011;106:946–54.

62. Vasen HF, Wasser M, van Mil A, et al. Magnetic resonance imaging surveillance detects early-stage pancreatic cancer in carriers of a p16-Leiden mutation. Gastroenterology 2011;140:850–6.

63. Zubarik R, Gordon SR, Lidofsky SD, et al. Screening for pancreatic cancer in a high-risk population with serum CA 19-9 and targeted EUS: a feasibility study. Gastrointest Endosc 2011;74:87–95.

64. Schneider R, Slater EP, Sina M, et al. German national case collection for familial pancreatic cancer (FaPaCa): ten years experience. Fam Cancer 2011;10:323–30.

65. Al-Sukhni W, Borgida A, Rothenmund H, et al. Screening for pancreatic cancer in a high-risk cohort: an eight-year experience. J Gastrointest Surg 2012;16:771–83.

66. Canto MI, Hruban RH, Fishman EK, et al. Frequent detection of pancreatic lesions in asymptomatic high-risk individuals. Gastroenterology 2012;142:796–804 [quiz: e14–5].

67. Shi C, Klein AP, Goggins M, et al. Increased Prevalence of Precursor Lesions in Familial Pancreatic Cancer Patients. Clin Cancer Res 2009;15:7737–43.

68. Cameron JL, He J. Two thousand consecutive pancreaticoduodenectomies. J Am Coll Surg 2015;220:530–6.

69. Gotoh M, Miyata H, Hashimoto H, et al. National Clinical Database feedback implementation for quality improvement of cancer treatment in Japan: from good to great through transparency. Surg Today 2015. [Epub ahead of print].

70. Naderi A, Couch FJ. BRCA2 and pancreatic cancer. Int J Gastrointest Cancer 2002;31:99–106.

71. Thompson D, Easton DF. Cancer Incidence in BRCA1 mutation carriers. J Natl Cancer Inst 2002;94:1358–65.

72. Hahn SA, Greenhalf B, Ellis I, et al. BRCA2 germline mutations in familial pancreatic carcinoma. J Natl Cancer Inst 2003;95:214–21.

73. Maisonneuve P, Marshall BC, Lowenfels AB. Risk of pancreatic cancer in patients with cystic fibrosis. Gut 2007;56:1327–8.

74. Roberts NJ, Jiao Y, Yu J, et al. ATM mutations in patients with hereditary pancreatic cancer. Cancer Discov 2012;2:41–6.

75. Neumann HP, Dinkel E, Brambs H, et al. Pancreatic lesions in the von Hippel-Lindau syndrome. Gastroenterology 1991;101:465–71.

76. Jones S, Hruban RH, Kamiyama M, et al. Exomic sequencing identifies PALB2 as a pancreatic cancer susceptibility gene. Science 2009;324:217.

77. Tischkowitz MD, Sabbaghian N, Hamel N, et al. Analysis of the gene coding for the BRCA2-interacting protein PALB2 in familial and sporadic pancreatic cancer. Gastroenterology 2009;137:1183–6.

Screening and Early Detection of Gastric Cancer

East Versus West

Yun-Suhk Suh, MD, MS, Han-Kwang Yang, MD, PhD*

KEYWORDS

• Gastric cancer • Treatment • Regional disparity • Screening

KEY POINTS

- Certain Asian countries including Korea and Japan shows much lower ratio of mortality over incidence of gastric cancer than other countries.
- Early detection after screening program and subsequent surgical treatment including appropriate lymph node dissection has been developed successfully in East Asian countries.
- Different ethnicity have not been reported as independent prognostic factors for gastric cancer yet.
- Molecular approaches for gastric cancer are expected as a new paradigm to characterize gastric cancer instead of conventional clinicopathologic or epidemiologic investigation.

GASTRIC CANCER EPIDEMIOLOGY: MORTALITY, INCIDENCE BETWEEN EAST AND WEST

Gastric cancer is the fifth most common malignancy in the world with about 1 million new cases estimated in 2012 (952,000 cases, 6.8% of the total).[1] Age-standardized incidence rates are about 6 times as high in Eastern Asia compared with North America, ranging from 4 in North America to 24.2 in Eastern Asia (41.8 in South Korea, the highest in the world) for both sexes. Regarding the cause of death, gastric cancer is the third leading cause of cancer death in the world (723,000 deaths; 8.8% of the total in 2012).

Considering a report from the United Nations in 2012, the life expectancy for gastric cancer patients does not seem to be related to incidence or morality among different countries (**Fig. 1**).[2] It should be noted that in general the mortality of gastric cancer is likely to show a high incidence in most countries. However, considering the ratio of mortality over incidence, Korea and Japan show a much lesser ratio than Western countries. This interesting phenomenon is more remarkable among gastric cancer prevalent areas. **Fig. 2** shows the incidence, mortality, and life expectancy for the

Department of Surgery, Cancer Research Institute, Seoul National University College of Medicine, 101 Daehang-Ro, Jongno-gu, Seoul 110-744, Korea
* Corresponding author.
E-mail address: hkyang@snu.ac.kr

Surg Clin N Am 95 (2015) 1053–1066
http://dx.doi.org/10.1016/j.suc.2015.05.012   surgical.theclinics.com

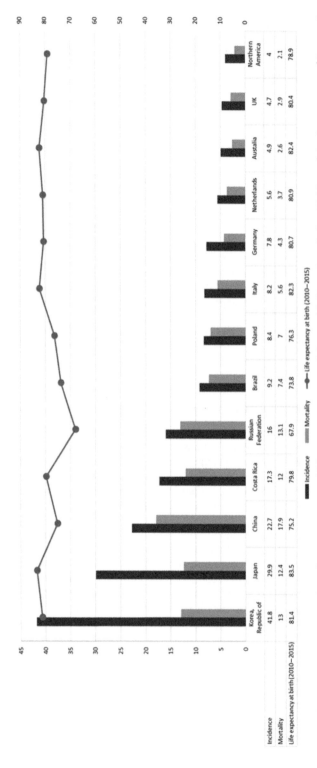

Fig. 1. The incidence and mortality of gastric cancer and life expectancy around the world. (*From* Population Division of the Department of Economic and Social Affairs of the United Nations Secretariat. World population prospects: the 2012 revision. New York: Population Division of the Department of Economic and Social Affairs of the United Nations Secretariat; 2013.)

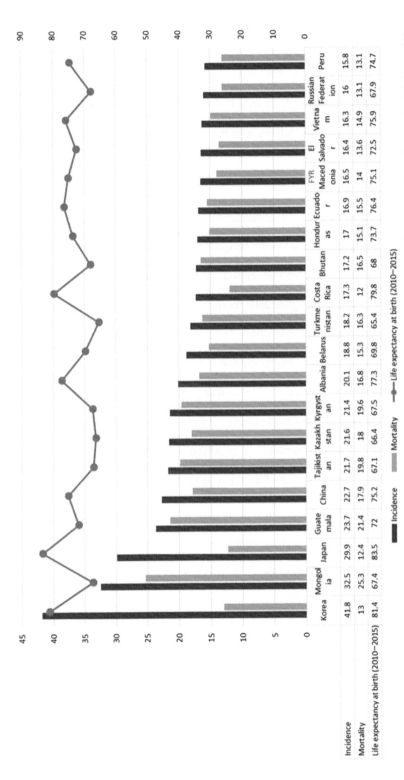

Fig. 2. The incidence and mortality of gastric cancer and life expectancy in the top 20 gastric–cancer prevalent areas. (*From* Population Division of the Department of Economic and Social Affairs of the United Nations Secretariat. World population prospects: the 2012 revision. New York: Population Division of the Department of Economic and Social Affairs of the United Nations Secretariat; 2013.)

20 countries with the highest gastric cancer prevalent. South Korea, where gastric cancer prevalence is the highest in the world, carries one of the lowest mortality rates (Age-standardized mortality rates per 100,000 = 13) among the 20 highest gastric cancer–prevalent countries in the world. In addition, in Japan where the age-standardized incidence rate is 29.9, which is one of the highest levels in the world, an age-standardized mortality rate of only 12.4 per 100,000 is reported.

If life expectancy of the population is not significantly different, low mortality compared with incidence is tentatively explained by early detection after screening, a difference in treatment strategy, or genetic disparity between the East and West.

RISK FACTORS
Helicobacter pylori

H pylori infection is known to be associated strongly with development and possible cofactor in the pathogenesis of gastric cancer, especially noncardiac gastric cancer.[3–6] According to the Asia-Pacific consensus guidelines on gastric cancer prevention, screening and eradication of H pylori can reduce gastric cancer incidence in high-risk populations and is also considered important in intermediate risk populations.[5] A previous, nonrandomized, interventional study revealed that a persistent H pylori infection group had significantly more gastric cancer patients after 3 years of follow-up compared with the H pylori eradication group (4.3% vs 1.5%).[7] Despite this finding, recent randomized trials have failed to show a benefit of eradication of H pylori on the prevention of gastric cancer, even though there was a protective tendency.[8,9] However, another other study that included patients with peptic ulcer disease or endoscopic resection showed a significant prophylactic effect of eradication of H pylori to prevent gastric cancer.[10,11] One metaanalysis with a total of 6695 participants reported that the relative risk for gastric cancer in treated patients was 0.65 (95% CI, 0.43–0.98) and H pylori eradication treatment "seems" to reduce gastric cancer risk.[12] Even though this approach is not currently acceptable in low-risk populations, such as in Western countries, a population-based evaluation of H pylori screening and treatment may offer a promising opportunity to lower mortality of gastric cancer even in Western countries such as Unites States.[13]

Diet and Smoking

Salty food and dietary nitrates are known potential carcinogens in gastric cancer. Basic functional studies using animal models have already revealed that a salty diet could be responsible for gastric cancer initiation as well as tumor promotion.[14,15] According to large cohort study of 2476 Japanese subjects, high dietary salt intake is a significant risk factor for gastric cancer and its association might be more strong in the presence of H pylori infection with atrophic gastritis.[16] Salty food in particular may synergize with gastric H pylori infection, which increases the risk of early gastric cancer.[17] Outside the East, the INTERSALT study using samples from 24 countries all over the world including the West also reported that salt intake is likely the rate-limiting factor of gastric cancer mortality at the population level.[18] Regarding smoking and gastric cancer, there already have been several systematic reviews with cohort studies or case control studies that revealed that smoking increases the risk of gastric cancer in Eastern as well as Western populations.[19–21] Cigarette smoking and H pylori infection are also synergistic significant risk factors.[22] These epidemiologic factors, including diet or smoking, are universal risk factors, irrespective of geography. Dietary modification to include less salted food or quitting smoking could be useful ways of preventing gastric cancer worldwide.

GASTRIC CANCER SCREENING EFFECT: EARLY DETECTION AND THE ASIAN EXPERIENCE

In Asia, population-based screening for gastric cancer has been performed in Korea, Japan, and the Matsu island of Taiwan.

Korea

In Korea, the National Cancer Control Committee was established in 1996. The committee developed a nationwide screening system and proposed the National Cancer Screening Program for gastric cancer in 1999. Currently, the National Cancer Screening Program recommends that individuals greater than 40 years of age undergo gastric cancer screening through either upper gastrointestinal series or endoscopy at least every 2 years. Because of the development of diagnostic tools, nationwide mass health screening has increased the detection of early gastric cancer (from 28.6% in 1995, to 47.4% in 2004, and 57.7% in 2009).[23,24] As the proportion of early gastric cancer has increased, the outcomes of gastric cancer patients, including mortality, has improved rapidly. According to a large retrospective analysis between 1985 and 2006 in Korea, the proportion of early gastric cancer has gradually increased from 24.8% to 48.9% (P<.001) and consequently the 5-year overall survival rate increased from 64.0% to 73.2% (P<.001), especially in patients aged older than 40 years.[25] After 2006, a single institution's report revealed that the proportion of patients in screening group increased from 45.1% in 2006 to 65.4% in 2011, and the percentages of patients with clinical stage I were 79.9% in screening group and 47.9% in the nonscreening group in Korea.[26] In terms of efficacy of screening, the repeated screening group showed a significantly greater proportion of early gastric cancer (96% vs 71% vs P = .01), smaller size of tumor (1.9 ± 1.2 vs 3.0 ± 1.6 cm; P = .01), greater proportion of intramucosal cancer (81% vs 50%; P = .02), and more frequent performance of endoscopic submucosal dissection as treatment (54% vs 23%, P = .007) compared with the infrequent screening group.[27] Recently, a large-scale, retrospective analysis from Korea using asymptomatic adults who underwent endoscopy during health checkups revealed that the proportion of early gastric cancer was 98.6% and 80.7% (P<.01) in annual and biennial screening group, respectively.[28] In addition, tumor size was also significantly smaller (1.7 vs 2.3 cm) and the proportion of intramucosal cancer was greater (75.0% vs 56.1%) in the annual compared with the biennial screening group.

Japan

Gastric cancer screening using photofluorography is recommended for population-based and opportunistic screening in Japan.[29] In Japan, conventional barium gastrography has been recommended for populations aged 40 years or over annually by the national cancer screening program for gastric cancer since 1983 under the Health Service Law for the Aged. In 2004, 4.4 million people participated in gastric cancer screening with about a 13% screening rate for gastric cancer.[29] In terms of reduction of mortality, the large prospective cohort study in Japan showed relative risk of 0.52 to 0.72[30–33] **(Table 1)**. Although overall incidence rate was not different between the screened and unscreened groups, the incidence of advanced gastric cancer was significant lower in screened group (relative risk, 0.75; 95% CI, 0.58–0.96).[32,33]

In addition, a previous population-based, case-control study showed that screening for gastric cancer might reduce mortality by 60% and that effect remains for at least 5 years.[34] On the other hand, low sensitivity of barium gastrography for detection of early gastric cancer (56.8%–88.5%) has been known as a weak point of that screening program.[29,35] Recently, alternative strategies for screening such as measurement of serum pepsinogen (PG) or H pylori antibody combined with eradication of H pylori have been

Table 1
Screening effect from Japan

Study	Population	Period	Sample Size	Age	Incidence	Relative Risk of Mortality
Japan Collaborative Cohort study (JACC) group[31]	JACC database	1988–1997	87,312	40–79	N/A	Male: 0.65 (0.45–0.95) Female: 0.75 (0.42–1.34)
Japan Public Health Center (JPHC)-based prospective study[32]	JPHC areas	1990–2003	42,150	40–59	1.06 (0.90–1.25)	0.52 (0.36–0.74)
Miyamoto et al,[33] 2007	Miyagi prefecture	1990–2001	41,394	40–64	0.94 (0.79–1.13)	0.54 (0.38–0.77)
Inaba et al,[30] 1999	Gifu prefecture	1992–1995	24,134	>40 y	N/A	Male: 0.72 (0.31–1.66) Female: 1.46 (0.43–4.90)

Abbreviation: N/A, not available.
Data from Refs.[30–33]

proposed.[36–38] Long-term results (15 years' follow-up) of a large-scale gastric cancer screening program using the serum PG test (PG I $\leq$ 70 ng/mL and PGI/II $\leq$ 3.0) among asymptomatic Japanese population (n = 101,892), detected gastric cancer using the PG test with subsequent planned gastroendoscopy in 0.48% of patients with a positive PG and 0.019% of patients with a negative PG ($P<.05$).[39] Importantly, using this method, 80% of detected gastric cancers were early gastric cancer. However, a study about racial differences of serum PG and gastric cancer incidence in Singapore showed that the prevalence of low PG (PG I < 25 ng/mL and PG I/II < 2.5) was the highest in Indian subjects in whom gastric cancer incidence was the lowest when compared with Chinese or Malay.[40] In addition, another study from Korea reported that the sensitivity and specificity of PG I/II ratio of $\leq$3.0 for the detection of dysplasia or cancer were relatively low (55.8%–62.3% and 61%).[41] Efficacy of a PG test would be different depending on gender, age, cancer histology, location, and cancer depth.[42] These inconsistent results suggest that PG test for screening of gastric cancer also may have limitations in terms of various ethnic or environmental disparity, and that biomarkers should be validated before they are used clinically in the screening for gastric cancer.

Taiwan

There have been 2 community-based screening programs for gastric cancer on the Matzu island of Taiwan. Between 1995 and 1999, a 2-stage screening program using PG and endoscopy was performed in a population of 2184 Matzu residents.[43] Endoscopic screening as a second-stage screening is performed in populations testing positive for anti H pylori (immunoglobulin G) or serum PG (PGI or PGI/II ratio) or population with a history of peptic ulcer or other upper gastrointestinal disease or with a family history of gastric cancer. This program revealed that only 2 patients were confirmed to have gastric cancer on endoscopic biopsy, with 43% of subjects who showed positive first-stage results and 30% who received endoscopy. To overcome this limited benefit, another population-based H pylori eradication program was performed between 2004 and 2008.[44] Participants greater than 30 years old were screened by use of the[13] carbon-urea breath test and those with positive results received endoscopy with subsequent *H pylori* eradication treatment. As a result, the 5-year average incidence of gastric cancer in this area declined from 40.3 to 30.4 per 100,000 person-years, which means the intervention effectiveness was 24.7%, but the 5-year average mortality owing to gastric cancer increased from 20.1 to 26.3 per 100,000 person-years.

West

Population-based screening for gastric cancer in Western societies has been rare and limited.[45–47] A previous review of 5-year survival rates in English-language publications from 1970 already suggested that diagnosis and treatment of the disease at an earlier stage will result in increase in 5-year survival rates, even outside Japan.[48] According to an 18-year experience at a single institution in from the West, many of the reported survival differences of gastric cancer may be owing to cohort differences, and not influenced by chronologic changes.[49] However, mass screening using endoscopy like in Korea might not be feasible in Western countries or even in highly developed Eastern countries such as Japan because of its cost effectiveness and a lack of experienced endoscopists.[50] In addition, the effect of open access endoscopy might also be compromised by delayed referral to specialized center, failure of endoscopists to detect early gastric cancer or prior treatment of H2 receptor antagonist masks disease with mucosal healing.[51] A nationwide screening system for gastric cancer usually requires significant financial as well as human resources for effective prevention results, and cost effectiveness is influenced by clinical outcomes, cost, incidence, and screening rates. According to a report from National Cancer Institute in the United States, where gastric cancer is the 16th common cancer (relevantly "rare"), approximately $1.8 billion might be spent on the management of gastric cancer in 2014, but only $11.2 million was used for gastric cancer related research, which was just 0.2% of total National Cancer Institute funding, and only 10% of this budget is used for prevention or early detection of gastric cancer in 2013.[52]

Recently, a cost-effectiveness analysis of the national gastric cancer screening program in South Korea revealed that, to increase 1 life-year, about $ 8104 to $8966 was additionally required for endoscopy, which was the most cost-effective strategy compared with upper gastrointestinal series or a nonscreening group in Korea.[53] A previous cost-effectiveness analysis using a Singaporean population (intermediate risk) and various other high-risk groups showed that screening of a high-risk group of Chinese men from 50 to 70 years old is highly cost effective with cost benefit of US$26,836 per quality-adjusted life-year[54] Another cost-effectiveness analysis between primary and secondary preventive strategy for gastric cancer in Taiwan revealed that early *H pylori* eradication once in lifetime seems more cost effective than a surveillance strategy.[55] These results should be validated depending on the risk of gastric cancer as well as *H pylori* infection, detectability of early gastric cancer using endoscopy, or timing of chemoprevention. In particular, even in low prevalence countries, health care providers should consider screening with primary prevention, including endoscopy for high-risk populations such as Asian immigrants.[56] To overcome these limitations, several state-of-the art technologies are now under development. Multitarget stool DNA testing could be considered as a noninvasive alternative in gastric cancer screening, as recently reported for colorectal cancer.[57]

DIFFERENCE OF TREATMENT STRATEGY

In addition to screening, there are clinically important differences in the treatment strategy, including surgery, especially the extent of lymphadenectomy, between the

East and the West. In the East, radical gastrectomy can be considered the primary choice of treatment for most operable gastric cancer as well as adenocarcinoma of esophagogastric junction, as opposed to neoadjuvant chemoradiotherapy. In addition, extensive lymphadenectomy (D2 lymph node dissection) is routinely performed for advanced gastric cancer.[58] However, only one-third of 18,043 resected gastric cancer patients had 16 or more lymph nodes according to the analysis using the US Surveillance, Epidemiology, and End Results (SEER) database.[59]

From the West, several randomized clinical trials were conducted to evaluate the effect of D1 and D2 lymphadenectomy. The 2 most well-known, large-scale trials include the MRC and Dutch trials, which both showed significantly greater morbidity and mortality, but similar 5-year survival rates in the D2 lymphadenectomy group, which was significantly worse than previous Eastern reports.[60–62] This difference of surgical strategy seems to be a continuing issue between the East and West. However, a recently conducted randomized clinical trial from Italy described that D2 lymph node dissection could be a better treatment choice for advanced gastric cancer.[63,64] In addition, a systemic review analyzing the long-term difference in survival after gastrectomy in randomized clinical trials between the East and West reported an association between gastrectomy performed in the East, improved 5-year survival (pooled odds ratio [OR], 4.83; 95% CI, 3.27–7.12) and reduced cancer recurrence (pooled OR, 0.33; 95% CI, 0.2–0.54) even after adjustment for confounding factors.[65] This study suggested that the disparity in operative techniques or strategies between the East and West could provide a potential explanation for such prognostic discrepancy. Interestingly, the Dutch trial, one of the most famous studies on the subject which advocates for a D1 dissection, reported their in long-term results that a D2 lymphadenectomy is associated with lesser locoregional recurrence and fewer gastric cancer-related deaths than D1 lymphadenectomy.[66] In addition, a principal investigator of the MRC trial, the other historical advocate for D1 dissection, addressed that the suggestion for D1 gastrectomy instead of D2 reflects the failure of the Western surgical community and the results of MRC trial are no longer a sustainable argument against D2 gastrectomy in modern surgery for invasive gastric cancer.[67]

Regarding D2 lymphadenectomy, not only the surgical treatment itself, but also the handling of surgical specimen can influence difference between Eastern and Western countries. A previous study from the West reported that optimal staging after D2 lymph node dissection combined with surgical ex vivo lymph node dissection resulted in all patients with greater than 16 examined lymph nodes, and D2 LN dissection group showed significant better overall survival than D1 LN dissection group.[68]

These disparities between the East and West may result in the different treatment outcomes of gastric cancer. According to the seventh American Joint Committee on Cancer TNM classification, 5-year survival rate at each stage among Korea,[69] Japan,[70] United States (SEER data 1973–2005 diagnosed in 1991–2000), China[71] is as follows: 95.1%, 94.2%, 70.8%, and 88.5% for stage Ia; 84.0%, 80.8%, 45.5%, and 71.5% for stage IIa; and 71.7%, 69.6%, 32.8%, and 66.8% for stage IIb. For stage IIIa in particular, the 5-year survival rate in Korea is 58.4%, whereas the SEER data show 19.8%.

GENETIC DISPARITY

According to a large comparative cohort study that included 711 gastric cancer patients treated in United States and 1646 patients treated in Korea, D2 lymphadenectomy was performed in 84% of patients in Korea and 89% of patients in the United States.[72] This study reported that overall survival was worse, stage for stage, in patients from the United States compared with Korean patients for TNM stages I, II, and III. After adjusting for clinically significant prognostic factors, Korean patients still had a 30% greater disease-specific survival than patients from the United States. As a possible explanation, in addition to technical issues of surgery, different ethnicity or tumor biology could be considered; however, differences in ethnicity or epigenetic differences have not been reported as independent prognostic factors for gastric cancer.[73–76] As an alternative, recently, molecular approaches for gastric cancer have been investigated as a new paradigm instead of conventional epidemiologic analysis. In 2011, cDNA arrays from 36 gastric cancer patients suggested that gastric cancer with epidemiologic difference can be classified by gene expression data, which was the first report regarding molecular classification of gastric cancer.[77] As of this writing, several basic science studies have been conducted for the molecular classification of gastric cancer in terms of prognostic factors, response to chemotherapy, distinct therapeutic targets, and diagnostic biomarkers.[78–81] However, most of these studies had a similar limitation of sample size or analyzing technique, and failed to show unique molecular characteristics that accounts for the epidemiologic or ethnic heterogeneity in clinical outcomes. Recently the Cancer Genome Atlas Research Network reported the comprehensive characterization of gastric cancer, which described the molecular evaluation of 295 primary gastric adenocarcinomas.[82] This study included samples from Canada, Germany, South Korea, Poland, Russia, Ukraine, the United States, and Vietnam. Although there were a few differences in terms of the frequency of molecular subtypes or pathway-level gene expression changes, this study also could not identify strong biologic differences between tumors of East Asian origin compared with non–East Asian tumors. On the other hand, hereditary diffuse gastric cancer, a familial gastric cancer syndrome has been known as molecular characterization by E-cadherin gene (CDH-1) mutation. The ethnicity of known hereditary diffuse gastric cancer families is diverse and Asian countries have reported only limited experience unlike sporadic gastric cancer.[76,83–85] Early hereditary diffuse gastric cancer is characterized by multiple microscopic foci of intramucosal signet ring cell carcinoma and the time to progression is variable and unpredictable.[86] Because of the multiple microscopic foci of carcinoma and high penetration rate, patients with a positive CDH1 mutation should be advised to consider prophylactic total gastrectomy regardless of endoscopic findings.[87]

SUMMARY

To evaluate the treatment outcome of gastric cancer, various differences including population-based screening, treatment strategy, and genetic disparity, should be considered. Early detection after screening program for gastric cancer and subsequent appropriate treatment has been developed successfully in areas with a high risk for gastric cancer, such as East Asian countries. Even in countries with a low prevalence of gastric cancer, a specific gastric cancer screening program is recommended for any high-risk population.

REFERENCES

1. Ferlay J, Soerjomataram I, Dikshit R, et al. Cancer incidence and mortality worldwide: sources, methods and major patterns in GLOBOCAN 2012. Int J Cancer 2015;136(5):E359–86.
2. Department of Economic and Social Affairs of the United Nations Secretariat. World population prospects: the 2012 revision. New York: Population Division

of the Department of Economic and Social Affairs of the United Nations Secretariat; 2013.

3. Parsonnet J, Friedman GD, Vandersteen DP, et al. *Helicobacter pylori* infection and the risk of gastric carcinoma. N Engl J Med 1991;325(16):1127–31.

4. Uemura N, Okamoto S, Yamamoto S, et al. *Helicobacter pylori* infection and the development of gastric cancer. N Engl J Med 2001;345(11):784–9.

5. Fock KM, Talley N, Moayyedi P, et al. Asia–Pacific consensus guidelines on gastric cancer prevention. J Gastroenterol Hepatol 2008;23(3):351–65.

6. Kamangar F, Dawsey SM, Blaser MJ, et al. Opposing risks of gastric cardia and noncardia gastric adenocarcinomas associated with *Helicobacter pylori* seropositivity. J Natl Cancer Inst 2006;98(20):1445–52.

7. Ogura K, Hirata Y, Yanai A, et al. The effect of *Helicobacter pylori* eradication on reducing the incidence of gastric cancer. J Clin Gastroenterol 2008;42(3):279–83.

8. Wong BC-Y, Lam SK, Wong WM, et al. *Helicobacter pylori* eradication to prevent gastric cancer in a high-risk region of China: a randomized controlled trial. JAMA 2004;291(2):187–94.

9. You W-C, Brown LM, Zhang L, et al. Randomized double-blind factorial trial of three treatments to reduce the prevalence of precancerous gastric lesions. J Natl Cancer Inst 2006;98(14):974–83.

10. Fukase K, Kato M, Kikuchi S, et al. Effect of eradication of *Helicobacter pylori* on incidence of metachronous gastric carcinoma after endoscopic resection of early gastric cancer: an open-label, randomised controlled trial. Lancet 2008;372(9636):392–7.

11. Wu CY, Kuo KN, Wu MS, et al. Early *Helicobacter pylori* eradication decreases risk of gastric cancer in patients with peptic ulcer disease. Gastroenterology 2009;137(5):1641–8.e1–2.

12. Fuccio L, Zagari RM, Eusebi LH, et al. Meta-analysis: can *Helicobacter pylori* eradication treatment reduce the risk for gastric cancer? Ann Intern Med 2009;151(2):121–8.

13. Herrero R, Parsonnet J, Greenberg ER. Prevention of gastric cancer. JAMA 2014;312(12):1197–8.

14. Tatematsu M, Takahashi M, Fukushima S, et al. Effects in rats of sodium chloride on experimental gastric cancers induced by N-methyl-N-nitro-N-nitrosoguanidine or 4-nitroquinoline-1-oxide. J Natl Cancer Inst 1975;55(1):101–6.

15. Furihata C, Ohta H, Katsuyama T. Cause and effect between concentration-dependent tissue damage and temporary cell proliferation in rat stomach mucosa by NaCl, a stomach tumor promoter. Carcinogenesis 1996;17(3):401–6.

16. Shikata K, Kiyohara Y, Kubo M, et al. A prospective study of dietary salt intake and gastric cancer incidence in a defined Japanese population: the Hisayama study. Int J Cancer 2006;119(1):196–201.

17. Lee S-A, Kang D, Shim K, et al. Original article effect of diet and *Helicobacter pylori* infection to the risk of early gastric cancer. J Epidemiol 2003;13(3):162–8.

18. Joossens JV, Hill M, Elliott P, et al. Dietary salt, nitrate and stomach cancer mortality in 24 countries. Int J Epidemiol 1996;25(3):494–504.

19. Nishino Y, Inoue M, Tsuji I, et al. Tobacco smoking and gastric cancer risk: an evaluation based on a systematic review of epidemiologic evidence among the Japanese population. Jpn J Clin Oncol 2006;36(12):800–7.

20. Ladeiras-Lopes R, Pereira AK, Nogueira A, et al. Smoking and gastric cancer: systematic review and meta-analysis of cohort studies. Cancer Causes Control 2008;19(7):689–701.

21. La Torre G, Chiaradia G, Gianfagna F, et al. Smoking status and gastric cancer risk: an updated meta-analysis of case-control studies published in the past ten years. Tumori 2009;95(1):13.

22. Shikata K, Doi Y, Yonemoto K, et al. Population-based prospective study of the combined influence of cigarette smoking and *Helicobacter pylori* infection on gastric cancer incidence. The Hisayama Study. Am J Epidemiol 2008;168(12):1409–15.

23. Information Committee of the Korean Gastric Cancer Association. 2004 Nationwide gastric cancer report in Korea. J Korean Gastric Cancer Assoc 2007;7:47–54.

24. Jeong O, Park Y-K. Clinicopathological features and surgical treatment of gastric cancer in South Korea: the results of 2009 nationwide survey on surgically treated gastric cancer patients. J Gastric Cancer 2011;11(2):69–77.

25. Ahn H, Lee HJ, Yoo MW, et al. Changes in clinicopathological features and survival after gastrectomy for gastric cancer over a 20-year period. Br J Surg 2011;98(2):255–60.

26. Kim YG, Kong S-H, Oh S-Y, et al. Effects of screening on gastric cancer management: comparative analysis of the results in 2006 and in 2011. J Gastric Cancer 2014;14(2):129–34.

27. Nam SY, Choi IJ, Park KW, et al. Effect of repeated endoscopic screening on the incidence and treatment of gastric cancer in health screenees. Eur J Gastroenterol Hepatol 2009;21(8):855–60.

28. Chung SJ, Park MJ, Kang SJ, et al. Effect of annual endoscopic screening on clinicopathologic characteristics and treatment modality of gastric cancer in a high-incidence region of Korea. Int J Cancer 2012;131(10):2376–84.

29. Hamashima C, Shibuya D, Yamazaki H, et al. The Japanese guidelines for gastric cancer screening. Jpn J Clin Oncol 2008;38(4):259–67.

30. Inaba S, Hirayama H, Nagata C, et al. Evaluation of a screening program on reduction of gastric cancer mortality in Japan: preliminary results from a cohort study. Prev Med 1999;29(2):102–6.

31. Mizoue T, Yoshimura T, Tokui N, et al. Prospective study of screening for stomach cancer in Japan. Int J Cancer 2003;106(1):103–7.

32. Lee KJ, Inoue M, Otani T, et al. Gastric cancer screening and subsequent risk of gastric cancer: a large-scale population-based cohort study, with a 13-year follow-up in Japan. Int J Cancer 2006;118(9):2315–21.

33. Miyamoto A, Kuriyama S, Nishino Y, et al. Lower risk of death from gastric cancer among participants of gastric cancer screening in Japan: a population-based cohort study. Prev Med 2007;44(1):12–9.

34. Fukao A, Tsubono Y, Tsuji I, et al. The evaluation of screening for gastric cancer in Miyagi Prefecture, Japan: a population-based case-control study. Int J Cancer 1995;60(1):45–8.

35. Yatake H, Takeda Y, Katsuda T, et al. Improved detection of gastric cancer during screening by additional radiographs as judged necessary by the radiographer. Jpn J Radiol 2011;29(3):177–86.

36. Kitahara F, Kobayashi K, Sato T, et al. Accuracy of screening for gastric cancer using serum pepsinogen concentrations. Gut 1999;44(5):693–7.

37. Miki K, Morita M, Sasajima M, et al. Usefulness of gastric cancer screening using the serum pepsinogen test method. Am J Gastroenterol 2003;98(4):735–9.

38. Asaka M, Kato M, Graham DY. Strategy for eliminating gastric cancer in Japan. Helicobacter 2010;15(6):486–90.

39. Miki K, Fujishiro M, Kodashima S, et al. Long-term results of gastric cancer screening using the serum pepsinogen test method among an asymptomatic middle-aged Japanese population. Dig Endosc 2009;21(2):78–81.

40. Ang TL, Fock KM, Dhamodaran S, et al. Racial differences in *Helicobacter pylori*, serum pepsinogen and gastric cancer incidence in an urban Asian population. J Gastroenterol Hepatol 2005;20(10):1603–9.
41. Kang JM, Kim N, Yoo JY, et al. The role of serum pepsinogen and gastrin test for the detection of gastric cancer in Korea. Helicobacter 2008;13(2):146–56.
42. Kim N, Jung HC. The role of serum pepsinogen in the detection of gastric cancer. Gut and liver 2010;4(3):307–19.
43. Liu C-Y, Wu C-Y, Lin J-T, et al. Multistate and multifactorial progression of gastric cancer: results from community-based mass screening for gastric cancer. J Med Screen 2006;13(suppl 1):2–5.
44. Lee Y-C, Chen TH-H, Chiu H-M, et al. The benefit of mass eradication of *Helicobacter pylori* infection: a community-based study of gastric cancer prevention. Gut 2013;62(5):676–82.
45. Christie J, Shepherd N, Codling B, et al. Gastric cancer below the age of 55: implications for screening patients with uncomplicated dyspepsia. Gut 1997; 41(4):513–7.
46. Roderick P, Davies R, Raftery J, et al. The cost-effectiveness of screening for *Helicobacter pylori* to reduce mortality and morbidity from gastric cancer and peptic ulcer disease: a discrete-event simulation model. Health Technol Assess 2003; 7(6):1–86.
47. Logan R, Langman M. Screening for gastric cancer after gastric surgery. Lancet 1983;322(8351):667–70.
48. Akoh J, Macintyre I. Improving survival in gastric cancer: review of 5-year survival rates in English language publications from 1970. Br J Surg 1992;79(4): 293–9.
49. Cunningham SC, Kamangar F, Kim MP, et al. Survival after gastric adenocarcinoma resection: eighteen-year experience at a single institution. J Gastrointest Surg 2005;9(5):718–25.
50. Leung WK, Wu M-S, Kakugawa Y, et al. Screening for gastric cancer in Asia: current evidence and practice. Lancet Oncol 2008;9(3):279–87.
51. Suvakovic Z, Bramble M, Jones R, et al. Improving the detection rate of early gastric cancer requires more than open access gastroscopy: a five year study. Gut 1997;41(3):308–13.
52. National Cancer Institute. A snapshot of stomach cancer. Available at: http://www.cancer.gov/researchandfunding/snapshots/stomach. Accessed February 7, 2015.
53. Cho E, Kang MH, Choi KS, et al. Cost-effectiveness outcomes of the national gastric cancer screening program in South Korea. Asian Pac J Cancer Prev 2013;14(4):2533–40.
54. Dan YY, So J, Yeoh KG. Endoscopic screening for gastric cancer. Clin Gastroenterol Hepatol 2006;4(6):709–16.
55. Lee Y-C, Lin J-T, Wu H-M, et al. Cost-effectiveness analysis between primary and secondary preventive strategies for gastric cancer. Cancer Epidemiol Biomarkers Prev 2007;16(5):875–85.
56. Taylor VM, Ko LK, Hwang JH, et al. Gastric cancer in Asian American populations: a neglected health disparity. Asian Pac J Cancer Prev 2014;15(24): 10565–71.
57. Imperiale TF, Ransohoff DF, Itzkowitz SH, et al. Multitarget stool DNA testing for colorectal-cancer screening. N Engl J Med 2014;370(14):1287–97.
58. Japanese Gastric Cancer Association. Japanese gastric cancer treatment guidelines 2010 (ver. 3). Gastric Cancer 2011;14(2):113–23.

59. Wang J, Dang P, Raut CP, et al. Comparison of a lymph node ratio–based staging system with the 7th AJCC system for gastric cancer: analysis of 18,043 patients from the SEER database. Ann Surg 2012;255(3):478–85.

60. Cuschieri A, Joypaul V, Fayers P, et al. Postoperative morbidity and mortality after D1 and D2 resections for gastric cancer: preliminary results of the MRC randomised controlled surgical trial. Lancet 1996;347(9007):995–9.

61. Cuschieri A, Weeden S, Fielding J, et al. Patient survival after D 1 and D 2 resections for gastric cancer: long-term results of the MRC randomized surgical trial. Br J Cancer 1999;79(9/10):1522.

62. Bonenkamp J, Hermans J, Sasako M, et al. Extended lymph-node dissection for gastric cancer. N Engl J Med 1999;340(12):908–14.

63. Degiuli M, Sasako M, Ponti A, et al. Survival results of a multicentre phase II study to evaluate D2 gastrectomy for gastric cancer. Br J Cancer 2004;90(9): 1727–32.

64. Degiuli M, Sasako M, Ponti A, et al. Randomized clinical trial comparing survival after D1 or D2 gastrectomy for gastric cancer. Br J Surg 2014;101(2):23–31.

65. Markar SR, Karthikesalingam A, Jackson D, et al. Long-term survival after gastrectomy for cancer in randomized, controlled oncological trials: comparison between West and East. Ann Surg Oncol 2013;20(7):2328–38.

66. Songun I, Putter H, Kranenbarg EM-K, et al. Surgical treatment of gastric cancer: 15-year follow-up results of the randomised nationwide Dutch D1D2 trial. Lancet Oncol 2010;11(5):439–49.

67. Cuschieri A, Hanna GB. Meta-analysis of d1 versus d2 gastrectomy for gastric adenocarcinoma: let us move on to another era. Ann Surg 2014;259(6):e90.

68. Schmidt B, Chang KK, Maduekwe UN, et al. D2 lymphadenectomy with surgical ex vivo dissection into node stations for gastric adenocarcinoma can be performed safely in Western patients and ensures optimal staging. Ann Surg Oncol 2013;20(9):2991–9.

69. Ahn H, Lee H, Hahn S, et al. Evaluation of the Seventh American Joint Committee on Cancer/International Union Against Cancer Classification of gastric adenocarcinoma in comparison with the sixth classification. Cancer 2010;116(24):5592–8.

70. Lee S-W, Nomura E, Bouras G, et al. Long-term oncologic outcomes from laparoscopic gastrectomy for gastric cancer: a single-center experience of 601 consecutive resections. J Am Coll Surg 2010;211(1):33–40.

71. Qiu M-Z, Wang Z-Q, Zhang D-S, et al. Comparison of 6th and 7th AJCC TNM staging classification for carcinoma of the stomach in China. Ann Surg Oncol 2011;18(7):1869–76.

72. Strong VE, Song KY, Park CH, et al. Comparison of gastric cancer survival following R0 resection in the United States and Korea using an internationally validated nomogram. Ann Surg 2010;251(4):640–6.

73. Nomura A, Stemmermann GN, Chyou PH, et al. *Helicobacter pylori* infection and gastric carcinoma among Japanese Americans in Hawaii. N Engl J Med 1991; 325(16):1132.

74. Yao JC, Tseng JF, Worah S, et al. Clinicopathologic behavior of gastric adenocarcinoma in Hispanic patients: analysis of a single institution's experience over 15 years. J Clin Oncol 2005;23(13):3094.

75. An C, Choi IS, Yao JC, et al. Prognostic significance of CpG island methylator phenotype and microsatellite instability in gastric carcinoma. Clin Cancer Res 2005;11(2):656.

76. Steinberg ML, Hwang BJ, Tang L, et al. E-cadherin gene alterations in gastric cancers in different ethnic populations. Ethn Dis 2008;18(2 Suppl 2). S2-70–S2-74.

77. Shah MA, Khanin R, Tang L, et al. Molecular classification of gastric cancer: a new paradigm. Clin Cancer Res 2011;17(9):2693–701.
78. Tan IB, Ivanova T, Lim KH, et al. Intrinsic subtypes of gastric cancer, based on gene expression pattern, predict survival and respond differently to chemotherapy. Gastroenterology 2011;141(2):476–85.e11.
79. Wang K, Kan J, Yuen ST, et al. Exome sequencing identifies frequent mutation of ARID1A in molecular subtypes of gastric cancer. Nat Genet 2011; 43(12):1219–23.
80. Deng N, Goh LK, Wang H, et al. A comprehensive survey of genomic alterations in gastric cancer reveals systematic patterns of molecular exclusivity and co-occurrence among distinct therapeutic targets. Gut 2012;61:673–84.
81. Wang G, Hu N, Yang HH, et al. Comparison of global gene expression of gastric cardia and noncardia cancers from a high-risk population in china. PLoS One 2013;8(5):e63826.
82. Network Genome Atlas Research Network. Comprehensive molecular characterization of gastric adenocarcinoma. Nature 2014;513(7517):202–9.
83. Yoon K-A, Ku J-L, Yang H-K, et al. Germline mutations of E-cadherin gene in Korean familial gastric cancer patients. J Hum Genet 1999;44(3):177–80.
84. Shinmura K, Kohno T, Takahashi M, et al. Familial gastric cancer: clinicopathological characteristics, RER phenotype and germline p53 and E-cadherin mutations. Carcinogenesis 1999;20(6):1127–31.
85. Yabuta T, Shinmura K, Tani M, et al. E-cadherin gene variants in gastric cancer families whose probands are diagnosed with diffuse gastric cancer. Int J Cancer 2002;101(5):434–41.
86. Blair V, Martin I, Shaw D, et al. Hereditary diffuse gastric cancer: diagnosis and management. Clin Gastroenterol Hepatol 2006;4(3):262–75.
87. Fitzgerald RC, Hardwick R, Huntsman D, et al. Hereditary diffuse gastric cancer: updated consensus guidelines for clinical management and directions for future research. J Med Genet 2010;47(7):436–44.

Hereditary Colorectal Cancer: Genetics and Screening

Lodewijk A.A. Brosens, MD, PhD[a,b,*], G. Johan A. Offerhaus, MD, PhD, MPH[a], Francis M. Giardiello, MD[c,d,*]

KEYWORDS

- Colorectal cancer • Hereditary nonpolyposis colorectal cancer • Lynch syndrome
- Familial adenomatous polyposis • MUTYH-associated polyposis

KEY POINTS

- Thirty percent of patients with CRC have a family history of CRC.
- Only 5% of CRCs arise in the setting of a mendelian inherited syndrome.
- Lynch syndrome is an autosomal dominant inherited disorder caused by germline mutation in one of the mismatch repair genes (*MLH1, MSH2, MSH6, PMS2*) or *EpCAM* gene and characterized by microsatellite unstable cancers.
- Patients with Lynch syndrome have a high risk of CRC (50%–80% lifetime risk) and extracolonic malignancies.
- Familial adenomatous polyposis (FAP) is an autosomal dominant inherited disorder caused by germline mutation of the *APC* (adenomatous polyposis coli) gene and characterized by hundreds to thousands of adenomatous polyps in the colorectum.
- If untreated, the lifetime risk of CRC in FAP is nearly 100%, and the average age of CRC diagnosis is 39 years.
- Attenuated FAP (AFAP) is characterized by fewer colorectal adenomatous polyps and a 70% lifetime risk of CRC.
- MUTYH-associated polyposis in an autosomal recessive inherited disorder caused by germline mutation in the *MUTYH* gene is characterized by a polyposis phenotype similar to AFAP and associated with an 80% lifetime risk of CRC.

Funding support: The John G Rangos Sr. Charitable Foundation; The Clayton Fund; NIH grant P50 CA62924; the Union for International Cancer Control (UICC) Yamagiwa-Yoshida Memorial International Cancer Study Grants; and the Nijbakker-Morra Stichting.

Disclosures and/or conflicts of interest: The authors have nothing to disclose.

[a] Department of Pathology, University Medical Center Utrecht (H04-312), Heidelberglaan 100, Utrecht 3584 CX, The Netherlands; [b] Department of Pathology, The Johns Hopkins University School of Medicine, CRB 2, Room 345, 1550 Orleans Street, Baltimore, MD 21231, USA; [c] Department of Medicine, Oncology Center, The Johns Hopkins University School of Medicine, 1830 East Monument Street, Room 431, Baltimore, MD 21205, USA; [d] Department of Pathology, The Johns Hopkins University School of Medicine, 1830 East Monument Street, Room 431, Baltimore, MD 21205, USA

* Corresponding authors.

E-mail addresses: l.a.a.brosens@umcutrecht.nl; fgiardi@jhmi.edu

Surg Clin N Am 95 (2015) 1067–1080
http://dx.doi.org/10.1016/j.suc.2015.05.004   surgical.theclinics.com
0039-6109/15/$ – see front matter © 2015 Elsevier Inc. All rights reserved.

INTRODUCTION

With more than 140,000 newly diagnosed patients each year, colorectal cancer (CRC) is the third most common cancer and the third leading cause of cancer death in men and women in the United States.[1] In 30% of these patients there is a family history of CRC, suggesting a heritable component, but only 5% of CRCs arise in the setting of a well-established mendelian inherited disorder such as Lynch syndrome (LS), familial adenomatous polyposis (FAP), mutY Homolog (MUTYH)-associated polyposis (MAP), juvenile polyposis, hereditary mixed polyposis, and Peutz-Jeghers syndrome.[2–4] In addition, serrated polyposis is a clinically defined syndrome characterized by multiple serrated polyps in the colorectum and an increased CRC risk, but the genetics are not yet known[5] (**Table 1**). Most familial CRCs (20%–30%) arise as so-called nonsyndromic familial CRC and likely have a multigenetic cause.[2,5] This article discusses genetic and clinical aspects of the 3 main hereditary CRC syndromes: LS, FAP, and MAP.

LYNCH SYNDROME
Clinical Features

LS (also known as hereditary nonpolyposis CRC [HNPCC]) is an autosomal dominantly inherited syndrome caused by germline mutation in one of the mismatch repair genes (*MLH1*, *MSH2*, *MSH6*, *PMS2*) or the *EpCAM* gene. Because of this genetic defect, LS tumors are characterized by microsatellite instability (MSI).[4]

CRC is the major clinical consequence of LS. The lifetime risk of CRC in LS has been variably estimated and seems to depend on the mismatch repair (MMR) gene mutated (**Table 2**). The average age of CRC diagnosis in patients with LS is 44 to 61 years, compared with 69 years in sporadic CRC. Tumors arise primarily (60%–80%) proximal to the splenic flexure.[6] A high rate of metachronous CRC (16% at 10 years; 41% at 20 years) is noted in patients with LS.[7–9] Compared with patients with attenuated FAP (AFAP) or MAP, patients with LS develop few colorectal adenomas by the age of 50 years (usually <3 adenomas).[10] The adenoma-carcinoma sequence seems to be more rapid in LS, with polyp to cancer times estimated at 35 months compared with 10 to 15 years in sporadic cancer.[10] The histopathology of LS CRC is often poorly differentiated, with signet cell histology, abundant extracellular mucin, tumor-infiltrating lymphocytes, and a lymphoid host response to tumor.[11] Patients with LS

Table 1 CRC syndromes		
Syndrome	**Genes**	**Mode of Inheritance**
LS	*MLH1, MSH2, MSH6, PMS2,* or *EpCAM*	Autosomal dominant
(Attenuated) FAP	*APC*	Autosomal dominant
MUTYH-associated polyposis	*MUTYH (MYH)*	Autosomal recessive
Peutz-Jeghers syndrome	*LKB1 (STK11)*	Autosomal dominant
Juvenile polyposis syndrome	*SMAD4* (~30%) *BMPR1A* (~20%)	Autosomal dominant
Hereditary mixed polyposis syndrome	*GREM1*	Autosomal dominant
Serrated polyposis syndrome	Unknown	Unknown

Table 2
Risk of CRC by age 70 years in LS

Gene Mutation Carriers	Risk (%)	Average Age of Diagnosis (y)
Sporadic CRC	5.5	69
MLH1 and *MSH2*	22–74	27–46
MSH6	10–22	54–63
PMS2	15–20	47–66

have improved survival from CRC stage for stage compared with patients with sporadic CRC.

In addition to CRC, patients with LS have increased risk for many extracolonic malignancies (**Table 3**). Endometrial cancer occurs in up to 54% of women with *MLH1* and *MSH2* mutations, with lower risk in those with *PMS2* (15%) mutations and much higher risk in women with *MSH6* mutations (71%). Later onset of colorectal and endometrial cancers is noted in patients with a *MSH6* mutation, compared with other MMR gene defects. In addition, tumors arising in the context of *MSH6* mutations can display low levels of MSI or even microsatellite stability.[6] Other neoplasms with lifetime risks ranging from 4% to 25% include transitional cell carcinoma of the urinary tract; adenocarcinomas of the ovary, stomach, hepatobiliary tract, and small bowel; brain cancer (glioblastoma); and cutaneous sebaceous neoplasms.[6,12] An increased risk of pancreas cancer in LS has been described by some investigators.[6] The relative risk of prostate cancer may be 2-fold to 2.5-fold higher than for the general population.[6] The relationship between LS and breast cancer is unclear. Also, laryngeal and hematological malignancies have been described but a definite association with LS is not established.[6] An association between sarcoma and LS probably exists but the magnitude of risk is unclear.[6]

Phenotypic stigmata of LS are rare but can include café-au-lait spots, cutaneous sebaceous gland tumors, and keratoacanthomas.[13] Café-au-lait spots are found in

Table 3
Risk of extracolonic cancer by age 70 years in LS

Cancer	Risk General Population (%)	Risk in LS (%)	Average Age of Diagnosis (y)
Endometrium	2.7	—	65
MLH1/MSH2	—	14–54	48–62
MSH6	—	17–71	54–57
PMS2	—	15	49
Stomach	<1	0.2–13	49–55
Ovary	1.6	4–20	43–45
Breast	12.4	5–18	52
Prostate	16.2	9–30	59–60
Urinary tract	<1	0.2–25	52–60
Small bowel	<1	0.4–12	46–49
Pancreas	1.5	0.4–4.0	63–65
Hepatobiliary tract	<1	0.02–4	54–57
Brain/central nervous system	<1	1–4	50
Sebaceous neoplasm	<1	1–9	n/a

a variant of LS known as constitutional mismatch repair deficiency syndrome, which is caused by biallelic mutations of MMR genes. In addition, these patients develop CRC or other LS cancers at a young age (childhood and teenage years), oligopolyposis in the small bowel and/or colon, brain tumors, and hematologic malignancies.[14]

Several sets of clinical criteria identify patients with LS. In 1990, the International Collaborative Group on Hereditary Nonpolyposis Colorectal Cancer established criteria (Amsterdam I Criteria) for HNPCC.[15] All of the following are required to diagnose HNPCC: (1) 3 or more relatives with histologically verified CRC, 1 of whom is a first-degree relative of the other 2 (FAP should be excluded); (2) CRC involving at least 2 generations; (3) 1 or more CRC cases diagnosed before the age of 50 years. More sensitive criteria, called Amsterdam II criteria, were established in 1999.[16] Amsterdam II criteria include some extracolonic tumors commonly seen in LS as qualifying cancers, in particular cancer of the endometrium, small bowel, or urothelium. Other LS-related tumors are now also included, such as cancer of the ovary, stomach, hepatobiliary tract, and brain.

The Revised Bethesda Guidelines are a third set of clinicopathologic criteria developed to identify individuals who deserve investigation for LS by evaluation of MSI and/or immunohistochemistry testing of their tumors.[17]

Genetic Defect

Germline mutations in one of several DNA mismatch repair genes, specifically *MLH1*, *MSH2*, *MSH6*, and *PMS2*, cause LS. These genes maintain fidelity of the DNA during replication by correction of nucleotide base mispairs and small insertions or deletions generated by misincorporations or slippage of DNA polymerase during DNA replication.[2,4] Mutations of the *EpCAM* gene, located just upstream from the *MSH2* gene, results in silencing of the *MSH2* gene in tissues that express *EpCAM* and produces a phenotype that is similar to LS.[18] Mutations in *MLH1* and *MSH2* account for up to 90% of patients with LS and up to 10% of LS patients have a *MSH6* mutation. A small minority of LS cases are caused by *PMS2* or *EpCAM* mutation.[4] Rare patients with a germline epimutation causing *MLH1* hypermethylation have been described.[19]

LS tumors are characterized by MSI, which is ubiquitous mutations at simple repetitive sequences (microsatellites) found in the tumor DNA (but not in DNA of adjacent normal colorectal mucosa) of individuals with MMR gene defects. MSI in a CRC indicates a defect in one of the MMR genes caused by either somatic inactivation (hypermethylation of the *MLH1* promoter in sporadic CRC) or a germline MMR gene defect (LS). MSI is found in most (>90%) colon malignancies in patients with LS and in 12% of patients with sporadic CRC. MSI is graded as MSI-high (MSI-H) (>30% of markers are unstable), MSI-low (<30% of markers are unstable), and MS-stable (no markers are unstable).[4]

Immunohistochemistry testing of CRC using antibodies to the MMR gene proteins MLH1, MSH2, MSH6, and PMS2 evaluates for the loss of MMR protein expression and assists in the identification of patients with LS. Deleterious alterations (either germline or somatic) in specific DNA MMR genes are indicated by loss or partial production of the MMR protein produced by that gene.[4]

Somatic mutations in the *BRAF* gene, largely at codon 600, are noted in 15% of sporadic CRCs but not in LS tumors.[20] Consequently, the presence of a *BRAF* mutation in an MSI-H CRC is evidence against the presence of LS.[4]

Genetic Testing

Identification of patients with LS can be done by application of the Amsterdam or Revised Bethesda Criteria, use of computer models of risk, tumor testing, or germline testing. Because the use of clinical criteria and modeling to identify patients with LS does not have optimal sensitivity and efficiency, universal screening for LS has also been endorsed by EGAPP (Evaluation of Genomic Application in Practice and Prevention) and by Healthy People 2020, the National Comprehensive Cancer Network (NCCN), and the Multi-Society Task Force on Colorectal Cancer (MSTF).[6,21] The MSTF recommends that this is done for all CRCs, or CRC diagnosed at age 70 years or earlier, and in individuals older than 70 years with a family history concerning for LS. Analysis may be done by immunohistochemical testing for the MLH1/MSH2/MSH6/PMS2 proteins and/or MSI testing. Tumors with loss of MLH1 should undergo analysis for *BRAF* mutation or *MLH1* promoter hypermethylation. If universal screening reveals evidence of LS, patients should be referred for genetic evaluation, which can involve germline testing for an MMR gene mutation (*MLH1, MSH2, MSH6, PMS2*) or the *EpCAM* gene. Also, patients with endometrial cancer before age 50 years, a known familial MMR gene mutation, fulfilling Amsterdam criteria or revised Bethesda guidelines, or a personal risk of greater than 5% of LS based on prediction models should undergo genetic evaluation for LS.

Management

Patients with LS are at increased risk of colorectal and extracolonic cancers at early ages. Although there is insufficient evidence to assess the benefit of annual history, physical examination, and patient and family education, expert opinion recommends this practice starting at 20 to 25 years of age.

A variety of screening recommendations exists for patients at risk (first-degree relatives of those affected) or affected with LS.[6] Screening for CRC by colonoscopy is recommended every 1 to 2 years, beginning at ages 20 to 25 years or 2 to 5 years before the youngest age of CRC diagnosis in the family if diagnosed before age 25 years. Screening for endometrial cancer should be offered to women by pelvic examination and endometrial sampling annually starting at age 30 to 35 years. Screening for ovarian cancer should be offered to women with LS by transvaginal ultrasonography annually starting at age 30 to 35 years. Hysterectomy and bilateral salpingo-oophorectomy should be recommended to women with LS who have finished childbearing or at age 40 years. Screening for gastric cancer should be considered in persons with LS by esophagogastroduodenoscopy with gastric biopsy of the antrum at age 30 to 35 years with *Helicobacter pylori* eradication when found. Subsequent surveillance every 2 to 3 years can be considered based on individual patient risk factors. Screening for cancer of the urinary tract should be considered with urinalysis annually starting at age 30 to 35 years.

Colectomy with ileorectal anastomosis is the primary treatment of patients with LS with CRC or colon neoplasia not removable by endoscopy. With partial colectomy a high 10-year cumulative risk of metachronous CRC (16%–19%) is reported, even in patients undergoing vigilant colonoscopic surveillance, and increases with longer observation.[7–9] This risk is substantially reduced if a subtotal or total colectomy is performed (0%–3.4%).[7–9] No difference in global quality of life was noted between patients with LS with partial or subtotal colectomy, although functional outcome (stool frequency, stool related aspects, social impact) was worse after subtotal colectomy.[22] Comparison of life expectancy gained performing total colectomy versus hemicolectomy in patients with LS at ages 27, 47, and 67 years by Markov modeling was 2.3, 1.0, 0.3 years, respectively.[23] These investigators concluded that total colectomy is the preferred treatment in LS but hemicolectomy may be an option in older patients. Although most LS CRCs are right sided, up to 20% occur in the rectum. When this happens, clinical decision making should include use of neoadjuvant chemoradiation and consideration of total proctocolectomy and ileal pouch–anal anastomosis (IPAA). Kalady and colleagues[24] found a risk of metachronous advanced neoplasia (cancer and severe dysplasia) of 51% in patients with HNPCC who had a low anterior resection for rectal cancer. Win and colleagues[9] found an overall risk of cancer of 24.5% and a cumulative risk to 30 years of 69%. Total proctocolectomy and IPAA is thus an important option to discuss with patients with LS with rectal cancer.

Growing but not conclusive evidence exists that use of aspirin is beneficial in preventing cancer in LS. Treatment of an individual patient with aspirin is a consideration after discussion of patient-specific risks, benefits, and uncertainties of treatment is conducted.[25]

FAMILIAL ADENOMATOUS POLYPOSIS
Clinical Features

FAP is an autosomal dominant inherited syndrome caused by germline mutation in the *APC* (adenomatous polyposis coli) gene.[26] Depending on the location of the mutation in the *APC* gene, FAP can manifest either in a classic form (classic FAP) or in the form of AFAP.[3,27] The prevalence of FAP is about 1 in 13,000.

Classic *FAP* is characterized by development in the teenage years of hundreds to thousands of adenomatous polyps (a minimum of 100) throughout the colorectum. About 50% of patients develop adenomas by age 15 years and 95% by age 35 years. If left untreated, patients with FAP develop CRC at an average age of 39 years (range, 35–43 years).[28]

AFAP is defined by the presence of an average of 30 polyps (oligopolyposis).[2] The diagnosis should be considered in patients 40 to 50 years old with 10 to 100 adenomas cumulatively. Patients with AFAP have a 70% lifetime risk of CRC, about 12 years later than in classic FAP.[2,28] Note that oligopolyposis can be an expression of a germline *APC* mutation or a biallelic *MUTYH* mutation (MUTYH-polyposis; discussed later).[29]

A variety of benign and malignant extracolonic manifestations have been described in FAP. Of concern are duodenal adenomas and duodenal cancer.[30] Duodenal adenomas are present in 30% to 70% of patients with FAP with a lifetime risk of almost 100%. The lifetime risk of duodenal adenocarcinoma is 4% to 10%. The Spigelman classification system is used to grade severity and guide clinical management of duodenal polyposis (**Tables 4** and **5**).[2,30,31] Adenomas in the jejunum and ileum occur sporadically. Most gastric polyps are benign fundic gland polyps, and are present in 50% of patients. Gastric adenomas occur in about 10% of patients with FAP, usually in the antrum. The lifetime risk of gastric cancer is low (0.6%–1%).[2,31]

Table 4
Spigelman classification for duodenal polyposis in FAP

Criteria	Points		
	1	2	3
Polyp number	1–4	5–20	>20
Polyp size (mm)	1–4	5–10	>10
Histology	Tubular	Tubulovillous	Villous
Dysplasia	Low grade	—	High grade

Stage 0, 0 points; stage I, 1 to 4 points; stage II, 5 to 6 points; stage III, 7 to 8 points; stage IV, 9 to 12 points.

From Spigelman AD, Williams CB, Talbot IC, et al. Upper gastrointestinal cancer in patients with familial adenomatous polyposis. Lancet 1989;2:784; with permission.

Table 5
Recommendations for management of duodenal polyposis in FAP, adjusted to the Spigelman stage of duodenal polyposis

Spigelman Stage	Endoscopic Frequency	Chemoprevention	Surgery
Stage 0	4 y	No	No
Stage I	2–3 y	No	No
Stage II	2–3 y	±	No
Stage III	6–12 mo	±	±
Stage IV	6–12 mo	±	Yes

Less frequent extraintestinal malignancies in FAP are hepatoblastoma and cancers of the thyroid, biliary tree, pancreas, and central nervous system.[3,28,32] The combination of colorectal polyposis and a primary central nervous system malignancy (medulloblastoma) is called Crail syndrome.

Desmoid tumors occur in about 10% of patients with FAP and are usually located in the small intestinal mesentery, abdominal wall or extremities.[33] Intra-abdominal desmoid tumors have a poor prognosis. Although desmoid tumors have no metastatic potential, local expansion and invasive growth with damage to intra-abdominal structures and perioperative complications are the cause of death in a significant proportion of patients with FAP.[3]

Benign extraintestinal manifestations can be used as diagnostic tools in the examination of first-degree relatives of patients with FAP.[3,34] Congenital hypertrophy of the retinal pigment epithelium (CHRPE) is discrete round-oval darkly pigmented areas in the ocular fundus ranging in size from 0.1 to 1 optic-disc diameter, and is found in greater than 90% of patients with FAP. CHRPE is asymptomatic but bilateral and/or multiple (>4) CHRPE is a clinical marker for asymptomatic carriers in families with FAP.[34,35]

Several oral and maxillofacial lesions can be found in patients with FAP. Occult radio-opaque jaw lesions are osteosclerotic bone lesions found on panoramic jaw radiographs and are used as predictors for polyp development in families with FAP with jaw lesions.[36] Oral mucosal vascular density may be a clinical marker of FAP and others at high risk for CRC.[37] Patients with FAP have an increased risk of jaw osteomas (in 46%–93% of patients with FAP), odontomas (in 9%–83% of patients with FAP), supernumerary teeth (in 11%–27% of patients with FAP), or unerupted (in 4%–38% of patients with FAP) teeth.[38] In addition, nasopharyngeal angiofibroma is 25 times more common in patients with FAP than in the general population.[39] Cutaneous lesions found in patients with FAP are lipomas, fibromas, and sebaceous and epidermoid cysts. In older literature, the combination of colorectal adenomatous polyposis and extraintestinal manifestations was designated as Gardner syndrome but it is now recognized that most patients with FAP have 1 or more extracolonic manifestations.[28]

Genetic Defect

The *APC* gene, a tumor suppressor gene on chromosome 5q21, was identified as the cause of FAP in 1991.[26] The *APC* gene has 15 exons and encodes a 2843-amino-acid protein with a key function in the Wnt signaling pathway. Germline mutations in the *APC* gene are found in 80% to 90% of patients with classic FAP and in 10% to 30% of patients with AFAP.[3] More than 300 different *APC* gene mutations have been reported. Most are frameshifts caused by insertions or deletions, or nonsense mutations, leading to truncated APC proteins. A high frequency of somatic *APC* mutations is found in the mutation cluster region in the 5′ part of exon 15, between codons 1286 and 1513, and in codon 1309.[28,40]

Genotype-phenotype studies showed that *APC* mutations in the central part of the gene (between codons 160 and 1393) result in classic FAP. Mutations between codon 1250 and codon 1464 cause profuse polyposis (>1000 colorectal polyps). In contrast, mutations in the 3′ and 5′ ends of the gene predispose to AFAP.[27,40] Genotype-phenotype correlations for duodenal polyposis in FAP are less clear, but may correlate with mutations distal to codon 1400 in exon 15.[30]

Several genotype-phenotype correlations have been reported. These correlations include multiplicity of extraintestinal lesions with mutations in codons 1465, 1546, and 2621 of the *APC* gene; ocular fundus lesions (CHRPE) with mutations between codons 463 and 1444; thyroid cancer with mutations in the 5′ part of exon 15 (outside codons 1286–1513) at codon 1061; and desmoid tumors with mutations at the 3′ end of codon 1444. *APC* mutation between codons 697 and 1224 has been linked with a 3-fold increased risk of brain tumors in general, and a 13-fold increased risk of medulloblastoma.[32] However, caution is needed in genetic counseling of patients with FAP because considerable intrafamilial and interfamilial phenotypic variability exists.

The *APC I1307K* gene mutation is found in 6% of Ashkenazi Jews. This T to A mutation at nucleotide 3920 leads to an extended mononucleotide tract of 8 consecutive adenine base pairs in one of the *APC* alleles. Although the predicted missense mutation itself does not lead to a dysfunctional APC protein, it leads to susceptibility to additional somatic mutations in this *APC* allele caused by polymerase slipping during DNA replication. The *I1307K* mutation confers a 2-fold increased risk of CRC and is associated with an increased number of adenomas (sometimes oligopolyposis as in AFAP) and CRCs per patient.[41]

Management

Colorectum

Patients with colorectal disorders at risk of FAP (first-degree relatives of patients with FAP) should be screened between the ages of 10 and 12 years. *APC* gene testing is the test of choice (**Box 1**). If no informative genetic test can be obtained, patients should have endoscopic screening with a yearly sigmoidoscopy or colonoscopy starting between the ages of 10 and 15 years. Each subsequent decade's screening frequency can be reduced by a year up to age 50 years, when patients should be screened every 3 years.[28]

For individuals suspected of AFAP, gene testing is recommended if 20 or more cumulative colorectal adenomas are found. Patients at risk for AFAP should receive endoscopic screening with colonoscopy at ages 12, 15, 18, and 21 years, and then every 2 years.[28] About 33% of patients with AFAP can be managed in the long term endoscopically by polypectomy.[2]

Box 1
Indications for *APC* gene testing

Greater than or equal to 100 colorectal adenomas

First-degree relatives of patients with FAP

Greater than or equal to 20 cumulative colorectal adenomas (suspected AFAP)

First-degree relatives of patients with AFAP

Prophylactic colectomy should be performed shortly after diagnosis of FAP to prevent CRC development. Surgical options include subtotal colectomy with ileorectal anastomosis, total proctocolectomy with Brooke ileostomy (or with continent ileostomy), and total proctocolectomy with mucosal proctectomy and ileoanal pull-through (with pouch formation). Lifelong endoscopic surveillance of any remaining rectal segment every 6 months is required because approximately 25% of these patients develop rectal cancer. From 16% to 33% of these patients eventually need proctocolectomy. Proctocolectomy with either ileostomy or restorative proctocolectomy is indicated for patients with dense polyposis and carcinoma at the time of subtotal colectomy in view of a very high risk of rectal cancer.[2,3]

Chemopreventive strategies, particularly with nonsteroidal antiinflammatory drugs (NSAIDs), have been studied in patients with FAP to delay adenoma development in the upper and lower gastrointestinal tract and to prevent adenoma recurrence in the retained rectum after rectal-sparing surgery. The NSAID sulindac and selective cyclooxygenase-2 inhibitor celecoxib reduced the number and size of colorectal polyps in the short term. Long-term use of sulindac reduced polyp number and prevented recurrence of high-grade adenomas in the retained rectal segment, although effects are variable and stringent endoscopic surveillance remains essential. The main benefit of NSAIDs may be more straightforward endoscopic surveillance because of decreased numbers and smaller polyps. Primary chemoprevention of adenomas in phenotypically unaffected *APC* gene mutation–positive patients did not prevent development of polyposis. Curcumin and eicosapentaenoic acid have shown efficacy in small chemoprevention trials and are being further studied.[42]

Upper gastrointestinal tract

Upper gastrointestinal endoscopy is indicated for patients with FAP between the ages of 25 and 30 years. Endoscopic surveillance regimens are best dictated by the Spigelman stage of duodenal polyposis[30,31] (see **Tables 4** and **5**). Endoscopic treatment of duodenal polyposis is troubled by high recurrence rates, varying from 50% to 100%. The benefit of endoscopic therapy is thus controversial, but may be useful in individual cases and to postpone surgery.[30] Surgery for duodenal polyposis is indicated in patients with Spigelman stage IV duodenal polyposis. Surgical options are local surgery (duodenotomy with polypectomy and/or ampullectomy), pancreas-preserving and pylorus-preserving duodenectomy, or classical pancreaticoduodenectomy. Morbidity and mortality of the type of surgery should be weighed against the risk of duodenal malignancy.[30]

Chemoprevention of duodenal polyps with NSAIDs seems less effective than in the colorectum. Although some groups find modest regression of small duodenal adenomas in patients treated with 400 mg of sulindac or 800 mg of celecoxib, most reports find no significant effect on duodenal polyposis.[30]

Desmoid tumors

Desmoid tumors are an important cause of morbidity and mortality in FAP. Surgery seems to be the treatment of choice for extra-abdominal and abdominal wall desmoids. The optimal treatment of intra-abdominal desmoids is less clear. Comparable outcomes have been reported for a conservative approach and surgery. Pharmacologic therapies with NSAIDs and antiestrogens showed comparable outcomes. Combination chemotherapy including doxorubicin seems to be the best option for progressively growing intra-abdominal desmoids.[3,43]

MUTYH-ASSOCIATED POLYPOSIS
Clinical Features

MAP is an autosomal recessively inherited syndrome caused by germline mutation of both alleles of the *MUTYH* gene (also known as the *MYH* gene).[44] The colonic phenotype mimics that of AFAP. Most patients have between 10 and a few hundred adenomas. Alternatively, biallelic germline *MUTYH* mutations have been found in some patients with early-onset CRC and few to zero polyps.[44] Although most polyps in MAP are adenomas, patients can present with serrated polyps or a mixture of adenomas and serrated polyps.[45] Colorectal polyps usually develop around the age of 40 years. The risk of CRC in MAP is 19% by age 50 years and 43% by age 60 years. The average age of CRC onset is 48 years. Relatives of patients with MAP with a heterozygous *MUTYH* mutation have a risk of CRC comparable with that of first-degree relatives of patients with sporadic CRC.[46]

Gastric and duodenal polyps occur in 11% to 17% of patients with MAP. The lifetime risk of duodenal cancer is about 4%.[47] A statistically nonsignificant trend toward an increased risk of gastric cancer is reported.[44,47]

Compared with the general population, patients with MAP have an almost doubled risk of extraintestinal malignancies, including ovarian, bladder, skin, and possibly breast cancer. However, based on the spectrum of cancers and the late age of onset, intensive surveillance measures for extraintestinal malignancies are not recommended.[47]

Genetic Defect

The *MUTYH* gene consists of 16 exons and is located on chromosome 1p34.3-p32.1. *MUTYH* encodes a DNA glycosylase involved in base excision repair of 8-oxo-7,8-dihydro-2′-deoxyguanosine:adenine mismatches caused by oxidative DNA damage.

Biallelic *MUTYH* mutations are found in about 30% of patients with 10 to 100 polyps and in 15% of patients with 100 to 1000 polyps. Especially in patients with more than 15 synchronous adenomas and CRC before age 50 years, there is a very high chance of finding biallelic *MUTYH* mutations.[44] **Box 2** summarizes indications for *MUTYH* germline testing.

More than 100 unique *MUTYH* gene mutations have been reported. Most of these are missense mutations, although small deletions, duplications, and insertions also occur. Y179C and G396D are hotspot mutations in white populations. At least 1 Y179C or G396D mutation is present in 90% of white patients with MAP and biallelic mutation of Y179C and/or G396D is present in 70%. However, there seems to be ethnic and regional differentiation in the *MUTYH* mutation spectrum.[44] Despite these population-specific mutations, the entire *MUTYH* gene should be screened for mutations.

Genotype-phenotype studies have shown that patients with homozygous G396D mutations or compound heterozygous G396D/Y179C mutations have a less severe

---

Box 2
Indications for *MUTYH* gene testing

Between 10 and 100 polyps (adenomas; can be mixed with serrated polyps)

Siblings of patients with biallelic *MUTYH* mutation

Consider: patients with early-onset CRC (<49–55 years) with or without polyps

Consider: children of monoallelic or biallelic *MUTYH* mutation carriers phenotype than patients with biallelic Y179C mutation. This finding is consistent with the greater reduction in glycosylase activity of Y179C mutations than G396D mutations. Patients with at least 1 G396D allele present later with MAP and have a significantly lower risk and later age of CRC diagnosis than patients with biallelic Y179C mutation. The mean ages of CRC diagnosis were 58 years (homozygous G396D), 52 years (compound heterozygous G396D/Y179C), and 46 years (homozygous Y179C) respectively.[48] Patients with a compound mutation of G396D and a mutation other than Y179C did not show a milder phenotype.

Management

Patients with MAP should undergo colonoscopy every 1 to 2 years. Subtotal colectomy is recommended if endoscopic management fails or if CRC develops. At present it is unclear whether patients with monoallelic *MUTYH* mutation should receive more intensive CRC screening than average-risk individuals.

Recommendations for screening and management of the upper gastrointestinal tract of patients with MAP are comparable with those for patients with FAP. Upper gastrointestinal tract screening should start around 30 years of age and, depending on the findings, be repeated at intervals similar to those used for FAP (see **Table 5**).

SUMMARY

CRC is the third most common cancer. Although most CRCs arise in a sporadic setting, without a clear familial or hereditary component, recognition of patients with a hereditary form of CRC is vital in view of the consequences for the patients and their families. Also, hereditary CRC syndromes are paradigms for gastrointestinal carcinogenesis in general. FAP was the first polyposis syndrome molecularly characterized by the discovery of the *APC* gene. Tumorigenesis in FAP is considered the prototype of the adenoma-carcinoma sequence in the large bowel caused by disrupted gatekeeper function of APC and subsequent Wnt activation accompanied by an accumulation of genetic changes and resultant clonal expansion.[26] Most (60%) CRCs follow this classic adenoma-carcinoma pathway characterized by Wnt activation and chromosomal instability.[49]

LS is the prototype of CRC caused by a caretaker defect (ie, deficiency of one of the MMR genes leading to cancers with MSI). About 15% of all CRCs are characterized by MMR deficiency and MSI. Most of these MSI CRCs are caused by somatic hypermethylation of the MMR gene *MLH1*, whereas a minority are caused by an inherited MMR gene defect, as in LS.[49]

For decades CRC was classified as either chromosomal instable or chromosomal stable/microsatellite unstable and all colorectal carcinomas were thought to arise from conventional adenomas via the suppressor pathway initiated with *APC* gene mutation (the classic Fearon-Vogelstein model). Elucidation of the serrated pathway to CRC in the past decade revealed that molecular classification of CRC is more complex and heterogeneous and that up to 25% of CRCs develop trough the serrated pathway. The recognition of the serrated pathway to CRC has shifted understanding of the molecular basis of CRC and changed clinical practice. Although polyps with a serrated architecture were previously considered harmless lesions, larger and right-sided serrated polyps are now recognized as bona fide CRC precursor lesions that should be removed like conventional adenomas. Although the genetics of serrated polyposis syndrome are not yet understood, studying this intriguing syndrome will undoubtedly further increase understanding of colorectal carcinogenesis in a similar way to studies on other inherited CRC syndromes.[26,49]

ACKNOWLEDGMENTS

The authors are indebted to Ms Linda Welch for technical support.

REFERENCES

1. Siegel R, Desantis C, Jemal A. Colorectal cancer statistics, 2014. CA Cancer J Clin 2014;64:104–17.
2. Jasperson KW, Tuohy TM, Neklason DW, et al. Hereditary and familial colon cancer. Gastroenterology 2010;138:2044–58.
3. Brosens LA, van Hattem WA, Jansen M, et al. Gastrointestinal polyposis syndromes. Curr Mol Med 2007;7:29–46.
4. Jansen M, Menko FH, Brosens LA, et al. Establishing a clinical and molecular diagnosis for hereditary colorectal cancer syndromes: Present tense, future perfect? Gastrointest Endosc 2014;80:1145–55.
5. Jass JR. Gastrointestinal polyposes: clinical, pathological and molecular features. Gastroenterol Clin North Am 2007;36:927–46, viii.
6. Giardiello FM, Allen JI, Axilbund JE, et al. Guidelines on genetic evaluation and management of Lynch syndrome: a consensus statement by the US Multi-Society Task Force on colorectal cancer. Gastroenterology 2014;147:502–26.
7. de Vos tot Nederveen Cappel WH, Nagengast FM, Griffioen G, et al. Surveillance for hereditary nonpolyposis colorectal cancer: a long-term study on 114 families. Dis Colon Rectum 2002;45:1588–94.
8. Parry S, Win AK, Parry B, et al. Metachronous colorectal cancer risk for mismatch repair gene mutation carriers: the advantage of more extensive colon surgery. Gut 2011;60:950–7.
9. Win AK, Parry S, Parry B, et al. Risk of metachronous colon cancer following surgery for rectal cancer in mismatch repair gene mutation carriers. Ann Surg Oncol 2013;20:1829–36.
10. Edelstein DL, Axilbund J, Baxter M, et al. Rapid development of colorectal neoplasia in patients with Lynch syndrome. Clin Gastroenterol Hepatol 2011;9: 340–3.
11. Peltomäki PT, Offerhaus GJ, Vasen HFA. Lynch syndrome. In: Bosman FT, Carneiro F, Hruban RH, et al, editors. WHO classification of tumours of the digestive system. Lyon (France): IARC Press; 2010. p. 152–5.
12. Bonadona V, Bonaiti B, Olschwang S, et al. Cancer risks associated with germline mutations in MLH1, MSH2, and MSH6 genes in Lynch syndrome. JAMA 2011; 305:2304–10.
13. Trimbath JD, Petersen GM, Erdman SH, et al. Cafe-au-lait spots and early onset colorectal neoplasia: a variant of HNPCC? Fam Cancer 2001;1:101–5.
14. Wimmer K, Kratz CP, Vasen HF, et al. Diagnostic criteria for constitutional mismatch repair deficiency syndrome: suggestions of the European consortium 'care for CMMRD' (C4CMMRD). J Med Genet 2014;51:355–65.
15. Vasen HF, Mecklin JP, Khan PM, et al. The International Collaborative Group on Hereditary Non-polyposis Colorectal Cancer (ICG-HNPCC). Dis Colon Rectum 1991;34:424–5.
16. Vasen HF, Watson P, Mecklin JP, et al. New clinical criteria for hereditary nonpolyposis colorectal cancer (HNPCC, Lynch syndrome) proposed by the International Collaborative group on HNPCC. Gastroenterology 1999;116:1453–6.
17. Umar A, Boland CR, Terdiman JP, et al. Revised Bethesda Guidelines for hereditary nonpolyposis colorectal cancer (Lynch syndrome) and microsatellite instability. J Natl Cancer Inst 2004;96:261–8.

18. Ligtenberg MJ, Kuiper RP, Chan TL, et al. Heritable somatic methylation and inactivation of MSH2 in families with Lynch syndrome due to deletion of the 3' exons of TACSTD1. Nat Genet 2009;41:112–7.
19. Hitchins MP, Ward RL. Constitutional (germline) MLH1 epimutation as an aetiological mechanism for hereditary non-polyposis colorectal cancer. J Med Genet 2009;46:793–802.
20. Domingo E, Niessen RC, Oliveira C, et al. BRAF-V600E is not involved in the colorectal tumorigenesis of HNPCC in patients with functional MLH1 and MSH2 genes. Oncogene 2005;24:3995–8.
21. Evaluation of Genomic Applications in Practice and Prevention (EGAPP) Working Group. Recommendations from the EGAPP Working Group: genetic testing strategies in newly diagnosed individuals with colorectal cancer aimed at reducing morbidity and mortality from Lynch syndrome in relatives. Genet Med 2009;11:35–41.
22. Haanstra JF, de Vos Tot Nederveen Cappel WH, Gopie JP, et al. Quality of life after surgery for colon cancer in patients with Lynch syndrome: partial versus subtotal colectomy. Dis Colon Rectum 2012;55:653–9.
23. de Vos tot Nederveen Cappel WH, Buskens E, van Duijvendijk P, et al. Decision analysis in the surgical treatment of colorectal cancer due to a mismatch repair gene defect. Gut 2003;52:1752–5.
24. Kalady MF, Lipman J, McGannon E, et al. Risk of colonic neoplasia after proctectomy for rectal cancer in hereditary nonpolyposis colorectal cancer. Ann Surg 2012;255:1121–5.
25. Burn J, Bishop DT, Mecklin JP, et al. Effect of aspirin or resistant starch on colorectal neoplasia in the Lynch syndrome. N Engl J Med 2008;359:2567–78.
26. Kinzler KW, Vogelstein B. Lessons from hereditary colorectal cancer. Cell 1996;87:159–70.
27. Spirio L, Olschwang S, Groden J, et al. Alleles of the APC gene: an attenuated form of familial polyposis. Cell 1993;75:951–7.
28. Trimbath JD, Giardiello FM. Review article: genetic testing and counselling for hereditary colorectal cancer. Aliment Pharmacol Ther 2002;16:1843–57.
29. Nielsen M, Hes FJ, Nagengast FM, et al. Germline mutations in APC and MUTYH are responsible for the majority of families with attenuated familial adenomatous polyposis. Clin Genet 2007;71:427–33.
30. Brosens LA, Keller JJ, Offerhaus GJ, et al. Prevention and management of duodenal polyps in familial adenomatous polyposis. Gut 2005;54:1034–43.
31. Spigelman AD, Williams CB, Talbot IC, et al. Upper gastrointestinal cancer in patients with familial adenomatous polyposis. Lancet 1989;2:783–5.
32. Attard TM, Giglio P, Koppula S, et al. Brain tumors in individuals with familial adenomatous polyposis: a cancer registry experience and pooled case report analysis. Cancer 2007;109:761–6.
33. Nieuwenhuis MH, De Vos Tot Nederveen Cappel W, Botma A, et al. Desmoid tumors in a Dutch cohort of patients with familial adenomatous polyposis. Clin Gastroenterol Hepatol 2008;6:215–9.
34. Giardiello FM, Offerhaus GJ, Traboulsi EI, et al. Value of combined phenotypic markers in identifying inheritance of familial adenomatous polyposis. Gut 1991;32:1170–4.
35. Traboulsi EI, Krush AJ, Gardner EJ, et al. Prevalence and importance of pigmented ocular fundus lesions in Gardner's syndrome. N Engl J Med 1987;316:661–7.
36. Offerhaus GJ, Levin LS, Giardiello FM, et al. Occult radiopaque jaw lesions in familial adenomatous polyposis coli and hereditary nonpolyposis colorectal cancer. Gastroenterology 1987;93:490–7.

37. Edelstein DL, Giardiello FM, Basiri A, et al. A new phenotypic manifestation of familial adenomatous polyposis. Fam Cancer 2011;10:309–13.
38. Wijn MA, Keller JJ, Giardiello FM, et al. Oral and maxillofacial manifestations of familial adenomatous polyposis. Oral Dis 2007;13:360–5.
39. Giardiello FM, Hamilton SR, Krush AJ, et al. Nasopharyngeal angiofibroma in patients with familial adenomatous polyposis. Gastroenterology 1993;105:1550–2.
40. Friedl W, Caspari R, Sengteller M, et al. Can APC mutation analysis contribute to therapeutic decisions in familial adenomatous polyposis? Experience from 680 FAP families. Gut 2001;48:515–21.
41. Laken SJ, Petersen GM, Gruber SB, et al. Familial colorectal cancer in Ashkenazim due to a hypermutable tract in APC. Nat Genet 1997;17:79–83.
42. Kim B, Giardiello FM. Chemoprevention in familial adenomatous polyposis. Best Pract Res Clin Gastroenterol 2011;25:607–22.
43. Nieuwenhuis MH, Mathus-Vliegen EM, Baeten CG, et al. Evaluation of management of desmoid tumours associated with familial adenomatous polyposis in Dutch patients. Br J Cancer 2011;104:37–42.
44. Nielsen M, Morreau H, Vasen HF, et al. MUTYH-associated polyposis (MAP). Crit Rev Oncol Hematol 2011;79:1–16.
45. Boparai KS, Dekker E, Van Eeden S, et al. Hyperplastic polyps and sessile serrated adenomas as a phenotypic expression of MYH-associated polyposis. Gastroenterology 2008;135:2014–8.
46. Jones N, Vogt S, Nielsen M, et al. Increased colorectal cancer incidence in obligate carriers of heterozygous mutations in MUTYH. Gastroenterology 2009;137: 489–94, 494.e1; [quiz: 725–6].
47. Vogt S, Jones N, Christian D, et al. Expanded extracolonic tumor spectrum in MUTYH-associated polyposis. Gastroenterology 2009;137:1976–85.e1–10.
48. Nielsen M, Joerink-van de Beld MC, Jones N, et al. Analysis of MUTYH genotypes and colorectal phenotypes in patients with MUTYH-associated polyposis. Gastroenterology 2009;136:471–6.
49. Jass JR. Classification of colorectal cancer based on correlation of clinical, morphological and molecular features. Histopathology 2007;50:113–30.

Personalized Approaches to Gastrointestinal Cancers

Importance of Integrating Genomic Information to Guide Therapy

Jin He, MD, PhD[a], Nita Ahuja, MD[b],*

KEYWORDS

- Tumor heterogeneity • Next-generation sequencing • Targeted therapy
- Biomarkers

KEY POINTS

- Cancer is such a heterogeneous disease that combining optimal use of targeted therapies in highly selected patients can achieve the best result.
- Early diagnosis of cancer or precancer lesions can lead to prophylactic surgery and eliminate the risk of certain types of cancer.
- Molecular profiling in cancer has allowed clinicians to correlate cancer genomics data with the cancer phenotype data.
- Fast-growing genomic technology, such as next-generation sequencing, now allow clinicians to obtain genomic profiles for patients with cancer, to guide their targeted chemotherapy, and to predict the response to chemotherapy. This ability will make personalized medical care possible.

If it were not for the great variability among individuals, medicine might as well be a science, not an art.

—*Sir William Osler, 1892*

INTRODUCTION
Tumor Heterogeneity

A tumor is composed of different subpopulations of cells. Most of those tumor cells are founder cells from which subclones are derived.[1] Each subclone has a distinct

[a] Department of Surgery, The Johns Hopkins University School of Medicine, 600 North Wolfe Street, Blalock 1202, Baltimore, MD 21287, USA; [b] Department of Surgery, The Johns Hopkins University School of Medicine, 600 North Wolfe Street, Blalock 685, Baltimore, MD 21287, USA
* Corresponding author.
E-mail address: nahuja1@jhmi.edu

Surg Clin N Am 95 (2015) 1081–1094
http://dx.doi.org/10.1016/j.suc.2015.05.002
0039-6109/15/$ – see front matter © 2015 Elsevier Inc. All rights reserved.
surgical.theclinics.com

genotype and phenotype, which then leads to divergent biological behavior. Tumor heterogeneity can explain the differential response to treatment and can be summarized into the following categories (**Fig. 1**):

- Intratumor heterogeneity,[2] which is defined as heterogeneity among the cells of the primary tumor. Genome-wide sequencing data demonstrate that most somatic mutations are present in all tumor cells and form the trunk of the somatic evolutionary tree. The mutations that cause the intratumor heterogeneity are in the branches. This heterogeneity is the foundation of the intermetastatic heterogeneity.
- Intermetastatic heterogeneity, which is defined as heterogeneity among different metastatic lesions. Patients with advanced cancer often present with multiple metastatic lesions in major organs. The heterogeneity among different metastatic lesions is often extensive, and can pose significant challenges for targeted therapy.
- Intrametastatic heterogeneity, which is defined as heterogeneity among the cells of each metastasis, and develops as the metastases grow.
- Intertumor or interpatient heterogeneity refers to heterogeneity among the tumors of different patients. No two patients with cancer have the same mutations

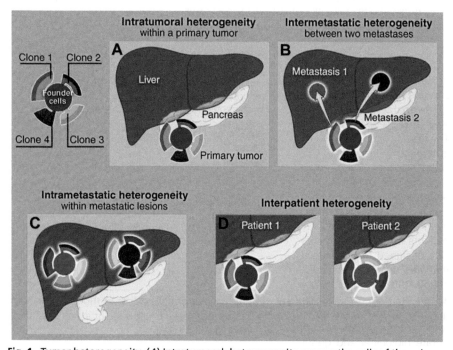

Fig. 1. Tumor heterogeneity. (*A*) Intratumoral: heterogeneity among the cells of the primary tumor. The differently colored regions in the subclones represent stages of evolution within a subclone. (*B*) Intermetastatic: heterogeneity among different metastatic lesions in the same patient. In the case illustrated here, each metastasis was derived from a different subclone. (*C*) Intrametastatic: heterogeneity among the cells of each metastasis develops as the metastases grow. (*D*) Interpatient: heterogeneity among the tumors of different patients. The mutations in the founder cells of the tumors of these 2 patients are almost completely distinct. (*From* Vogelstein B, Papadopoulos N, Velculescu VE, et al. Cancer genome landscapes. Science 2013;339;1552; with permission.)

in the founder cells of their cancers. This heterogeneity is one of the major drivers for clinicians to design a personalized approach to treat different patients with cancer. The intertumor heterogeneity can be used to classify tumors into subgroups based on genetic mutations, copy changes, and expression profiles.

The most popular theory to explain tumor heterogeneity is the clonal evolution model, which was proposed by Nowell[3] in 1976. Heterogeneity happens as a tumor evolves from a benign to a malignant/metastatic lesion by acquiring a series of mutations over time. In the past decade, cancer genomic studies have revealed mutations in about 140 genes that can drive tumor growth.[1] The limited number of driver genes can have complicated mutation patterns or frequency or epigenetic changes, which lead to tumor heterogeneity. Understanding tumor heterogeneity and developing rapid tests to comprehensively identify the genetic alterations is critical for successful targeted therapy.

CURRENT CONCERNS AND LIMITATIONS OF DIAGNOSIS AND THERAPY

Cancer treatments are based on results from randomized control trials and cohort studies using TNM (tumor, node, metastasis) staging. The traditional TNM staging is defined as follows:

- T: size or direct extent of the primary tumor
- N: degree of spread to regional lymph nodes
- M: presence of distant metastasis

This TNM staging is determined by clinical and pathologic factors and still dictates management of patients with gastrointestinal cancer. Genetic variability of individual cancers has not been considered in the traditional staging and treatment model.

The goal of traditional adjuvant chemotherapy was to eliminate micrometastatic disease after so-called curative resections to prevent future metastases and recurrence. The ideal target for adjuvant therapy for any particular malignancy is one that is exclusive to the cancer cell, and does not exist on healthy cells, thereby isolating the cancer without collateral damage. Such a perfect therapy remains elusive. A less ideal, but more attainable, target has been the identification of a protein that is overexpressed on, or displays higher activity in, cancer cells.

In most cases, chemotherapy is more an extender of survival than it is a cure. Moreover, the toxic side effects associated with chemotherapy can be inhibitory, because patients often cannot tolerate the dosage or duration prescribed. Targeted therapy was designed to improve the survival of patients with cancer by delivering therapy that was unique to cancer cells. Targeted therapy would then potentially be more effective in killing cancer cells and the specificity of the therapeutic action should lessen the systemic toxicity associated with these personalized drugs.[4,5] As whole-genome sequencing approaches become feasible in small biopsy samples along with the concomitant decrease in cost of these technologies, there is a need to incorporate biological and genetic information into clinical decision making, allowing a more personalized approach in targeted therapies. It is imperative to know whether the cancer harbors the mutations that the medication targets before any targeted medication is given.[6,7] Ideally, patients would receive the targeted therapy matched to the genomic profile of the tumor. However, prospective clinical trials are still needed to determine the benefit of matching therapy to genomic alterations. Ongoing exemplary trials, including the National Cancer Institute (NCI) MATCH (Molecular Analysis for Therapy Choice Program) trial and the European Organization for Research and Treatment of Cancer (EORTC) MINDACT (Microarray In Node-Negative and 1 to

3 Positive Lymph Node Disease May Avoid Chemotherapy) trial, will provide evidence of whether such approaches will bear results.[8,9]

The MATCH trial is a group of phase II trials that will enroll adults with advanced solid tumors. In these trials, tumor biopsy samples will undergo next-generation DNA sequencing to identify genetic abnormalities that may respond to targeted drugs. Patients will be treated based not on their type of cancer but on the genetic abnormality that is thought to be driving their cancer. The primary end point for the MATCH trials will be tumor response. Patients whose cancers progress during the first assigned treatment may be able to go on another MATCH trial arm if they have a second actionable molecular target in their tumors. In addition, any patient whose cancer initially shrinks and then progresses during the trial will be eligible to have their tumors rebiopsied and, if they have a genetic change that is targeted by another drug being tested in MATCH, they may be eligible to enroll in one of the other phase II MATCH trials.

MINDACT was designed to test whether genetic testing is more effective than clinical assessment in determining the need for chemotherapy in treating women with breast cancer that is either node negative or involves no more than 3 lymph nodes. The feasibility study of using the 70-gene panel (TargetPrint) in the MINDACT trial was recently published. TargetPrint was assessed for its concordance with standard immunohistochemistry/fluorescence in situ hybridization assessments of ER, PR, and HER2 status. TargetPrint and local assessment of ER, PR, and HER2 showed high concordance in the first 800 MINDACT patients.[9]

At present, most genetic testing is still being performed as single-gene tests, in which a patient who is identified as high risk, because of family history or otherwise, is tested for a specific mutation. It is unusual to test multiple genetic mutations that have not previously been described in a specific tumor type. However, with the rapid advance of biotechnology and the collective understanding of the human genome, clinicians and patients have the ability to screen for hundreds of potentially cancer-causing genetic mutations (including deletions, insertions, alterations, and translocations, as well as exome-based substitutions) associated with cancer, with reports of up to a 99% positive predictive value.[10,11] The fast-growing next-generation sequencing technology is a typical example. Frampton and colleagues[10] reported their experience on the use of massive parallel DNA sequencing to characterize base substitutions, short insertions and deletions (indels), copy number alterations, and selected fusions across 287 cancer-related genes from formalin-fixed and paraffin-embedded (FFPE) clinical specimens. Using a validation strategy with reference samples of 53 pooled cell lines that model key determinants of accuracy, their test sensitivity was 95% to 99% across alteration types, with high specificity (positive predictive value >99%). Their test revealed clinically actionable mutations in 76% of tested tumors, which is 3 times more sensitive than current diagnostic tests. Roychowdhury and colleagues[12] reported their pilot experience in integrating sequencing data into clinical practice. They were able to generate meaningful sequencing data in a clinically relevant time frame of 3 to 4 weeks. The data were then discussed in the multidisciplinary Sequencing Tumor Board. Their early experience in 4 patients showed the feasibility of using individual mutational landscape to facilitate biomarker-driven clinical trials in oncology.

Liang and colleagues[13] reported whole-genome sequencing (WGS) findings in paired tumor/normal samples collected from 3 separate patients with pancreatic cancer. One-hundred and forty-two somatic coding events, including point mutations, insertion/deletions, and chromosomal copy number variants, were identified. The KRAS signaling pathway was the most heavily affected pathway, along with tumor-stroma interactions and tumor suppressive pathways.

However, the current genome-wide sequencing technologies are not perfect. Biankin and colleagues[14] used massively parallel sequencing to analyze the exomes of 99 primary pancreatic cancer samples. The sequencing data were then compared with the mutational data of a set of pancreatic cancer cell lines and xenografts in which mutations had previously been identified using conventional Sanger sequencing. Only 159 (63%) of the expected 251 driver gene mutations were identified in the primary tumors studied by next-generation sequencing alone, indicating a false-negative rate of 37%. The limit of current sequencing technology can be caused by some regions of the genome being difficult to be sequenced. Moreover, tissue sampling bias is inevitable, as are challenges of sample purity whereby the stromal cells can dilute tumor DNA and reduce the probability of finding a mutation.

Personalized approaches in gastrointestinal cancers can be broadly summarized into the following aspects:

1. Early diagnosis of patients with a hereditary mutation leads to prophylactic surgery and then eliminates the risk of certain types of cancer.
2. The unique genetic profile of each tumor is generated and then used to develop targeted chemotherapy options.
3. Using the genomic profile as a predictive biomarker for the response to chemotherapy and guide clinical decision making.

The recent advance of these personalized approaches in different types of gastrointestinal cancers is discussed later.

PERSONALIZED TREATMENT OF PANCREATIC CANCERS

It is estimated that around 46,000 people will be diagnosed with pancreatic cancer in 2014, 85% of whom will die of pancreatic cancer. The overall outcome of pancreatic cancer has not changed in the last 3 decades. Recent advances have shown that the commonly mutated genes in pancreatic cancer include an oncogene, KRAS, and 3 tumor suppressor genes: TP53, p16/CDKN2A, and SMAD4.[15,16]

Understanding of the mutations in a patient can help to identify individual cancer-specific molecular characteristics, which can then guide individualized treatment. There is a significant genetic component contributing to the risk of developing pancreatic cancer. It is necessary to tailor the treatments to the individual cancer-specific molecular characteristics that arise from genetic mutations. Genome-wide analysis through sequencing of the exome or the whole genome is becoming possible with the rapidly growing technology and decreasing cost.

The next-generation in-depth sequencing of pancreatic cancer could uncover genetic mutations that have not been detected by standard testing. The identification of these mutations from genomic data allows clinicians to be able to correlate the phenotype of the cancer, and to guide clinical decision making. This ability will further lead to the patients receiving treatments in clinical trials that otherwise would not have been considered or available. These clinical trials also allow management strategies to be matched to individual patients based on the genetic makeup of their cancers. Recently, Liang and colleagues[13] reported WGS findings in paired tumor/normal samples collected from 3 separate patients with pancreatic cancers. They identified 142 somatic coding events, including point mutations, insertion/deletions, and chromosomal copy number variants. As expected, the KRAS signaling pathway was the most heavily affected pathway, along with tumor-stroma interactions and tumor suppressive pathways.

One example is using poly(ADP-ribose) polymerase (PARP) inhibitor to treat a subset of patients with pancreatic cancers that express mutations in BRCA1, BRCA2, or

PALB2.[8] The BRCA1 and BRCA2 genes encode large proteins that coordinate the homologous recombination repair double-strand breaks (DSBs) pathway. PARPs are a family of nuclear enzymes that regulate the repair of DNA single-strand breaks through the base-excision repair (BER) pathway. In the presence of BRCA mutation, the BER rescue pathway for DNA repair is not affected and thus can be used for DNA repair. PARP inhibitors (PARPi) can be used to target BRCA1/2-mutated tumors, which cannot use homologous recombination to repair DSBs, to shut down their BER rescue pathway, thus leading to accumulation of DNA damage, genomic instability, and cell death.[17] The indirect effect of PARPi on mutated tumor suppressor genes, BRCA1, BRCA2, or PALB2 has shown promising benefit in clinical case reports.[18,19] Villarroel and colleagues[20] reported on a patient with advanced, gemcitabine-resistant pancreatic cancer who was later treated with the DNA-damaging agent, mitomycin C. This patient, who has inactivation of the PALB2 gene, had more than 36 months of tumor response.

PERSONALIZED TREATMENT OF GASTROINTESTINAL STROMAL TUMORS

Gastrointestinal stromal tumors (GIST) are sarcomas arising from the interstitial cells of Cajal. The treatment of GIST is a classic successful example of personalized treatment. Most GISTs (>95%) express the CD117 antigen, derived from the c-KIT proto-oncogene, which is abnormally activated in GIST. This activated proto-oncogene leads to unregulated oncogenic cell signaling. The most common mutation occurs in exon 11, although mutations in a variety of exons have been reported. Exon 11 deletions have been associated with more aggressive tumors and poorer prognosis than other mutation patterns.[21] GISTs, which lack c-KIT mutation and are CD117 negative, most commonly arise from a mutation within platelet-derived growth factor receptor alpha (PDGFRα), another member of tyrosine kinase family. Regardless of the mutation, both types of GIST respond to tyrosine kinase inhibitors (TKIs) such as imatinib and sunitinib. There are a few KIT/PDGFRα-negative (also known as wild-type) GISTs, some of which are associated with germline mutations in the succinyl dehydrogenase subunits (Carney-Stratakis syndrome).[22] These wild-type GISTs do not respond well to TKIs; are often multicentric; and are, coincidentally, less aggressive tumors following a more indolent course.

- TKIs
  - Imatinib (Gleevec)
  - Sunitinib (Sutent)
  - Regorafenib (Stivarga)

The TKIs act on the active site of the tyrosine kinase receptor, decreasing the activity of the particular kinase, but not affecting other tyrosine kinases required for cellular function. Imatinib was initially found to act on the Abelson (abl) domain of the (bcr-abl) proto-oncogene of Philadelphia chromosome and was first formulated for use in chronic myelogenous leukemia with great success. It was thereafter found to have effect on the tyrosine kinase activity of the c-KIT and PDGFRα proto-oncogenes as well. Its usefulness in GISTs was first noted with a complete response in a single patient with metastatic disease.[23] Since then, several randomized trials showed broad efficacy for these tumors as primary therapy and in the adjuvant setting.[24,25] Optimal duration of adjuvant therapy with imatinib has been debated. In low-risk, completely resected GIST, current recommendations include observation or 1 year of adjuvant imatinib. In patients with intermittent to high-risk GIST,[26] the recommendations are for 3 years of adjuvant therapy based on the study by Joensuu and colleagues.[27]

For patients who are advanced or metastatic, continuous therapy until tumor progression is recommended. Although the side effects are generally well tolerated, the cost of these therapies has recently been debated as being prohibitive.[28]

For patients who progress on, or cannot tolerate, imatinib, sunitinib is the second-line therapy agent that has been shown to be most effective in patients with c-KIT exon 9 or PDGFRα mutations,[29] as well as acting on vascular endothelial growth factors, rearranged during transfection (RET) proto-oncogene, and many other tyrosine kinase receptors. Because of its broader targeting, its side effects are more extensive than those of imatinib.

The third-line therapy for GIST is regorafenib, which was recently shown in a randomized trial to significantly improve progression-free survival in patients who no longer responded to first-line or second-line therapy.[30] In this international, multicenter, randomized phase 3 trial, 199 patients with GIST who failed imatinib and sunitinib were randomized to receive regorafenib (n = 133) or matching placebo (n = 66). Median progression-free survival was 4.8 months (interquartile range, 1.4–9.2) for regorafenib and 0·9 months (0.9–1.8) for placebo (hazard ratio, 0·27; 95% confidence interval, 0.19–0.39; $P<.0001$).

PERSONALIZED TREATMENT IN COLORECTAL CANCER

Most colorectal cancers are sporadic and result from progressive accumulations of mutations with loss of functions of tumor suppressor genes and activation of oncogenes. A subset of colorectal cancers (15%), such as those with hereditary nonpolyposis colorectal cancer, can also have inherited defects in the mismatch repair genes resulting in microsatellite instability (**Table 1**). Most (up to 40%) colorectal cancers have mutations in the *K-ras* oncogene.[31] Those colorectal cancers, which lack *K-ras* mutations, the so-called *K-ras* wild type (WT), have shown promising response to therapies targeted to the anti–epidermal growth factor receptor (EGFR).

- EGFR inhibitors
  - Cetuximab (Erbitux)
  - Panitumumab (Vectibix)

Cetuximab was the first EGFR inhibitor to be used for colorectal cancer. It binds on the extracellular portion of the EGFR, which then blocks cell division via several mitogen-activated protein kinases (MAPKs). Cetuximab was used as a combination therapy in patients who had failed first-line and second-line therapy for metastatic colorectal cancer[32,33] (**Fig. 2**).

K-ras acts as an intracellular downstream mediator of the MAPK cell-signaling pathway.[34] A mutation in *K-ras*, therefore, would render upstream EGFR inhibition useless.[35,36] In similar fashion, it has been shown that mutations in *B-raf*, the intracellular target of ras, also render anti-EGFR therapies useless.[37] With improved patient selection based on these mutation statuses, EGFR inhibitors have shown promise as targeted

Table 1
Somatic mutations identified in human colorectal cancer

Oncogenes	Tumor Suppressor Genes	Mismatch Repair
ras (H, K, N)	p53	MLH-1
raf (B)	APC	MSH-2
PIK3CA	DCC	MSH-6
PTEN	—	—

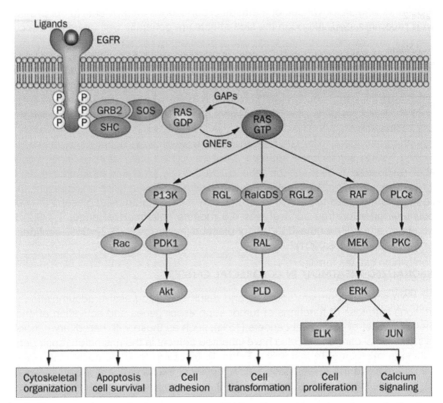

Fig. 2. Targeting therapy in the rat sarcoma (RAS) pathway. Ligands such as cetuximab can bind on the extracellular portion of the EGFR, which then blocks cell division via several MAPKs. Any mutation of RAS or downstream rapidly accelerated fibrosarcoma (RAF) genes renders upstream EGFR inhibition useless. (*From* Normanno N, Tejpar S, Morgillo F, et al. Implications for KRAS status and EGFR-targeted therapies in metastatic CRC. Nat Rev Clin Oncol 2009;6(9):521; with permission.)

therapies in combination with standard chemotherapy regimens for *K-ras/B-raf* WT patients, as shown by several trials (**Table 2**). Panitumumab acts in similar fashion to cetuximab, and showed modest benefit in the PRIME (Panitumumab Randomized Trial in Combination with Chemotherapy for Metastatic Colorectal Cancer to Determine Efficacy) trial as combination first-line therapy with a platinum-based regimen.[38]

The BMP/Wnt pathway is highly activated in mutant KRAS-dependent colon cancer cells, pointing to its downstream effector MAP3K7 (TAK1) as a promising drug target in this recalcitrant form of colorectal cancer. The induction of apoptosis by RNA interference (RNAi)–mediated depletion or pharmacologic inhibition of TAK1 is linked to its suppression of hyperactivated Wnt signaling, which is evident in both endogenous and genetically reconstituted cells. Therefore TAK1 inhibition is a potential therapeutic strategy for a treatment-refractory subset of colon cancers showing aberrant KRAS and Wnt pathway activation.[39]

PERSONALIZED TREATMENT IN GASTRIC CANCER

Early diagnosis of susceptibility of gastric cancer can lead to prophylactic surgery and eliminate the cancer risk. Similar to prophylactic surgery for patients with *BRCA1*

Table 2 Trials involving cetuximab as first-line or second-line therapy		
Trial Name and Year	**Treatment**	**Primary End Point**
BOND,[33] 2004	Adjuvant cetuximab ± irinotecan as second-line therapy	PFS, RR
EPIC,[51] 2008	Adjuvant irinotecan ± cetuximab as second-line therapy	PFS, RR
CYSTAL,[52] 2011	Adjuvant FOLFIRI ± cetuximab as first-line therapy	OS, PFS, RR
OPUS,[53] 2011	Adjuvant FOLFOX ± cetuximab as first-line therapy	PFS, RR
COIN,[54] 2011	Adjuvant oxaliplatin ± cetuximab as first-line therapy	Negative PFS/OS
NORDIC,[55] 2012	Adjuvant oxaliplatin ± cetuximab as first-line therapy	Negative PFS

Abbreviations: OS, overall survival; PFS, progression-free survival; RR, response rate.
Data from Refs.[33,51–55]

mutation (which causes a hereditary breast-ovarian cancer syndrome) and *APC* mutation (which causes familial adenomatous polyposis, an inherited condition that progresses into colon cancer if untreated), patients with *CDH1* mutation may benefit from early gastrectomy.

Approximately 10% of gastric cancers are attributed to a germline mutation of the *CDH1* gene. Such patients have about an 87% lifetime risk of hereditary diffuse gastric cancer. A recent study from Pandalai and colleagues[40] showed the results of prophylactic total gastrectomy for 10 patients with *CDH1* mutation. Nine patients had 77 foci of noninvasive cancer and 2 patients had foci of T1 invasive cancer on final pathology.

Another example of a personalized approach is mesenchymal-epithelial transition (MET) amplification in gastric cancer. MET, also known as the hepatocyte growth factor receptor, is a receptor tyrosine kinase that is overexpressed and activated in a subset of gastric cancer. MET amplification and expression are associated with invasive phenotype and correlated with poor prognosis in this subset of gastric cancer.[41] Crizotinib (dual c-Met/ALK inhibitor), which was recently approved for lung cancers with ALK rearrangement, showed therapeutic potential in a subset of gastric cancers.[42]

PROGNOSIS

In the past, adjuvant chemotherapy was given after curative surgery to eliminate micrometastasis. However, the benefit of this adjuvant chemotherapy was limited to a small group of patients. A panel of molecular biomarkers has been developed to identify subpopulations of patients who are most likely to benefit from standard adjuvant chemotherapy.

Oncotype DX

Oncotype consists of a panel of 12 genes to categorize the risk of recurrence for patients with stage II colon cancer who usually do not get adjuvant chemotherapy. Frozen tumor tissue is required for the real-time reverse transcription polymerase chain reaction–based Oncotype assay. A high recurrence score means potential benefit from adjuvant chemotherapy to patients despite their negative lymph node status; stage II colon cancer with high Oncotype score behaves like stage III disease. This assay could then guide a personalized approach for stage II patients.[43]

Srivastava and colleagues[44] evaluated the impact of recurrence score (RS) results from Oncotype on physician recommendations regarding adjuvant chemotherapy in patients with T3, mismatch repair–proficient (MMR-P) stage II colon cancer. They enrolled 141 patients in this multicenter, prospective study. Treatment recommendations changed for 63 (45%; 95% confidence interval, 36%–53%) of these 141 T3 MMR-P patients, with intensity decreasing for 47 (33%) and increasing for 16 (11%). Recommendations for chemotherapy decreased from 73 patients (52%) to 42 (30%). Compared with traditional clinicopathologic assessment, incorporation of the RS results into clinical decision making was associated with treatment recommendation changes for 45% of patients with T3 MMR-P stage II colon cancer in this prospective multicenter study. Use of the RS assay may lead to overall reduction in adjuvant chemotherapy use in this subgroup of patients with stage II colon cancer.

ColoPrint

ColoPrint uses a panel of 18 genes to identify high-risk patients with stage 2 colon cancer who may benefit from adjuvant chemotherapy. Use of FFPE tissue is acceptable for the ColoPrint assay.

Maak and colleagues[45] used the ColoPrint assay to study 135 patients who underwent curative resection for stage II colon cancer. Most of the stage II patients (73.3%) were classified as low risk by the assay. The 5-year distant metastasis–free survival was 94.9% for low-risk patients and 80.6% for high-risk patients. In multivariable analysis, ColoPrint was the only significant parameter to predict the development of distant metastasis, with a hazard ratio of 4.28 (95% confidence interval, 1.36–13.50; $P = .013$). Clinical risk parameters from the American Society of Clinical Oncology recommendation did not add power to the ColoPrint classification. ColoPrint was able to predict the development of distant metastasis of patients with stage II colon cancer and facilitates the identification of patients who may be safely managed without chemotherapy.

Both Oncotype and ColoPrint assays are examples of how genomic profiles can be used to guide the decision making for delivery of chemotherapy. Such biomarker approaches may allow clinicians to avoid toxic chemotherapy in patients who will not benefit from chemotherapy and target aggressive therapy to those who will derive a benefit. These genetic profiling tests are being prospectively validated in clinical trials.

Circulating Tumor Cells

Circulating tumor cells (CTCs) are another example of personalized approach for early diagnosis. The most commonly used version, CTC-Chips, relies on blood flow through a specialized chamber coated with antibody to the epithelial marker epithelial cell adhesion molecule (EpCAM) to capture CTCs with high efficiency.[46,47] The number of captured CTCs correlates with clinical evidence of tumor response. The CTC capture can be used in early detection of cancer, monitoring tumor genotypes over the course of treatment, and biological characterization of CTCs.[48,49]

Recent study of pancreatic CTCs showed that expression of WNT2 in pancreatic cancer cells increases metastatic propensity in vivo.[50] Expression of WNT2 in pancreatic cancer cells suppresses anoikis, and enhances anchorage-independent sphere formation. This effect is correlated with fibronectin upregulation. Suppressing this pathway by inhibition of MAP3K7 kinase (also known as TAK1) may reduce metastatic potential in pancreatic cancer cells.

SUMMARY

Cancer is such a heterogeneous disease that combining optimal use of targeted therapies in highly selected patients can achieve the best result.

Early diagnosis of cancer or precancer lesions can lead to prophylactic surgery and eliminate the risk of certain types of cancer.

Molecular profiling in cancer has allowed clinicians to correlate cancer genomics data wit the cancer phenotype data. Fast-growing genomic technology, such as next-generation sequencing, now allows clinicians to obtain genomic profiles for patients with cancer, to guide their targeted chemotherapy, and to predict the response to chemotherapy. This ability will make personalized medical care possible.

REFERENCES

1. Vogelstein B, Papadopoulos N, Velculescu VE, et al. Cancer genome landscapes. Science 2013;339(6127):1546–58.
2. Swanton C. Intratumor heterogeneity: evolution through space and time. Cancer Res 2012;72(19):4875–82.
3. Nowell PC. The clonal evolution of tumor cell populations. Science 1976; 194(4260):23–8.
4. Robert C, Karaszewska B, Schachter J, et al. Improved overall survival in melanoma with combined dabrafenib and trametinib. N Engl J Med 2015;372(1):30–9.
5. Thorpe LM, Yuzugullu H, Zhao JJ. PI3K in cancer: divergent roles of isoforms, modes of activation and therapeutic targeting. Nat Rev Cancer 2014;15(1):7–24.
6. Schilsky RL. Implementing personalized cancer care. Nat Rev Clin Oncol 2014; 11(7):432–8.
7. Simon R, Roychowdhury S. Implementing personalized cancer genomics in clinical trials. Nat Rev Drug Discov 2013;12(5):358–69.
8. Conley BA, Doroshow JH. Molecular analysis for therapy choice: NCI MATCH. Semin Oncol 2014;41(3):297–9.
9. Viale G, Slaets L, Bogaerts J, et al. High concordance of protein (by IHC), gene (by FISH; HER2 only), and microarray readout (by TargetPrint) of ER, PgR, and HER2: results from the EORTC 10041/BIG 03-04 MINDACT trial. Ann Oncol 2014;25(4):816–23.
10. Frampton GM, Fichtenholtz A, Otto GA, et al. Development and validation of a clinical cancer genomic profiling test based on massively parallel DNA sequencing. Nat Biotechnol 2013;31(11):1023–31.
11. Park JY, Kricka LJ, Fortina P. Next-generation sequencing in the clinic. Nat Biotechnol 2013;31(11):990–2.
12. Roychowdhury S, Iyer MK, Robinson DR, et al. Personalized oncology through integrative high-throughput sequencing: a pilot study. Sci Transl Med 2011; 3(111):111ra21.
13. Liang WS, Craig DW, Carpten J, et al. Genome-wide characterization of pancreatic adenocarcinoma patients using next generation sequencing. PLoS One 2012;7(10):e43192.
14. Biankin AV, Waddell N, Kassahn KS, et al. Pancreatic cancer genomes reveal aberrations in axon guidance pathway genes. Nature 2012;491(7424):399–405.
15. Iacobuzio-Donahue CA, Velculescu VE, Wolfgang CL, et al. Genetic basis of pancreas cancer development and progression: insights from whole-exome and whole-genome sequencing. Clin Cancer Res 2012;18(16):4257–65.
16. Iacobuzio-Donahue CA. Genetic evolution of pancreatic cancer: lessons learnt from the pancreatic cancer genome sequencing project. Gut 2012;61(7): 1085–94.
17. Yuan Y, Liao YM, Hsueh CT, et al. Novel targeted therapeutics: inhibitors of MDM2, ALK and PARP. J Hematol Oncol 2011;4:16.

18. Lowery MA, Kelsen DP, Stadler ZK, et al. An emerging entity: pancreatic adenocarcinoma associated with a known BRCA mutation: clinical descriptors, treatment implications, and future directions. Oncologist 2011;16(10):1397–402.

19. Fogelman DR, Wolff RA, Kopetz S, et al. Evidence for the efficacy of iniparib, a PARP-1 inhibitor, in BRCA2-associated pancreatic cancer. Anticancer Res 2011;31(4):1417–20.

20. Villarroel MC, Rajeshkumar NV, Garrido-Laguna I, et al. Personalizing cancer treatment in the age of global genomic analyses: PALB2 gene mutations and the response to DNA damaging agents in pancreatic cancer. Mol Cancer Ther 2011;10(1):3–8.

21. Andersson J, Bumming P, Meis-Kindblom JM, et al. Gastrointestinal stromal tumors with KIT exon 11 deletions are associated with poor prognosis. Gastroenterology 2006;130(6):1573–81.

22. Janeway KA, Kim SY, Lodish M, et al. Defects in succinate dehydrogenase in gastrointestinal stromal tumors lacking KIT and PDGFRA mutations. Proc Natl Acad Sci U S A 2011;108(1):314–8.

23. Joensuu H, Roberts PJ, Sarlomo-Rikala M, et al. Effect of the tyrosine kinase inhibitor STI571 in a patient with a metastatic gastrointestinal stromal tumor. N Engl J Med 2001;344(14):1052–6.

24. Blanke CD, Rankin C, Demetri GD, et al. Phase III randomized, intergroup trial assessing imatinib mesylate at two dose levels in patients with unresectable or metastatic gastrointestinal stromal tumors expressing the kit receptor tyrosine kinase: S0033. J Clin Oncol 2008;26(4):626–32.

25. Dematteo RP, Ballman KV, Antonescu CR, et al. Adjuvant imatinib mesylate after resection of localised, primary gastrointestinal stromal tumour: a randomised, double-blind, placebo-controlled trial. Lancet 2009;373(9669):1097–104.

26. Joensuu H. Risk stratification of patients diagnosed with gastrointestinal stromal tumor. Hum Pathol 2008;39(10):1411–9.

27. Joensuu H, Eriksson M, Sundby Hall K, et al. One vs three years of adjuvant imatinib for operable gastrointestinal stromal tumor: a randomized trial. JAMA 2012; 307(12):1265–72.

28. Experts in Chronic Myeloid Leukemia. The price of drugs for chronic myeloid leukemia (CML) is a reflection of the unsustainable prices of cancer drugs: from the perspective of a large group of CML experts. Blood 2013;121(22):4439–42.

29. Heinrich MC, Maki RG, Corless CL, et al. Primary and secondary kinase genotypes correlate with the biological and clinical activity of sunitinib in imatinib-resistant gastrointestinal stromal tumor. J Clin Oncol 2008;26(33): 5352–9.

30. Demetri GD, Reichardt P, Kang YK, et al. Efficacy and safety of regorafenib for advanced gastrointestinal stromal tumours after failure of imatinib and sunitinib (GRID): an international, multicentre, randomised, placebo-controlled, phase 3 trial. Lancet 2013;381(9863):295–302.

31. Tortola S, Marcuello E, Gonzalez I, et al. p53 and K-ras gene mutations correlate with tumor aggressiveness but are not of routine prognostic value in colorectal cancer. J Clin Oncol 1999;17(5):1375–81.

32. Lenz HJ, Van Cutsem E, Khambata-Ford S, et al. Multicenter phase II and translational study of cetuximab in metastatic colorectal carcinoma refractory to irinotecan, oxaliplatin, and fluoropyrimidines. J Clin Oncol 2006;24(30):4914–21.

33. Cunningham D, Humblet Y, Siena S, et al. Cetuximab monotherapy and cetuximab plus irinotecan in irinotecan-refractory metastatic colorectal cancer. N Engl J Med 2004;351(4):337–45.

34. Normanno N, Tejpar S, Morgillo F, et al. Implications for KRAS status and EGFR-targeted therapies in metastatic CRC. Nat Rev Clin Oncol 2009;6(9):519–27.
35. Lievre A, Bachet JB, Le Corre D, et al. KRAS mutation status is predictive of response to cetuximab therapy in colorectal cancer. Cancer Res 2006;66(8): 3992–5.
36. Amado RG, Wolf M, Peeters M, et al. Wild-type KRAS is required for panitumumab efficacy in patients with metastatic colorectal cancer. J Clin Oncol 2008; 26(10):1626–34.
37. Di Nicolantonio F, Martini M, Molinari F, et al. Wild-type BRAF is required for response to panitumumab or cetuximab in metastatic colorectal cancer. J Clin Oncol 2008;26(35):5705–12.
38. Douillard JY, Siena S, Cassidy J, et al. Randomized, phase III trial of panitumumab with infusional fluorouracil, leucovorin, and oxaliplatin (FOLFOX4) versus FOLFOX4 alone as first-line treatment in patients with previously untreated metastatic colorectal cancer: the PRIME study. J Clin Oncol 2010;28(31):4697–705.
39. Singh A, Sweeney MF, Yu M, et al. TAK1 inhibition promotes apoptosis in KRAS-dependent colon cancers. Cell 2012;148(4):639–50.
40. Pandalai PK, Lauwers GY, Chung DC, et al. Prophylactic total gastrectomy for individuals with germline CDH1 mutation. Surgery 2011;149(3):347–55.
41. Peng Z, Zhu Y, Wang Q, et al. Prognostic significance of MET amplification and expression in gastric cancer: a systematic review with meta-analysis. PLoS One 2014;9(1):e84502.
42. Okamoto W, Okamoto I, Arao T, et al. Antitumor action of the MET tyrosine kinase inhibitor crizotinib (PF-02341066) in gastric cancer positive for MET amplification. Mol Cancer Ther 2012;11(7):1557–64.
43. Clark-Langone KM, Sangli C, Krishnakumar J, et al. Translating tumor biology into personalized treatment planning: analytical performance characteristics of the Oncotype DX Colon Cancer Assay. BMC Cancer 2010;10:691.
44. Srivastava G, Renfro LA, Behrens RJ, et al. Prospective multicenter study of the impact of oncotype DX colon cancer assay results on treatment recommendations in stage II colon cancer patients. Oncologist 2014;19(5):492–7.
45. Maak M, Simon I, Nitsche U, et al. Independent validation of a prognostic genomic signature (ColoPrint) for patients with stage II colon cancer. Ann Surg 2013;257(6):1053–8.
46. Haber DA, Velculescu VE. Blood-based analyses of cancer: circulating tumor cells and circulating tumor DNA. Cancer Discov 2014;4(6):650–61.
47. Karabacak NM, Spuhler PS, Fachin F, et al. Microfluidic, marker-free isolation of circulating tumor cells from blood samples. Nat Protoc 2014;9(3):694–710.
48. Bardia A, Haber DA. Solidifying liquid biopsies: can circulating tumor cell monitoring guide treatment selection in breast cancer? J Clin Oncol 2014;32(31): 3470–1.
49. Yu M, Bardia A, Aceto N, et al. Cancer therapy. Ex vivo culture of circulating breast tumor cells for individualized testing of drug susceptibility. Science 2014;345(6193):216–20.
50. Yu M, Ting DT, Stott SL, et al. RNA sequencing of pancreatic circulating tumour cells implicates WNT signalling in metastasis. Nature 2012;487(7408):510–3.
51. Sobrero AF, Maurel J, Fehrenbacher L, et al. EPIC: phase III trial of cetuximab plus irinotecan after fluoropyrimidine and oxaliplatin failure in patients with metastatic colorectal cancer. J Clin Oncol 2008;26(14):2311–9.
52. Van Cutsem E, Kohne CH, Lang I, et al. Cetuximab plus irinotecan, fluorouracil, and leucovorin as first-line treatment for metastatic colorectal cancer: updated

analysis of overall survival according to tumor KRAS and BRAF mutation status. J Clin Oncol 2011;29(15):2011–9.

53. Bokemeyer C, Bondarenko I, Hartmann JT, et al. Efficacy according to biomarker status of cetuximab plus FOLFOX-4 as first-line treatment for metastatic colo-rectal cancer: the OPUS study. Ann Oncol 2011;22(7):1535–46.

54. Maughan TS, Adams RA, Smith CG, et al. Addition of cetuximab to oxaliplatin-based first-line combination chemotherapy for treatment of advanced colorectal cancer: results of the randomised phase 3 MRC COIN trial. Lancet 2011; 377(9783):2103–14.

55. Tveit KM, Guren T, Glimelius B, et al. Phase III trial of cetuximab with continuous or intermittent fluorouracil, leucovorin, and oxaliplatin (Nordic FLOX) versus FLOX alone in first-line treatment of metastatic colorectal cancer: the NORDIC-VII study. J Clin Oncol 2012;30(15):1755–62.

Index

Note: Page numbers of article titles are in **boldface** type.

Surg Clin N Am 95 (2015) 1095–1104
http://dx.doi.org/10.1016/S0039-6109(15)00130-9
0039-6109/15/$ – see front matter © 2015 Elsevier Inc. All rights reserved.

surgical.theclinics.com

United States Postal Service

Statement of Ownership, Management, and Circulation
(All Periodicals Publications Except Requester Publications)

1. Publication Title	2. Publication Number	3. Filing Date
Surgical Clinics of North America	5 2 9 - 8 0 0 0	9/18/15

4. Issue Frequency	5. Number of Issues Published Annually	6. Annual Subscription Price
Feb, Apr, Jun, Aug, Oct, Dec	6	$370.00

7. Complete Mailing Address of Known Office of Publication (Not printer) (Street, city, county, state, and ZIP+4®)

Elsevier Inc.
360 Park Avenue South
New York, NY 10010-1710

Contact Person: Stephen R. Bushing
Telephone (Include area code): 215-239-3688

8. Complete Mailing Address of Headquarters or General Business Office of Publisher (Not printer)

Elsevier Inc., 360 Park Avenue South, New York, NY 10010-1710

9. Full Names and Complete Mailing Addresses of Publisher, Editor, and Managing Editor (Do not leave blank)

Publisher (Name and complete mailing address)

Linda Belfus, Elsevier Inc., 1600 John F. Kennedy Blvd., Suite 1800, Philadelphia, PA 19103

Editor (Name and complete mailing address)

John Vassallo, Elsevier Inc., 1600 John F. Kennedy Blvd., Suite 1800, Philadelphia, PA 19103-2899

Managing Editor (Name and complete mailing address)

Adrianne Brigido, Elsevier Inc., 1600 John F. Kennedy Blvd., Suite 1800, Philadelphia, PA 19103-2899

10. Owner (Do not leave blank. If the publication is owned by a corporation, give the name and address of the corporation immediately followed by the names and addresses of all stockholders owning or holding 1 percent or more of the total amount of stock. If not owned by a corporation, give the names and addresses of the individual owners. If owned by a partnership or other unincorporated firm, give its name and address as well as those of each individual owner. If the publication is published by a nonprofit organization, give its name and address.)

Full Name	Complete Mailing Address
Wholly owned subsidiary of	1600 John F. Kennedy Blvd. Ste. 1800
Reed/Elsevier, US holdings	Philadelphia, PA 19103-2899

11. Known Bondholders, Mortgagees, and Other Security Holders Owning or Holding 1 Percent or More of Total Amount of Bonds, Mortgages, or Other Securities. If none, check box ☐ None

Full Name	Complete Mailing Address
N/A	

12. Tax Status (For completion by nonprofit organizations authorized to mail at nonprofit rates) (Check one)
The purpose, function, and nonprofit status of this organization and the exempt status for federal income tax purposes:
☐ Has Not Changed During Preceding 12 Months
☐ Has Changed During Preceding 12 Months (Publisher must submit explanation of change with this statement)

13. Publication Title	14. Issue Date for Circulation Data Below
Surgical Clinics of North America	August 2015

15.	Extent and Nature of Circulation	Average No. Copies Each Issue During Preceding 12 Months	No. Copies of Single Issue Published Nearest to Filing Date
a.	Total Number of Copies (Net press run)	1729	1243
b. Legitimate Paid and/Or Requested Distribution (By Mail and Outside the Mail)	(1) Mailed Outside-County Paid/Requested Mail Subscriptions stated on PS Form 3541. (Include paid distribution above nominal rate, advertiser's proof copies and exchange copies)	718	457
	(2) Mailed In-County Paid/Requested Mail Subscriptions stated on PS Form 3541. (Include paid distribution above nominal rate, advertiser's proof copies and exchange copies)		
	(3) Paid Distribution Outside the Mails Including Sales Through Dealers And Carriers, Street Vendors, Counter Sales, and Other Paid Distribution Outside USPS®	458	503
	(4) Paid Distribution by Other Classes of Mail Through the USPS (e.g. First-Class Mail®)		
c.	Total Paid and/or Requested Circulation (Sum of 15b (1), (2), (3), and (4))	1176	960
d. Free or Nominal Rate Distribution (By Mail and Outside the Mail)	(1) Free or Nominal Rate Outside-County Copies included on PS Form 3541	45	40
	(2) Free or Nominal Rate In-County Copies included on PS Form 3541		
	(3) Free or Nominal Rate Copies mailed at Other classes Through the USPS (e.g. First-Class Mail®)		
	(4) Free or Nominal Rate Distribution Outside the Mail (Carriers or Other means)	45	40
e.	Total Nonrequested Distribution (Sum of 15d (1), (2), (3) and (4))	45	40
f.	Total Distribution (Sum of 15c and 15e)	1221	1000
g.	Copies not Distributed (See instructions to publishers #4 (page 43))	508	243
h.	Total (Sum of 15f and g)	1729	1243
i.	Percent Paid and/or Requested Circulation (15c divided by 15f times 100)	96.31%	96.00%

* If you are claiming electronic copies go to line 16 on page 3. If you are not claiming Electronic copies, skip to line 17 on page 3.

16. Electronic Copy Circulation	Average No. Copies Each Issue During Preceding 12 Months	No. Copies of Single Issue Published Nearest to Filing Date
a. Paid Electronic Copies		
b. Total paid Print Copies (Line 15c) + Paid Electronic copies (Line 16a)		
c. Total Print Distribution (Line 15f) + Paid Electronic Copies (Line 16a)		
d. Percent Paid (Both Print & Electronic copies) (16b divided by 16c X 100)		

☐ I certify that 50% of all my distributed copies (electronic and print) are paid above a nominal price

17. Publication of Statement of Ownership
If the publication is a general publication, publication of this statement is required. Will be printed in the *October 2015* issue of this publication.

18. Signature and Title of Editor, Publisher, Business Manager, or Owner

Stephen R. Bushing – Inventory Distribution Coordinator

Stephen R. Bushing

Date: September 18, 2015

I certify that all information furnished on this form is true and complete. I understand that anyone who furnishes false or misleading information on this form or who omits material or information requested on the form may be subject to criminal sanctions (including fines and imprisonment) and/or civil sanctions (including civil penalties).

PS Form 3526, July 2014 (Page 1 of 3 (Instructions Page 3)) PSN 7530-01-000-9931 PRIVACY NOTICE: See our Privacy policy in www.usps.com

PS Form 3526, July 2014 (Page 3 of 3)

Moving?

Make sure your subscription moves with you!

To notify us of your new address, find your **Clinics Account Number** (located on your mailing label above your name), and contact customer service at:

Email: journalscustomerservice-usa@elsevier.com

800-654-2452 (subscribers in the U.S. & Canada)
314-447-8871 (subscribers outside of the U.S. & Canada)

Fax number: 314-447-8029

Elsevier Health Sciences Division
Subscription Customer Service
3251 Riverport Lane
Maryland Heights, MO 63043

*To ensure uninterrupted delivery of your subscription, please notify us at least 4 weeks in advance of move.

Printed and bound by CPI Group (UK) Ltd, Croydon, CR0 4YY

07/10/2024

01040498-0020